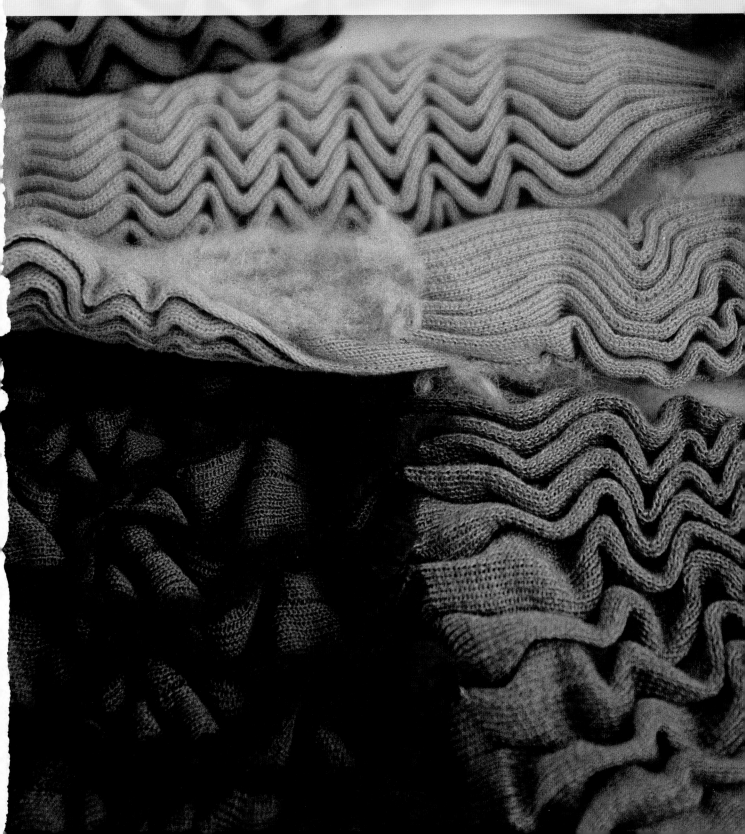

KNITWEAR IN FASHION

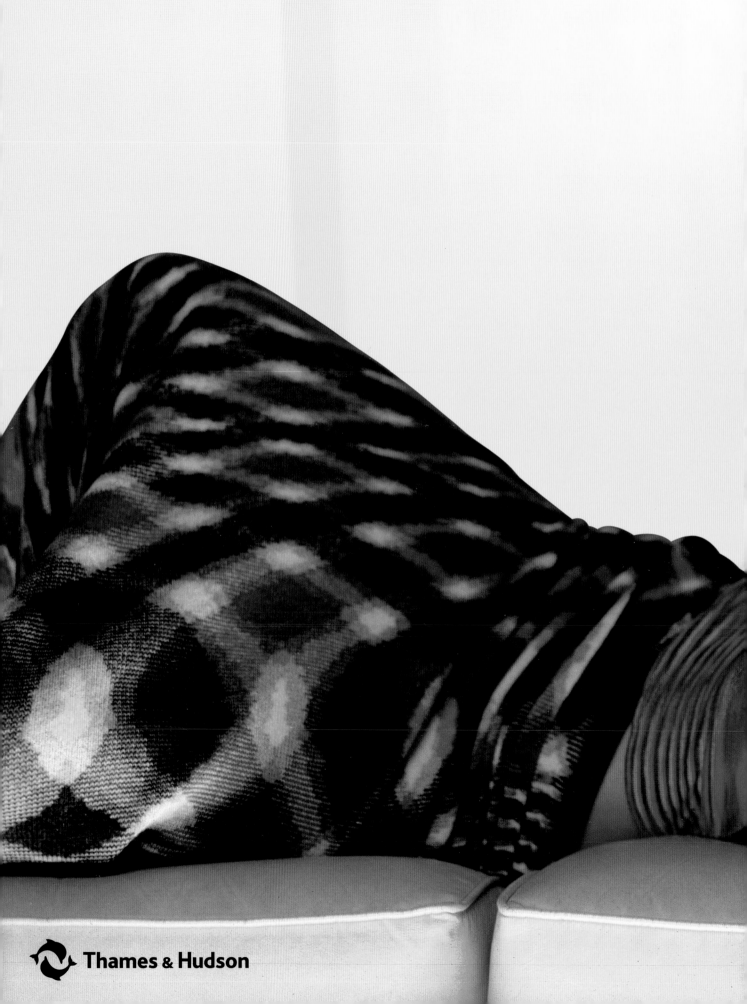

Thames & Hudson

Sandy Black

KNITWEAR IN FASHION

300 illustrations, 285 in color

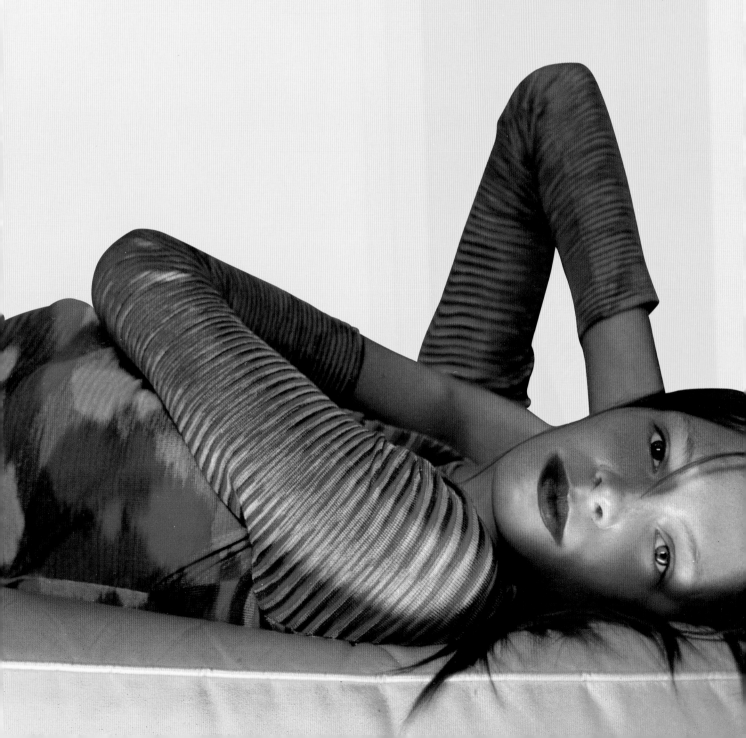

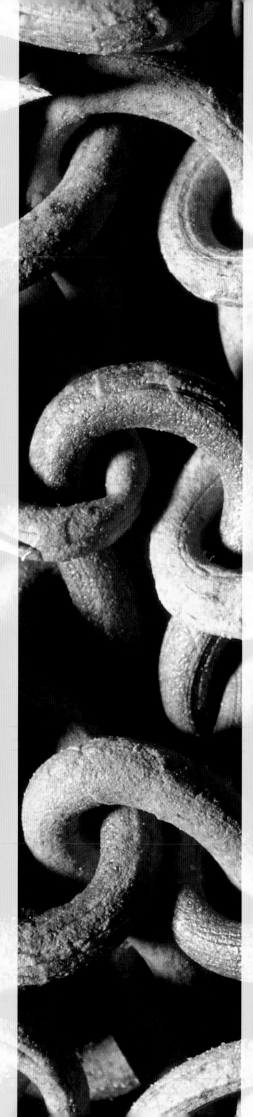

First published in the United States of America in 2002
by Thames & Hudson Inc., 500 Fifth Avenue,
New York, New York 10110

thamesandhudsonusa.com

Library of Congress Catalog Card Number 2001099694
ISBN 0-500-51084-9

Printed and bound in Singapore by
Star Standard Industries

p. 1 Mie Iwatsubo, knitted fabric, 2001

pp. 2-3 Missoni, sweater and skirt; autumn/winter 1997/98

pp. 4-5 Georgina Naish, flexible clay knit, 1998

CONTENTS

INTRODUCTION
– REINVENTING THE ART 6

1 KNITWEAR IN FASHION
– FASHION IN KNITWEAR
Reinventing the Classics 10
Decades of Change 28
Creative Fashion Accessories 52

2 INNOVATION AND EXPERIMENT
– MAKING THE FUTURE
Materials, Structures and Processes 66
Radical Knitwear 90
The Seamless Revolution 118

3 BLURRING THE BOUNDARIES
– CONTEMPORARY ART AND DESIGN
Artworks and Sculptural Form 132
Knitwear in Performance 152
Design for Interiors 162

INFORMATION
The Technology of Knitting 174
Developments in Design 178
Yarns and Fibres 179
Designer Biographies 181
Glossary of Technical Terms 189
Further Reading and Resources 190
Picture Credits and Acknowledgments 191
Index 192

Opposite Marcia Windebank, panel, 1999. Utilizing the filigree effect of lace knitting, Windebank creates abstract textural compositions that are dyed and treated with paper pulp to stiffen and fix them in striking shapes for interior decoration.

In the climate of accelerated technological change which has prevailed over the past twenty-five years, new technologies and new fibres have transformed knitting from a homely discipline into the most innovative and exciting textile medium, and knitwear has gained a place at the forefront of contemporary fashion. Never before have so many designers and artists experimented with knit as a basis for their work, exploring structures and finishes, materials and meaning, and exploiting the unique sculptural qualities of knitted construction. A new generation of fashion designers who are pushing the boundaries have reinvented the art. By presenting a wide spectrum of hand-knitting, hand-frame knitting and industrial production, *Knitwear in Fashion* offers a fresh look at this 'common art' in the context of current creative fashion and design.

Fashion has emerged during recent years as a discipline worthy of study in its own right; as a socio-cultural, economic and high-profile design phenomenon, expressive and reflective of constant change, and open to multiple readings and interpretations. This fashion discourse has been conducted through a growing range of publications, both popular and academic, and increasingly through exhibitions. Given that the attention of the academy to fashion as a discipline is so relatively recent, knitwear as an element of fashion has received even less attention, perhaps due to its specialist nature and its hybrid position as both clothing and textile.

Knitwear is universal – everyone wears it in some form, either as underwear, hosiery or outerwear – but its domestic and mass-market connotations have until recently consigned it to a minor role in fashion and textile study. Museum collections have tended to overlook knitwear items and many historical pieces of everyday wear have simply worn out. However, the last few years have seen a change in attitude and knitwear has at last begun to be featured in fashion exhibitions, which now occur more frequently. As the introduction to the knit section of the 'Jouer la Lumière' textiles exhibition at the Louvre in 2001 confirms: '... often little understood in museums, and also badly understood by textile historians, knitting today plays a major role and reveals itself to be capable of a stunning diversity.' It is this diversity that has led me to present this anthology of knitwear and knitting, together with a love of materials and construction, and a desire to celebrate this 'little understood' technique for its unique capabilities: the way in which it can engineer both two- and three-dimensional shape; its affinity with the body through innate characteristics of stretch-to-fit; and its infinite structural and patterning potential.

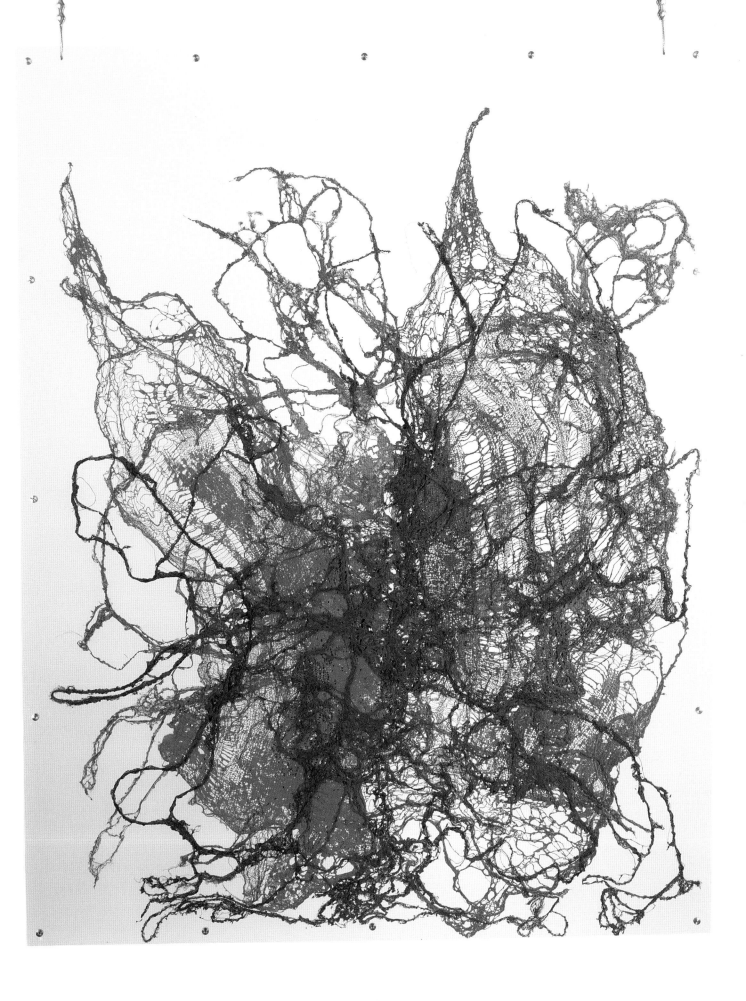

Hand-knitting became mechanized in 1589, with the invention of the stocking knitting frame by William Lee of Nottinghamshire. This gave greater speed of production but necessitated the use of flat fabric, and temporarily the ability to create complete garments in the round was forsaken. Technical developments continued steadily throughout the eighteenth, nineteenth and twentieth centuries, giving rise to a range of fundamental knitted fabric structures. It has, however, taken until recent years for the most sophisticated industrial machinery to be able to replicate the garment-making skills achievable by hand in the round on four or five needles and practised for centuries.

Knitted construction is versatile: it can be made as flat fabric or tubular fabric, both of which require 'cut and sew' production, or as garment-shaped, 'fully fashioned' pieces. The familiar, domestic hand- and machine-knitting, and the industrial knitting mostly used for clothing, is 'weft' knitting, produced from one thread that interloops in horizontal 'rows'. A second type of industrial knitting is 'warp' knitting, which is usually used to produce furnishing fabrics but has been developed for clothing, most famously by the Missoni family. This technology is almost a cross between knitting and weaving, and uses a warp of many threads to create vertical chains linked together to form a fabric. Within all techniques the wide range of yarn choices and machine gauges gives infinite possibilities of weight and fabric characteristics. This versatility gives tremendous creative potential when designers and technologists work together, and the designer can develop sufficient technical understanding to envisage the possibilities. Design and technology are inextricably linked, especially in the case of knitwear, which can do so much more than mimic woven cloth. In the 1970s and '80s it was clear that design developments led technological progress, but now designers and technologists struggle to keep up with the opportunities afforded by the latest technology.

Education systems around the world differ in their approach to fashion and textile design, and the relationship (or lack of one) between fashion and textiles. Although woven and printed fabric design is commonplace and can cross into fine art spheres, knit is not always included and has often developed as a separate expertise via apprenticeship through industrial production or by building on handcraft skills. Fashion designers consequently have very little technical knowledge of knitwear (with notable exceptions) and depend upon knitwear designers and technologists to interpret their ideas, in the same way as they depend on pattern-cutters. However, as the technology has become more accessible and more responsive to new ideas, so fashion designers have increasingly exploited the technology of knitting within their collections. Witness, for example, the increasing use of internal shaping (in effect the same as darts in dressmaking) in sweaters we see in the mainstream market, and the extraordinary range of pattern and construction now available in tights and stockings.

Knitwear can be sexy, cosy, decorative, classic, oversized, micro, clinging, enveloping, chunky, see-through, sophisticated or theatrical, amongst many other things, though the perception which persists – in Britain at least – is frozen in wartime memories of 'make do and mend', knitting for victory, knitting for economy and women's work. The knitting industry is relatively young but knitting as a domestic activity is embedded in our social history and collective consciousness, and still evokes highly emotional responses and memories. It is constantly called upon to perform its metaphorical role in literature – from Dickens and his *tricoteuses* at the guillotine in *A Tale of Two Cities* to E. Annie Proulx's Aunt Agnis in *The Shipping News*.

The once-familiar expression of love shown through knitting for a sweetheart, a baby or a family member has declined so much that the local wool shop is now a rarity in Britain. But walk along the fashionable rue Franc Bourgeois in the ever-burgeoning Marais area of Paris, where Issey Miyake has opened his first A-POC store outside Japan, and you will see a wool shop – Anny Blatt Yarns. It is many years since the same brand was able to sustain a presence in the comparable Covent Garden in London, which points to a significant difference in attitude towards the domestic activity of hand-knitting and its closer relationship to fashion in France than in Britain. The wool shop in most British cities was always a feature of suburbia rather than newly trendy city centres, except perhaps during the 'designer knitting' boom of the 1980s, pioneered by Patricia Roberts, which was taken up by department stores.

Key developments in design helped to put knitwear back on the fashion map from the early 1980s onwards. This book illustrates some of those important developments. The following chapters survey contemporary fashion knitwear and international fashion designers who have made a significant contribution to knitwear design, reinventing the stereotypes, taking knitting in new directions and giving it a new identity.

Convergence of disciplines is taking place across many areas of design and art practice, including graphic, product, interior and fashion design, and fashion intelligence is now applied across many fields and industries (such as the car industry) to stimulate change (and consumption). Artists are increasingly utilizing the knitting medium to harness its rich metaphorical power, and clothing features more frequently in the gallery context. Designers are capitalizing on the visual and light-filtering qualities of knitted fabrics in unusual materials with innovative ideas for modern interiors. Much new contemporary design incorporates knitted structures as a fundamental element within sculptural jewelry and lighting. A final section of the book looks at some of the alternative uses of knitwear and knitted textiles in evidence in contemporary creative practice.

Designing for knitwear and knitted textiles requires an interplay between craft, design, technology, fashion and aesthetics. Technological developments, coupled to the computer revolution, have been crucial to the reinvention of industrial knitting from its somewhat bland beginnings. Sophisticated knitting technology has enabled innovative design – previously achievable only by manual craft production – to be realized commercially. Integration of electronics with textiles is also underway and knit is increasingly used in technical and medical textiles. Looking to the future, the new technologies offer exciting potential for new forms of industrial knitting which have yet to be fully exploited.

Opposite A new look for an old classic. A narrow fitting beaded cashmere cardigan by Whistles complements a jewelled skirt by Moschino Cheap & Chic, creating an urban romanticism for spring/summer 2001. The decorated cardigan was an all-important accessory during the 1990s and, given new proportions and styling, has become a reinvented classic, breaking down old distinctions between day and evening wear.

Knitwear has been part of fashion since elaborate hand-knitted silk stockings replaced the woven linen hose worn by Elizabethan noblemen and courtiers from Spain and France, the better to accentuate their shapely legs. These men were fashion leaders and inspired a thriving stocking trade, in which England played a major part.

Historically, knitwear was first used to provide practical clothing for warmth, protection and ease of movement, starting with coverings for the extremities – head, feet and hands – and then for the body. As underclothing, it gave rise to 'shirts', underpants and 'combinations', and the 'gansey' or 'jersey' worn by fishermen. Gradually, the fashionable multiple layers of nineteenth-century clothing became more streamlined and relaxed for outdoor activities, and knitted underwear transmuted into outerwear: the bathing suit scandalously created a transition, being worn next to the body but on public display. The masculine 'sweater' (originally for absorbing the sweat generated by exercise) was adopted by women, and the knitted cardigan and jacket also became highly fashionable. During both First and Second World Wars, women (and men) patriotically knitted socks and comforts for the soldiers, and domestic economies meant that much family clothing was of necessity home-made. Patterns were available for everything from knee-warmers and socks to dresses and suits.

In the late nineteenth and early twentieth centuries, it was sporting activities and the burgeoning emancipation of women that again put knitwear into a fashionable arena. The key factors of comfort and freedom were perfectly met by the inherent qualities of knitted fabric, in stark contrast to the constricting and complex garments of the time. Coco Chanel pioneered this change with casual and practical pieces created from knitted jersey fabrics which had previously been confined to underwear. This fashion revolution, together with the designs of Poiret, Patou and Vionnet, heralded freedom from corsets and restrictive dress. A direct influence can be traced from Chanel's jersey dressing and sweaters of the 1920s through to the casual knitted clothing of today.

During the post-war years, the international knitwear industry developed rapidly, particularly in Italy, but the highest quality knitwear, including cashmere, was manufactured in Scotland, whose factories supplied both American and French design houses in addition to exporting their own classics to Japan and South America. Design and styling were not strengths of the British knitwear industry, which valued the efficiency of long production runs over changing styles. However, Pringle, one of the oldest Scottish factories, took a lead from Continental fashion and in the 1930s was the first manufacturer to appoint a designer – Otto Weiz from Austria.

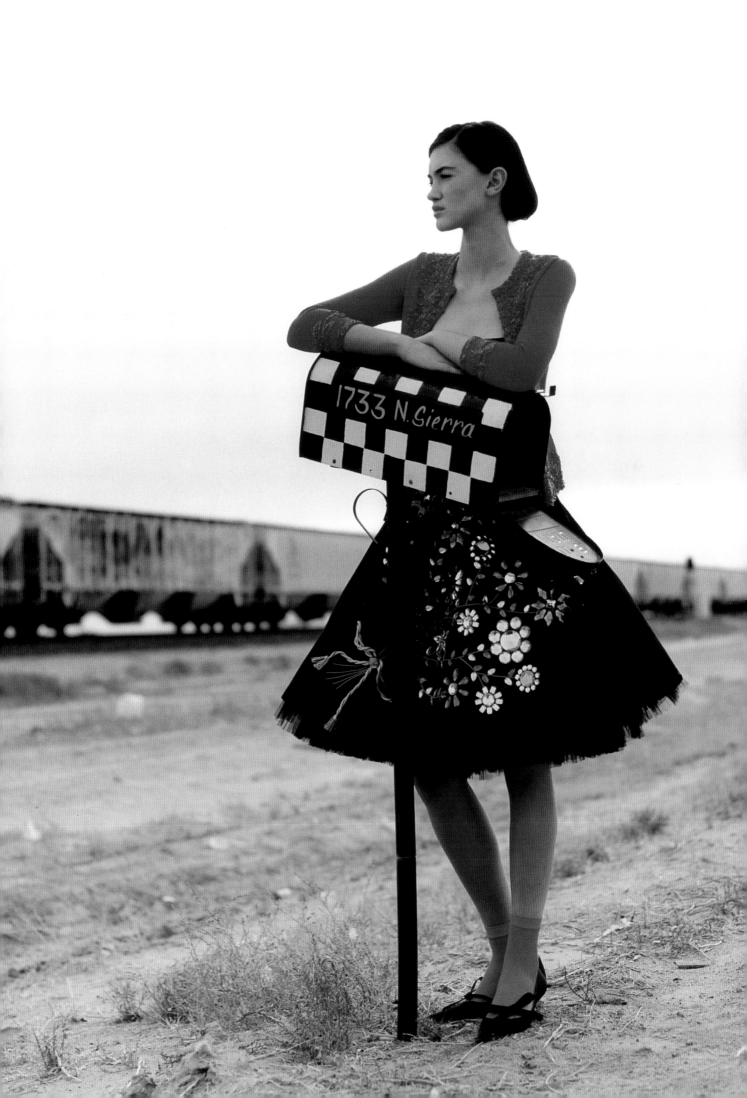

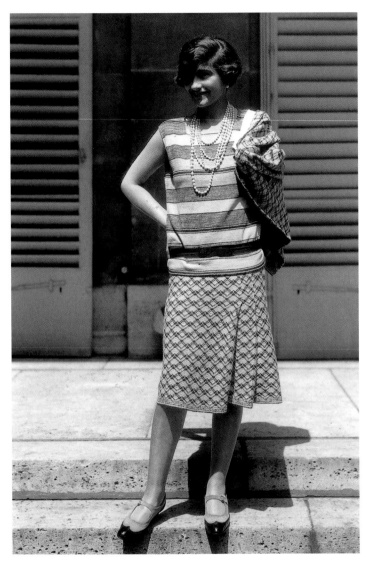

Above Coco Chanel, 1929. Chanel was the embodiment of her own fashion philosophy of relaxed, comfortable but smart clothing. Here she wears a version of her classic three-piece suit, consisting of cardigan, pullover (literally pulled over the head) and skirt in striped and patterned jersey fabric specially created for her collections, together with her signature strings of pearls.

For many years knitwear was confined to sensible, plain and functional garments of good quality. Middle-class values led to the adoption of the twinset (cardigan and sweater, with or without pearls), invented by Pringle in the 1930s, as the classic, neat, understated and moderately sophisticated look. The country weekend dress of the British landed gentry was promoted as a role model for classic taste, and was ably supplied by the English and especially Scottish knitwear industries – a look which was, and still is, exported around the world.

In the 1940s and '50s came the 'sweater girls', invented by the Hollywood glamour machine. Their garments exploited the stretch properties of knitted fabric to the full, tantalisingly revealing the body, or rather its underpinning, whilst simultaneously shielding it. Similarly, the elastic qualities of ribbed knitting gave rise to the figure-hugging 'skinny rib' sweater of the 1960s. In the same era the avant-garde black poloneck became iconic.

Meanwhile, Italian knitwear was continuing to develop its strengths of quality and craftsmanship, and Italian style became a recognized commodity on the international fashion circuit, particularly for a new casual but sophisticated style of clothing. By the 1970s Milan had become a fashion capital, assisted by the highly individual knitwear of the Missonis and international promotion in *Vogue*.

In Europe and America the knitwear tradition had embraced both knitted separates and eveningwear with elaborate, printed, embroidered and beaded sweaters. Chic and sophisticated 'knit dressing', consisting of dresses, long cardigans and layered outfits, was established by French houses such as Sonia Rykiel and Dorothée Bis, and Italian designers Laura Biagiotti and Krizia, who also created a signature range of animal and pictorial knitwear. At the lower market level, Benetton pioneered its basic but colourful sweater ranges from the 1960s onwards.

During the craft revival of the 1970s a new generation rediscovered a love of the handmade and of individual expression through materials, partly in reaction to the uniformity and basic quality of mass manufacture. British 'designer knitwear' of this period found an international market, particularly in America and Japan. The explosion of new ideas created a shift, as knitwear markets polarized into the older age-group buying classic and traditional knitwear and the growing younger, fashion-oriented consumer buying 'items' for impact – often a colourful, hand-knitted, patterned sweater. Many of the British designers of this decorative knitwear, such as Susan Duckworth and Sasha Kagan, were self-taught or came from a crafts or arts background; others such as Patricia Roberts, Sarah Dallas and Marion Foale trained in fashion. 'Designer knitwear' had a great influence on industrial production worldwide, opening up fashion markets to the mainstream knitwear industry and stimulating new technological developments.

During the 1980s decorative sweaters became the norm for casual clothing but power dressing took over the smart wardrobe, leaving little place for knitwear either on or off the catwalk. A decade later, fashion sensibilities had turned away from hard minimalism to comfort and

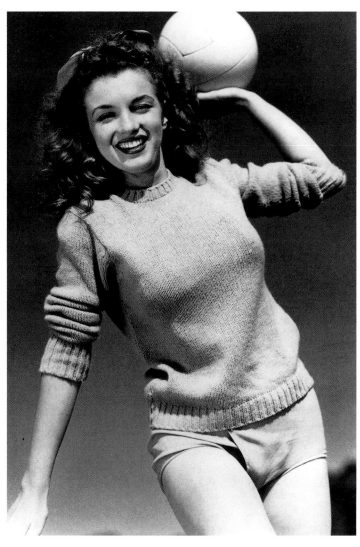

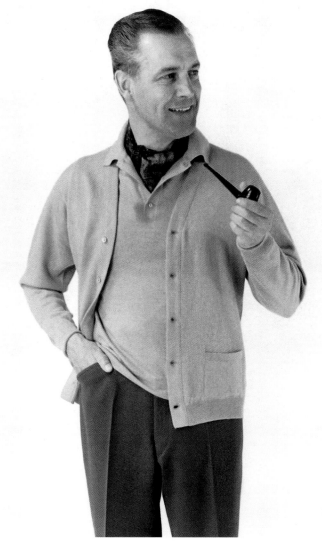

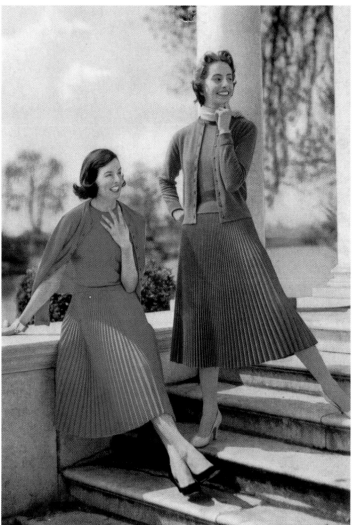

Above left Norma Jean Baker. A pre-Marilyn Monroe promotional picture showing Norma Jean's attributes in a precursor to the 'sweater girl' look – simultaneous sexuality and innocence. The classic plain woollen sweater achieved almost iconic status through the allure of film stars promoted as 'sweater girls'.

Left Pringle twinsets, 1956. The twinset became popular in America and Britain in the 1930s. Pringle claim to have invented it when they created a set consisting of short-sleeved sweater with classic round collar and ribbed edgings, and round-neck cardigan in exactly matching colour and fabric. The vogue for co-ordinated clothing was later augmented by a matching pleated skirt for the ultimate chic, or a tweed skirt woven from the same yarns.

Above Twinset, 1965. Promotional photograph from the former International Wool Secretariat (now Woolmark), epitomizing the confident professional who relaxes at the weekend in casual sportswear (and cravat). The twinset for men was common at this time. The fit is close to the body, and the proportions, such as length of cardigan and depth of trims, serve to date the look to modern eyes. The model is shown in typical, rugged, 'knitting pattern' pose – ripe for pastiche.

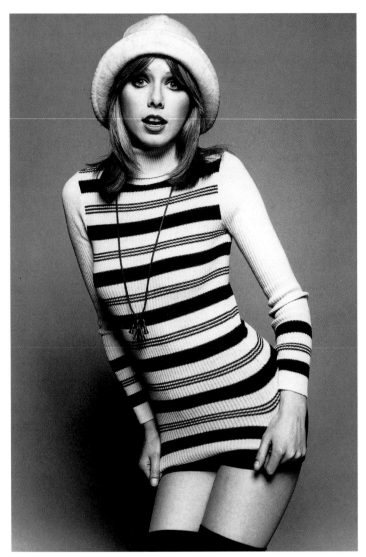

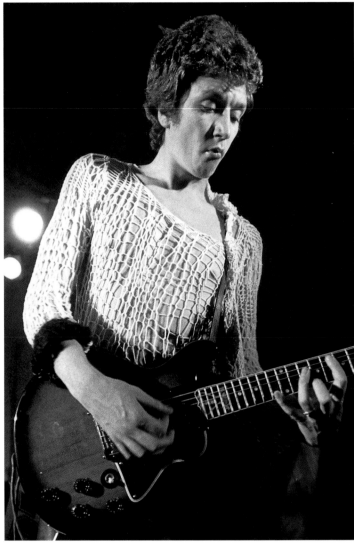

Above left Skinny rib sweater and hot pants, 1971. Promotional image from Courtaulds Fibres, capturing the fashion mood of the moment. Young fashion had become a force to be reckoned with, in marketing terms, and the skinny rib was a trend definitely targeted at the young, slim and carefree. The simple all-over rib structure was easily manufactured for the mainstream market.

Above right Steve Jones, Sex Pistols 'Anarchy in the UK' tour, 1976. Jones wears a then-shocking, string vest-like, hand-knitted sweater – large, loose knitting easily distorted and quickly made for maximum visual impact. The underground movement of punk was expressed through clothing as much as through music. Subversion of the norms was evidenced in slashed, frayed and destroyed clothing, like this sweater, which displayed more holes than fabric. Vivienne Westwood was the high priestess of punk, setting the tone with her deliberately outrageous outfits and imagery.

quality. The new desire for cocooning in luxury fibres was perfectly fulfilled by simple but well-designed knitwear, often in cashmere, and a new set of comfortable classics was created.

Traditional knitwear manufacturers have been instrumental in working with new designers, in the process developing their own brand identity. Ballantyne, Pringle and old-established English company John Smedley have all revamped their lines to appeal to a younger clientèle and to reposition themselves in a fashion-forward market. Vivienne Westwood has set free the classic argyll pattern, working with John Smedley, and Clements Ribeiro have restyled and recoloured traditional cashmere knitwear with signature stripes and spots, in conjunction with Barrie. Shirin Guild has taken traditional sweater elements and completely reworked them with new and greatly oversized, square proportions, fashioned from luxury and unusual yarns.

More attention is now given to fit and proportion. Edgings and trims have been streamlined and in many cases have disappeared, creating a more modern feel. The twinset has been reinvented with new styles, materials, patterns and proportions. At the turn of the new millennium, the cashmere cardigan worn over the shoulders and the neat sweater teamed with a skirt or trousers once again became a staple of international fashion, as shown in the ladylike collections of Prada and Louis Vuitton by Marc Jacobs. The little decorated cardigan over a printed tea dress also quickly spread to the mainstream. Mens' knitwear has received similar design and styling input – not least in colour. Comme des Garçons consistently produce brightly coloured and patterned knitwear for men with intricate details or layers of patchwork and printing. Dries Van Noten and Kenzo use asymmetric details which subvert the traditional sweater or cardigan. The new classics have been established.

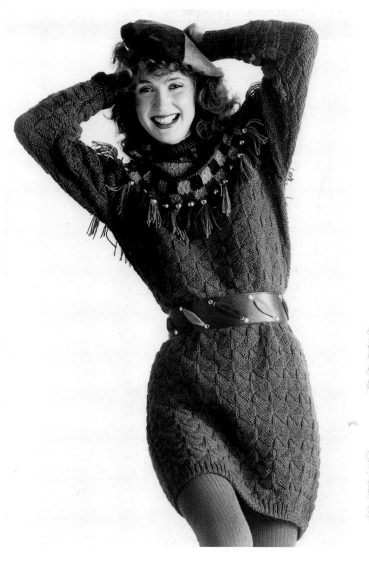

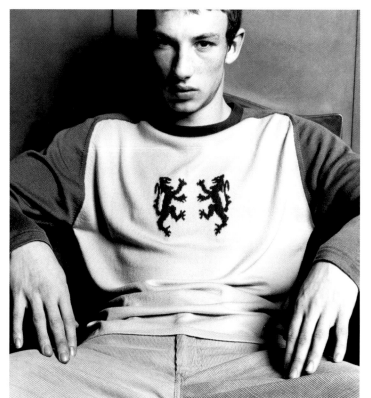

Above Artwork, autumn/winter 1981/82. A signature look with fringing and studs decorating the patterned yoke of a classic wool sweater dress, hand-knitted in basketweave stitch. The sweater dress, reliant on stretch and a minimum amount of shaping to the body, is a simple, comfortable item of clothing – basically an elongated sweater – which has periodically been in (and out of) fashion.

Left Pringle menswear, autumn/winter 2001/02. A look that relaunched the Pringle label as a brand appealing particularly to young men. Adoption of the trademark lion as a design motif has been a key factor, developed each season, each time with more intricacy – one design, for example, featured nine lions. Mock intarsia is used for cost-effective production on Shima Seiki machines.

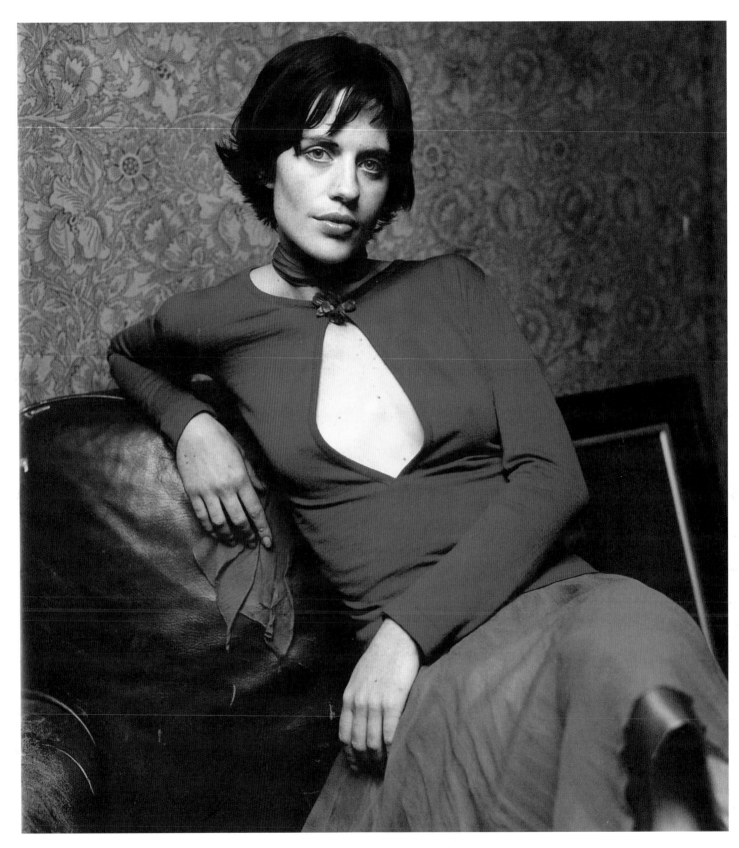

Above Image from John Smedley advertising campaign, autumn/
winter 2000/01. John Smedley have manufactured knitwear for
top-name fashion houses throughout their long history. With
stylish photography and updated designs, they are also positioning
the label as a brand in its own right. The flagship London retail
outlet and trendy advertising campaigns firmly place the products
in a fashion context.

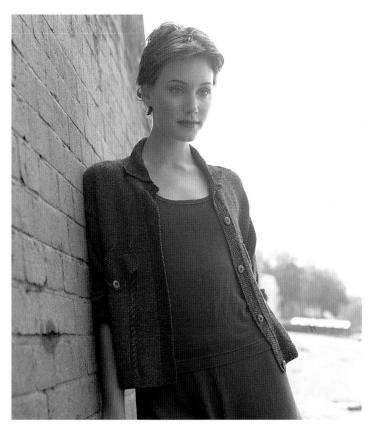

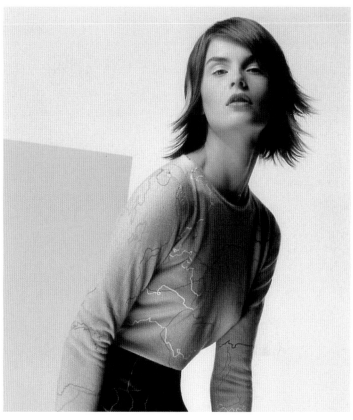

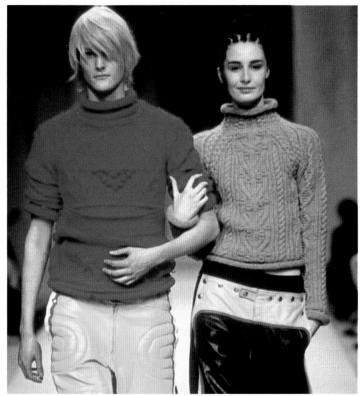

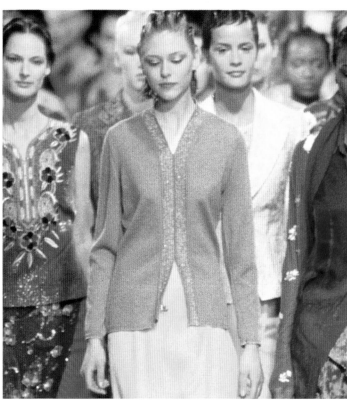

Top Artwork, spring/summer 1998. The classic denim jacket reinterpreted in hand-knitwear using indigo-dyed cotton yarn, which fades with washing in the same manner as woven denim.

Above Jean Paul Gaultier, autumn/winter 1999/2000. Aran hand-knitting features regularly throughout Gaultier's work. In this collection, entitled 'The Couple', co-ordinating outfits included sweaters based on classics but with new details. Other couples wore sequinned argyll sweaters or Norwegian patterned sweaters.

Top Tse New York, autumn/winter 2000/01. Printed classic cashmere sweater and printed skirt, designed by Hussein Chalayan for Tse.

Above Dries Van Noten, autumn/winter 1996/97. This catwalk finale shows Van Noten's love of fabric, colour and pattern in clothes which fuse influences from his travels in India and the Far East. Knitwear was not a major feature but an eclectic factor, which perhaps reflects the real way in which people wear a mix of clothes from a variety of sources.

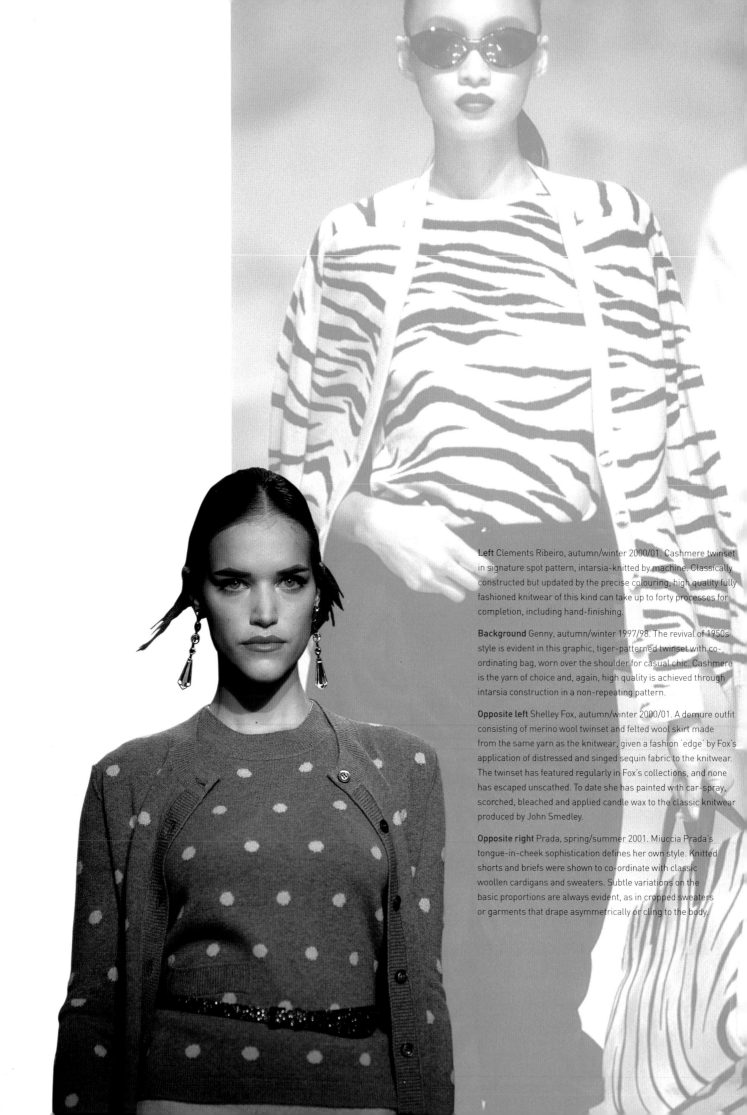

Left Clements Ribeiro, autumn/winter 2000/01. Cashmere twinset in signature spot pattern, intarsia-knitted by machine. Classically constructed but updated by the precise colouring, high quality fully fashioned knitwear of this kind can take up to forty processes for completion, including hand-finishing.

Background Genny, autumn/winter 1997/98. The revival of 1950s style is evident in this graphic, tiger-patterned twinset with co-ordinating bag, worn over the shoulder for casual chic. Cashmere is the yarn of choice and, again, high quality is achieved through intarsia construction in a non-repeating pattern.

Opposite left Shelley Fox, autumn/winter 2000/01. A demure outfit consisting of merino wool twinset and felted wool skirt made from the same yarn as the knitwear, given a fashion 'edge' by Fox's application of distressed and singed sequin fabric to the knitwear. The twinset has featured regularly in Fox's collections, and none has escaped unscathed. To date she has painted with car-spray, scorched, bleached and applied candle wax to the classic knitwear produced by John Smedley.

Opposite right Prada, spring/summer 2001. Miuccia Prada's tongue-in-cheek sophistication defines her own style. Knitted shorts and briefs were shown to co-ordinate with classic woollen cardigans and sweaters. Subtle variations on the basic proportions are always evident, as in cropped sweaters or garments that drape asymmetrically or cling to the body.

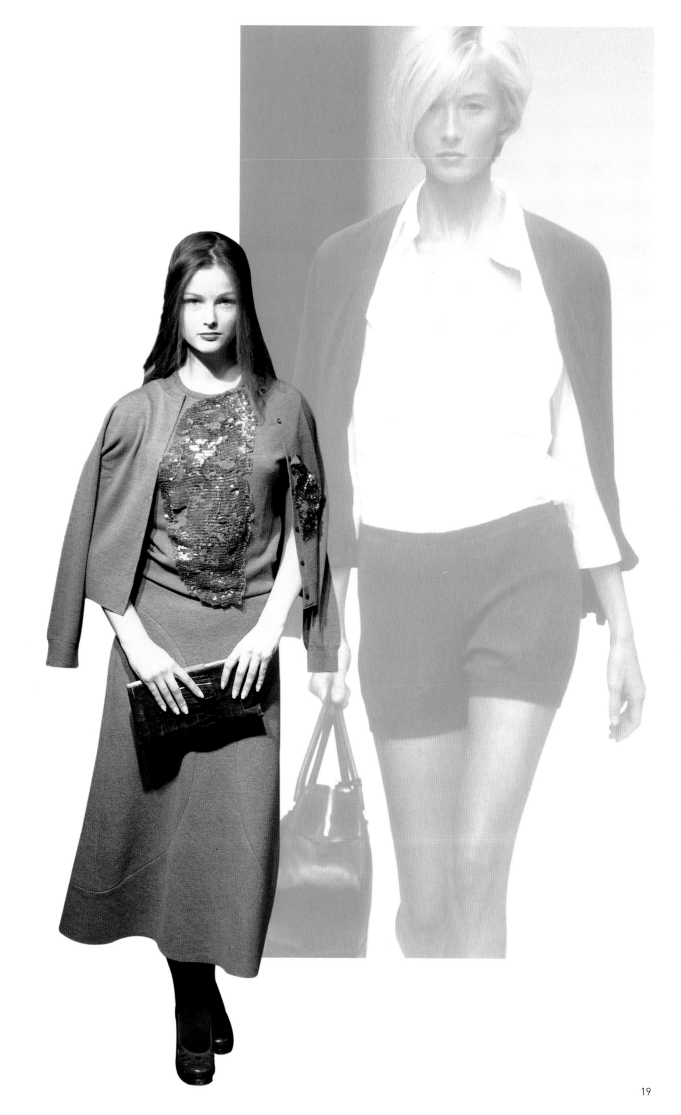

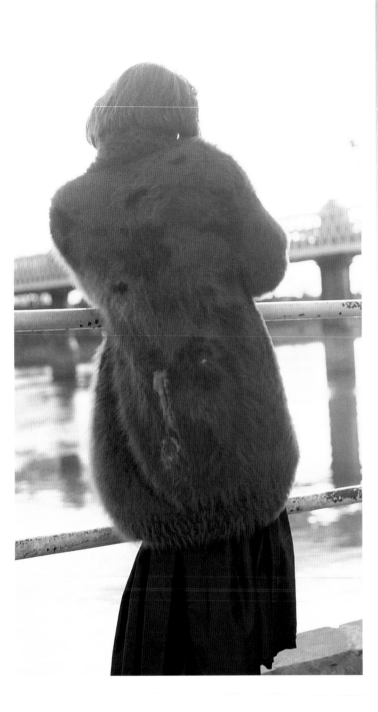

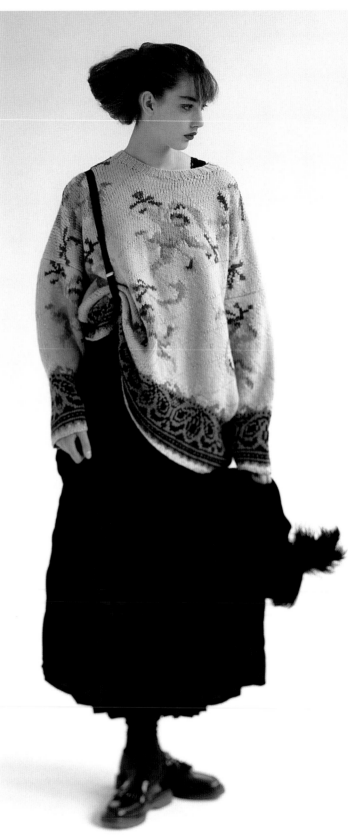

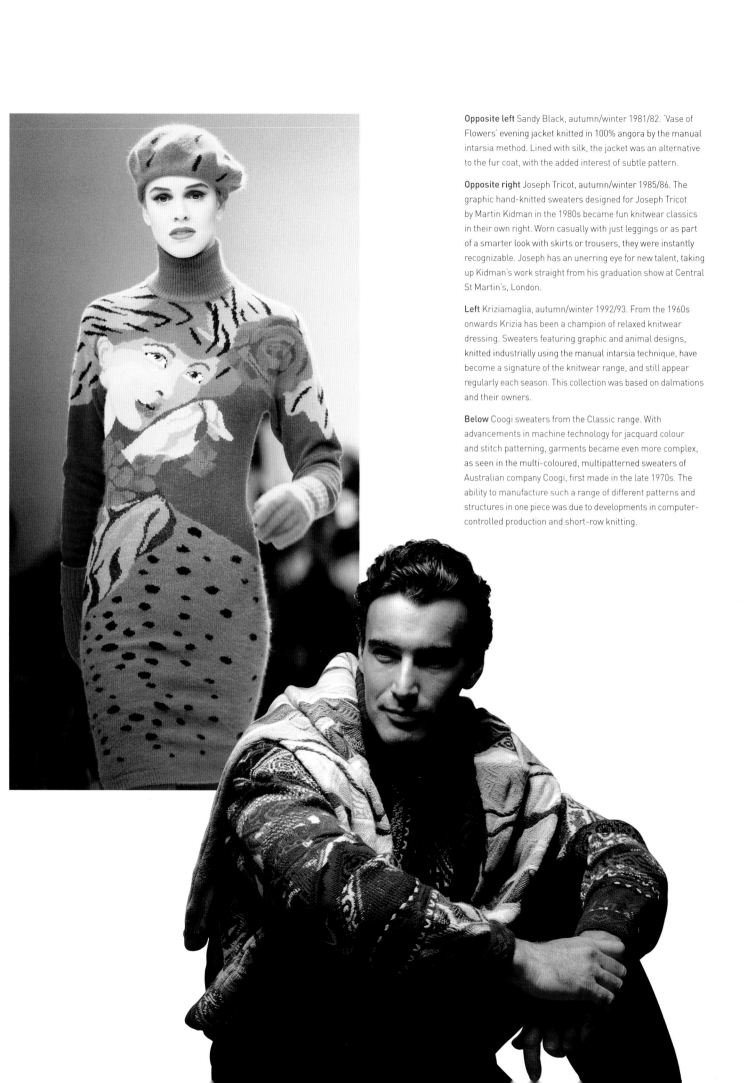

Opposite left Sandy Black, autumn/winter 1981/82. 'Vase of Flowers' evening jacket knitted in 100% angora by the manual intarsia method. Lined with silk, the jacket was an alternative to the fur coat, with the added interest of subtle pattern.

Opposite right Joseph Tricot, autumn/winter 1985/86. The graphic hand-knitted sweaters designed for Joseph Tricot by Martin Kidman in the 1980s became fun knitwear classics in their own right. Worn casually with just leggings or as part of a smarter look with skirts or trousers, they were instantly recognizable. Joseph has an unerring eye for new talent, taking up Kidman's work straight from his graduation show at Central St Martin's, London.

Left Kriziamaglia, autumn/winter 1992/93. From the 1960s onwards Krizia has been a champion of relaxed knitwear dressing. Sweaters featuring graphic and animal designs, knitted industrially using the manual intarsia technique, have become a signature of the knitwear range, and still appear regularly each season. This collection was based on dalmations and their owners.

Below Coogi sweaters from the Classic range. With advancements in machine technology for jacquard colour and stitch patterning, garments became even more complex, as seen in the multi-coloured, multipatterned sweaters of Australian company Coogi, first made in the late 1970s. The ability to manufacture such a range of different patterns and structures in one piece was due to developments in computer-controlled production and short-row knitting.

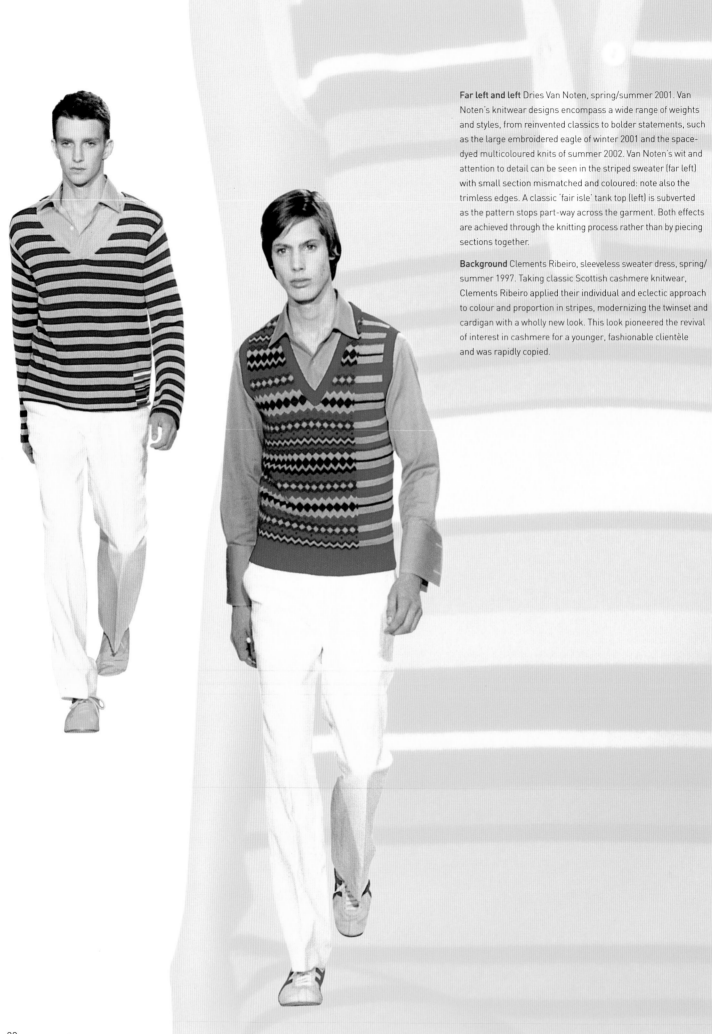

Far left and left Dries Van Noten, spring/summer 2001. Van Noten's knitwear designs encompass a wide range of weights and styles, from reinvented classics to bolder statements, such as the large embroidered eagle of winter 2001 and the space-dyed multicoloured knits of summer 2002. Van Noten's wit and attention to detail can be seen in the striped sweater (far left) with small section mismatched and coloured: note also the trimless edges. A classic 'fair isle' tank top (left) is subverted as the pattern stops part-way across the garment. Both effects are achieved through the knitting process rather than by piecing sections together.

Background Clements Ribeiro, sleeveless sweater dress, spring/summer 1997. Taking classic Scottish cashmere knitwear, Clements Ribeiro applied their individual and eclectic approach to colour and proportion in stripes, modernizing the twinset and cardigan with a wholly new look. This look pioneered the revival of interest in cashmere for a younger, fashionable clientèle and was rapidly copied.

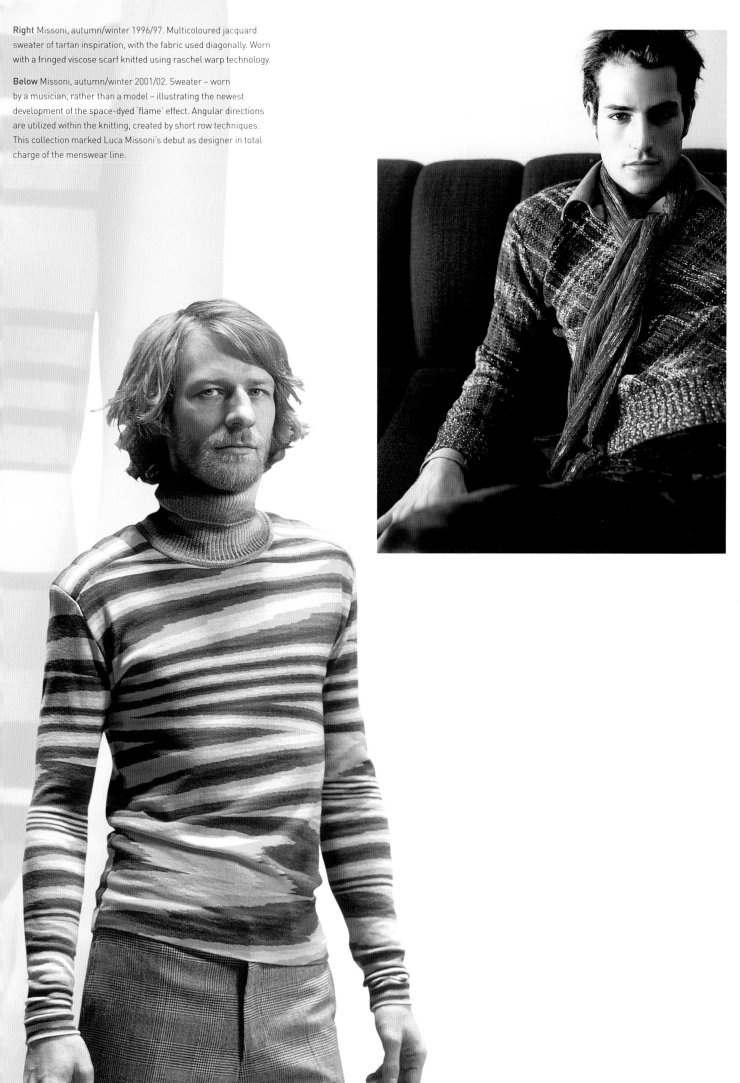

Right Missoni, autumn/winter 1996/97. Multicoloured jacquard sweater of tartan inspiration, with the fabric used diagonally. Worn with a fringed viscose scarf knitted using raschel warp technology.

Below Missoni, autumn/winter 2001/02. Sweater – worn by a musician, rather than a model – illustrating the newest development of the space-dyed 'flame' effect. Angular directions are utilized within the knitting, created by short row techniques. This collection marked Luca Missoni's debut as designer in total charge of the menswear line.

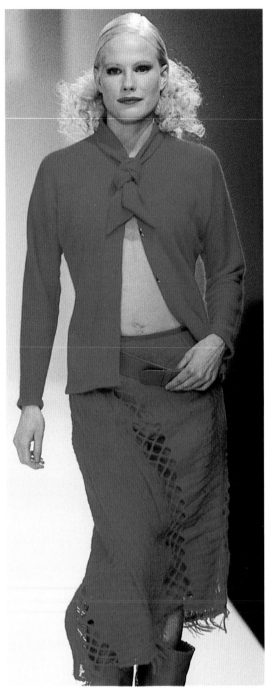

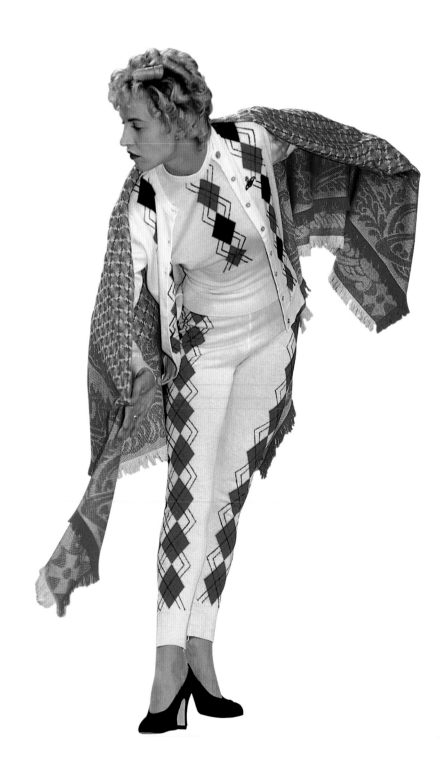

Above Betty Jackson, autumn/winter 2001/02. Jackson's recent collections have been directed towards a younger customer, hence the deconstructed look of this collection. The classic knitted tie-neck cardigan is contrasted with a raw-edged, warp-knitted fabric skirt. Jackson uses a wide range of knitted constructions as a staple part of the range, often sourced from freelance textile designers.

Right Vivienne Westwood, 'Voyage to Cythera' collection, autumn/ winter 1989/90. One of the first designers to reinterpret argyll-patterned classic knitwear for fashion, Westwood appropriated the twinset and the long johns manufactured by John Smedley, and combined them into a suit, with great commercial success. Argyll knitwear has remained a constant element of many Westwood collections, including the 'boiled wool' versions of autumn/winter 2001/02 roughly cut and sewn, moving away from the fully fashioned classics.

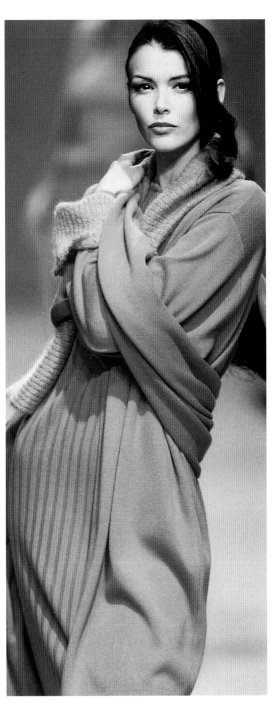

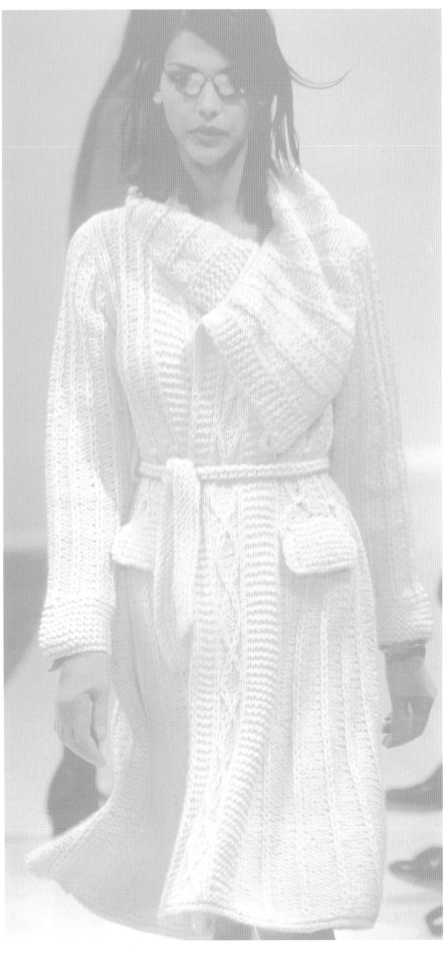

Above Joaquim Verdu, autumn/winter 1994/95. Verdu specializes in knitwear, creating fluid shapes and total looks from layering subtle variations of knit fabrics, in preference to patterned knitwear. He combines fashionable sophistication with the feeling of comfort and luxury created by easy-to-wear clothing.

Right Marina Spadafora, autumn/winter 1996/97. Hand-knitted alpaca/wool blend coat, showing Spadafora's easy style. She favours handmade production for a large part of her varied collections. However, there are always surprises and experiments. She is likely to team this classic coat with leather-effect trousers, achieved by spraying wool fabric with lacquer.

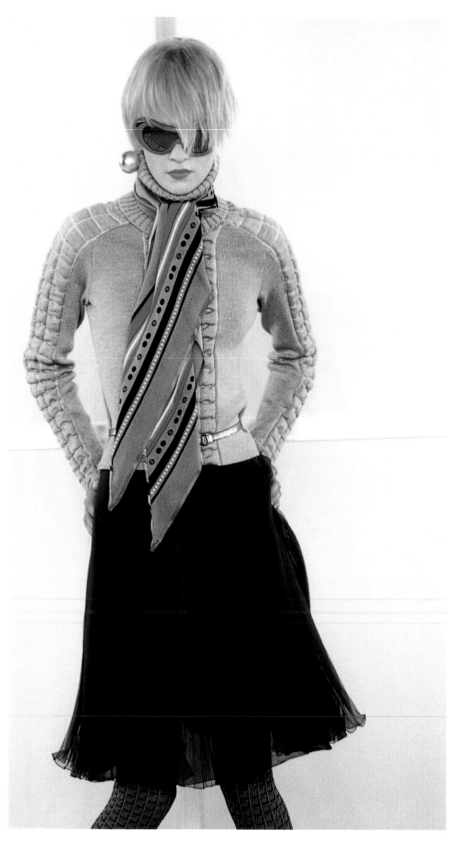

1 Knitwear in Fashion – Fashion in Knitwear

Left Chanel, autumn/winter 2000/01. Engineered knitwear using double-bed, quilt-effect fabric to accentuate the unusual design of the sweater. As part of the same collection, skirts with quilted borders at the hems were produced, creating a shape which stands away from the body due to the thickness of the fabric.

Opposite left Shirin Guild, autumn/winter 2001/02. Cashmere twinset showing the drape resulting from Guild's use of oversized proportions, particularly the width of garments. Volume of fabric and generous sizing mean that the clothes are flattering to women of any size or stature. Guild's knitted dresses are really oversized sweaters but with variations, such as shaped, curved hems to flatter the body, showing typically meticulous attention to detail.

Opposite right Twincinc by Cinc, autumn/winter 2001/02. A label exclusively creating new twinsets for men – together with integral ties and scarves – from a wide range of knitted double jersey fabrics, including printed and reversible fake fur, fake reversible chamois and jacquards. Cut-and-sew production mimics the detailing of unstructured tailoring as a replacement for the traditional shirt and jacket.

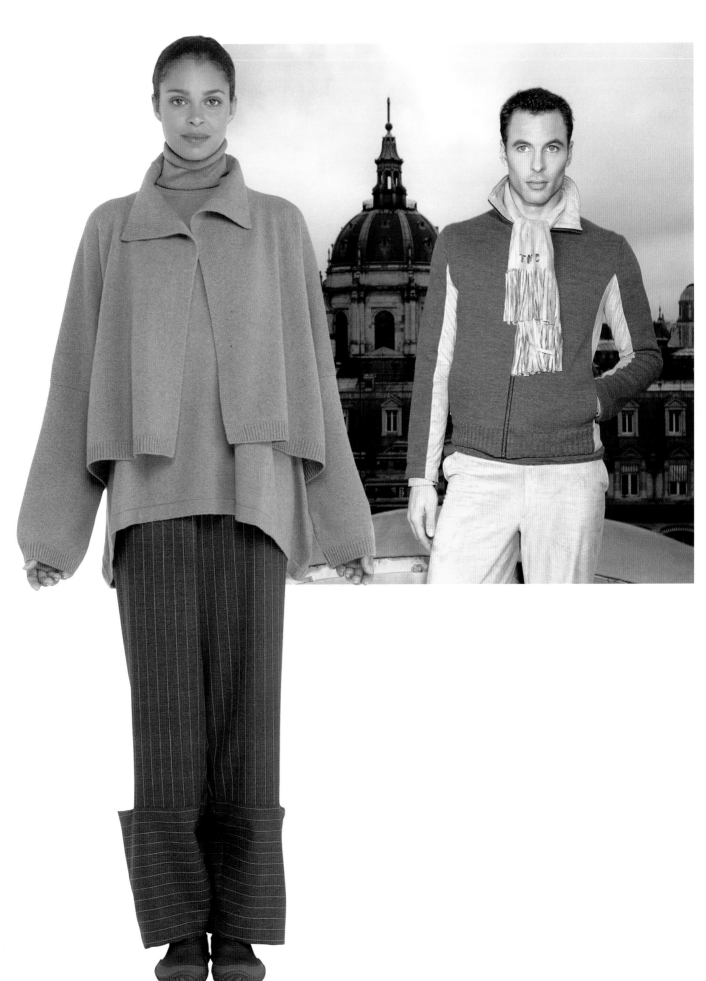

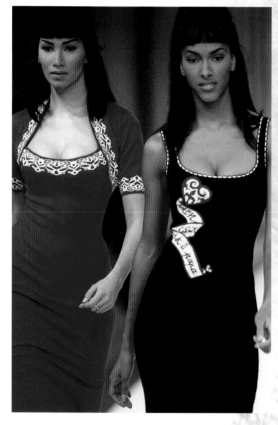

Above Azzedine Alaïa, spring/summer 1992. Knitted fabric in the hands of Alaïa becomes a vehicle for body sculpture, in which he moulds the female form. His groundbreaking stretch Lycra dresses create the perfect vehicle for display and even humour (the knitted jacquard scroll on the right reads 'my heart belongs to papa'; another dress features jacquard pubic hair). Adoring and adored by supermodels and stars, Alaïa himself is referred to as 'papa'.

Opposite left and background Azzedine Alaïa, autumn/winter 1991/92. A dress created from a velvet-like speciality viscose chenille yarn. When knitted, this produces a dense fabric which appears woven but has the essential stretch and give of knitwear. Alaïa's famous body-contouring is evident in the decorative seaming he has developed. Although the body is completely covered, it is nevertheless utterly revealed.

Opposite right Azzedine Alaïa, autumn/winter 1991/92. Another Alaïa classic: this leopard-patterned, jacquard-knitted stretch fabric was applied to coats, sweaters, leggings, bodysuits and dresses. Jacquard is still a favourite technique. The short or long pleated skirt, which has regularly featured in Alaïa's collections, was developed for 2001 by incorporating a floral design into the triangular shapes which form the one-piece skirt.

Classic knitwear transcends fashionability to sit alongside current trends as the product of a parallel industry. The popularity of knitwear in designer collections cycles through fashion every few years, and each time it returns elements remain to become classics in their own right. The loose, comfortable sweater, decorated with all manner of imagery, became a basic wardrobe item in the early 1980s. The fine-knit, lace-trimmed tank and cardigan, overdyed in all colours, and the beaded or ribbon-trimmed cardigan worn over a print dress featured prominently from the mid-1990s onwards. When fashion turns to a handcrafted ethos, large-scale knitting appears, as seen in the late '90s knitwear revival. For winter 2001 heavier, cosy knitwear returned to the fashion pages, but with a glamorous and sensual edge.

Catwalk fashion – especially the more visually newsworthy pieces – may not always translate directly into items for sale in stores, but nevertheless it remains hugely influential, as global communications have improved and shows are beamed around the world within minutes of their taking place. Therefore a focus on the innovations at designer level certainly indicates the drivers for change in mainstream fashion, even though the dictatorial power of both design houses and magazines has declined. From the vast array of choices, certain ideas catch hold and become commercially successful. Technical considerations play their role in this – for example, 'trimless' edges are much more commercially viable than labour-intensive finishing processes. The base level of design evident in both knitted fabric and knitwear construction has advanced tremendously over the past thirty years, as can be seen from the predominance of fully fashioned knitwear and engineered shape in the marketplace compared with the cut-and-sew technology favoured in earlier years. Knitwear is regularly an 'invisible' but staple element of many collections – not often shown on the catwalk but a significant turnover nevertheless.

There are a variety of approaches to knitwear at all points on the fashion spectrum, from mass market to couture. A minority of collections are knitwear-led, and most incorporate knitwear occasionally as a design feature or statement. There are a small number of predominantly knitwear design houses creating the total knit look (a position difficult to sustain), but most knitwear is sold as separates – sweaters and cardigans – to complement the main collection or as freestanding ranges. At couture and top designer level, knitwear often includes hand crafted, one-off pieces, and regularly appears on the catwalk in collections such as Lacroix, Dior, Comme des Garçons and Gaultier.

Craft skills are still very important to the commercial industry: hand-operated, semi-industrial machines are utilized in design studios to feed ideas to industrial production,

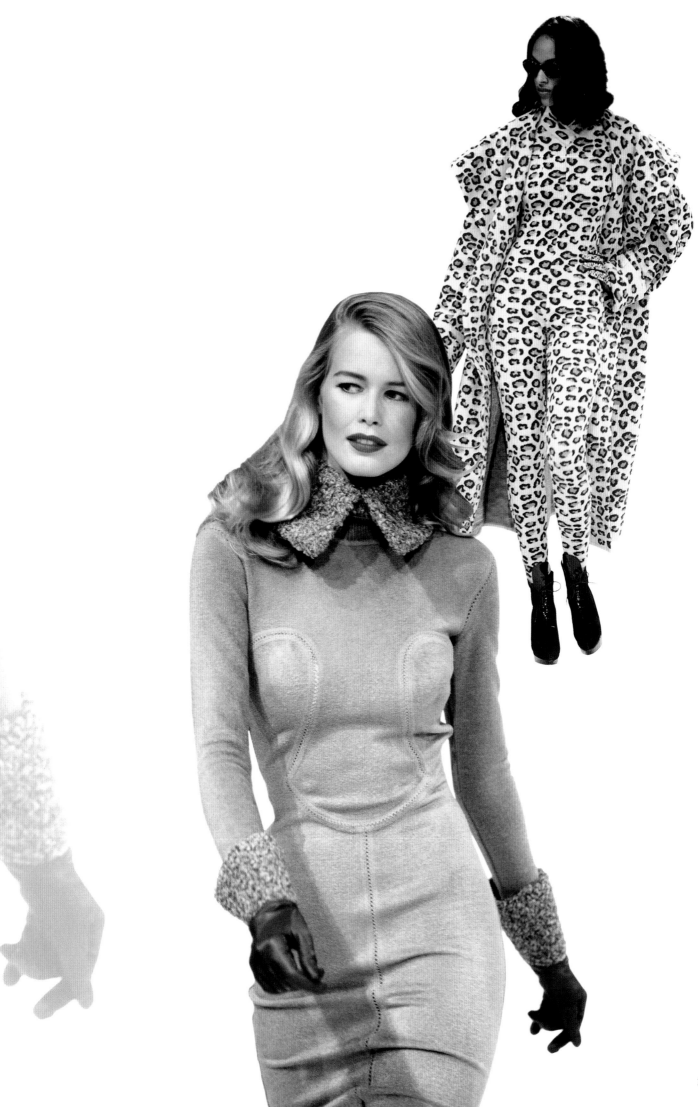

Below Missoni, autumn/winter 2001/02. A body-sculpted silhouette with graphic 'flame' effect in stark yellow and black. This collection – the first under the sole direction of Angela Missoni – included tops with contrasting panels of patchwork patterns, paying homage to the pieced 'tapestries' of Ottavio Missoni in his eightieth year.

Opposite left Missoni, autumn/winter 1996/97. A classic Missoni look from the 1970s which has been restyled for the 1990s. This was the major collection to relaunch the Missoni line to a younger audience, with the important contribution of photographer Mario Testino. The dress features the intricate zigzag fabric knitted on warp machinery that has become an enduring trademark of the company.

Opposite right Missoni, spring/summer 1998. A 'barely there' wisp of a garment, illustrating the move towards a more sexy, glamorous look that reveals the body. The floating strands are in fact the disconnected vertical chain-stitch 'warps' of the knitting process which, when interlinked, form the more solid fabric areas.

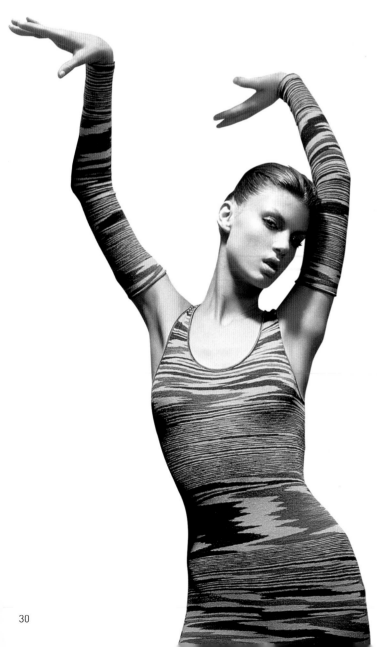

and hand-embroidered or hand-painted swatches can provide inspiration for an entire knitwear line. So the cycles of ideas and production evolve through design education, design studios, international trade fairs, sourcing of swatches by design houses and manufacturers, and interpretation by fashion designers and factories.

In Italy knitwear businesses have evolved in two ways – via a strong handcraft tradition which now supplies the couture market and specialist production, and via the planned industrial growth and regional development of the post-war era when individual entrepreneurs set up small factories – often family-based businesses, which are still able to operate effectively. The example *par excellence* of this growth from small beginnings is the Missoni design house, and there are many others, such as Marina Spadafora, who is one of three sisters in the business. Many factories now manufacture for the international designer market, offering a uniquely valuable service of design interpretation – design champions (often formidable women) who work with the technicians to realize new concepts. Design has a more central position in Italian production: more factories are prepared to accept new challenges and push the boundaries to invest in experimental design ideas, and consequently Italian production is much sought-after.

The Missoni family occupy a unique position in Italian and international knitwear design. Ottavio and Rosita Missoni started producing their colourful knitwear in the 1950s. It was soon taken up by fashion editor Anna Piaggi and became an international fashion sensation by the 1970s. However, as fashion changed around them and their customers grew older, it was not until the mid-1990s that their signature multicolour zigzags and stripe patterns, made using a mix of old and new technology, looked just right again.

In France the couture led fashion until post-war economies and social change resulted in the formation of the ready-to-wear industry. The women who set up the first knitwear-led empires started modestly. Sonia Rykiel started with one sweater she designed for herself (which incidentally had inside-out seams visible). Her signature stripes and slogan sweaters and dresses have since featured continuously in the collections, updated in colour and styling. Capitalizing on the recent vogue for vintage, she has reissued a series of designs spanning the life of the company under the label 'modern vintage'.

Over the past thirty years, the interest of fashion designers has turned increasingly to knitwear. In the UK and America the focus was on decorative sweaters and separates to make a statement rather than merely accessorize. In contrast, notably in France and Italy, a total knitwear dressing look developed for the professional woman, which became a chic but practical wardrobe, usually in understated, sophisticated layers of neutral colours with an occasional flash of stronger tones. In the UK, this relaxed look came to be represented by Betty Jackson and Nicole Farhi. This genre was given an early injection of freshness, fun and colour by Kenzo, who wrapped the fashion-conscious women of the 1970s in brightly coloured layers of knits

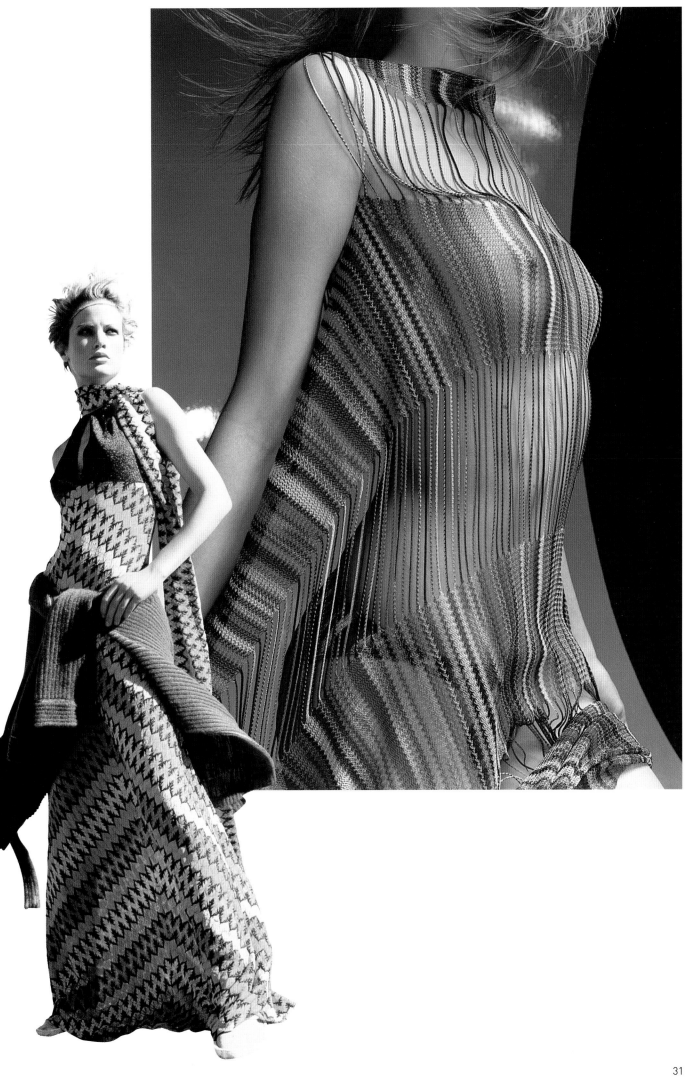

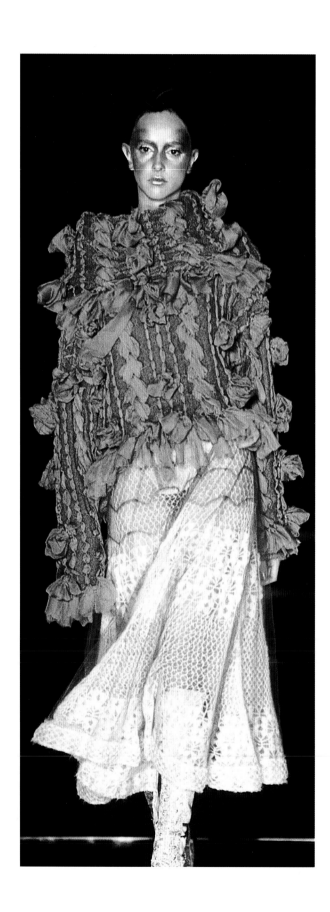

from top to toe and created the highly influential Jungle Jap label. Following huge success in Paris, entrepreneur Joseph Ettedgui introduced Kenzo to the UK in 1971, at the same time starting his own retail career. Over the intervening period Kenzo refined and developed his look, mixing global influences with his own Japanese heritage and a joyful celebration of pattern and colour to create eclectic collages, highly intricate multicolour jacquard fabrics and signature floral prints. Knitwear remains a high proportion of the collections, which for winter 2001 featured heavy embroidery, lace and metallic pleats.

Perhaps the greatest revolution in knitted fabrics over the last twenty years has come from the integration of new stretch fibres with enhanced performance factors. The rise of body-consciousness and the fitness boom of the 1980s translated directly into fashion and the British duo Body Map (Stevie Stewart and David Holah) created a fresh impact in 1983 with their lively presentations and revealing designs. Using specially developed Lycra jersey blends, hand-knits and prints by Hilde Smith, they rode on the wave of new energy and London club culture, eventually developing into a predominantly sportswear line.

In recent years proportions and symmetries of garments have been changed and edgings foregone to give a cleaner silhouette, or allowed to curl naturally to make their own finish. Trimless knitwear has become the new norm. A key development is the ability of machinery to create internal shaping, rather than just shaping the edges of a garment (the traditional 'fully fashioning'). The effect is very similar to a sewn dart but, when combined with ribbed structure, gives a highly effective surface and constructional pattern of contour lines (see p. 71). Hence designers can create more original and interesting shapes within what is ostensibly a plain garment.

The dress has also received a great deal of new exposure as a knitwear item partly due to the early work of Givenchy designer Julien Macdonald for Lagerfeld and Chanel, and Irish knitwear designer Lainey Keogh, who created sensuality through luxurious, body-revealing textures and a fantasy, almost pre-Raphaelite mood. The knitted dress now exists on a polarized spectrum of sexy, glamorous veil and, at the other extreme, cosy cover-up, based on the elongated sweater.

Transparency has been a catwalk ploy used increasingly over the past fifteen years and has virtually lost its capacity to shock in this context. Knitwear has played its part in the game by simultaneously covering and yet revealing, the extent determined by the yarn choice, knitting gauge or density, and stitch structure. With the rise of 'deconstructed' fashion and grunge in the early 1990s, a new genre of chaotic knitted and crochet webs came into existence, showing once again how knitwear both reflects and contributes to the prevailing fashion mood.

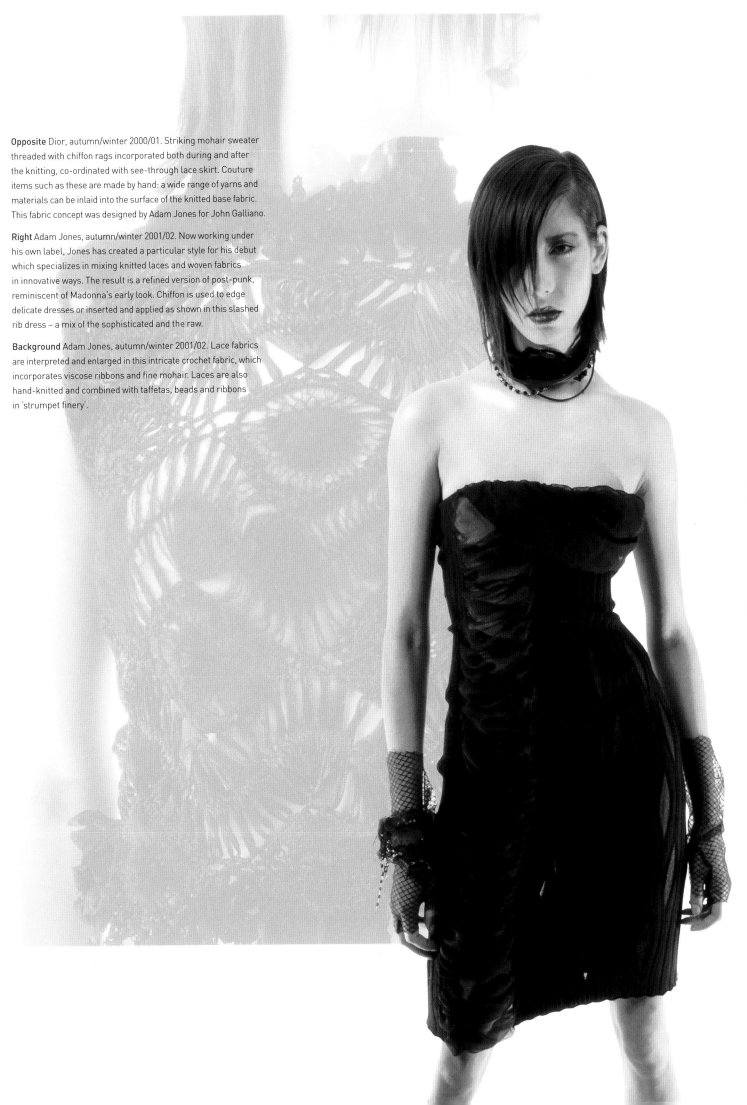

Opposite Dior, autumn/winter 2000/01. Striking mohair sweater threaded with chiffon rags incorporated both during and after the knitting, co-ordinated with see-through lace skirt. Couture items such as these are made by hand: a wide range of yarns and materials can be inlaid into the surface of the knitted base fabric. This fabric concept was designed by Adam Jones for John Galliano.

Right Adam Jones, autumn/winter 2001/02. Now working under his own label, Jones has created a particular style for his debut which specializes in mixing knitted laces and woven fabrics in innovative ways. The result is a refined version of post-punk, reminiscent of Madonna's early look. Chiffon is used to edge delicate dresses or inserted and applied as shown in this slashed rib dress – a mix of the sophisticated and the raw.

Background Adam Jones, autumn/winter 2001/02. Lace fabrics are interpreted and enlarged in this intricate crochet fabric, which incorporates viscose ribbons and fine mohair. Laces are also hand-knitted and combined with taffetas, beads and ribbons in 'strumpet finery'.

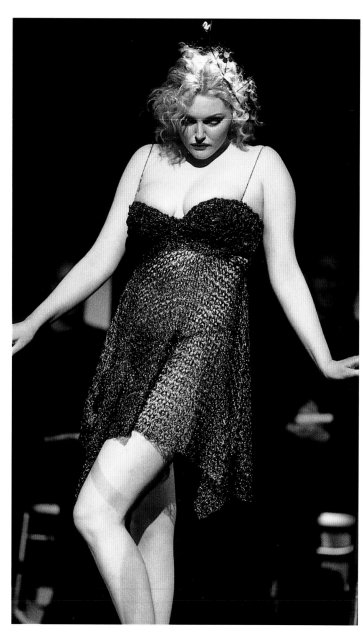

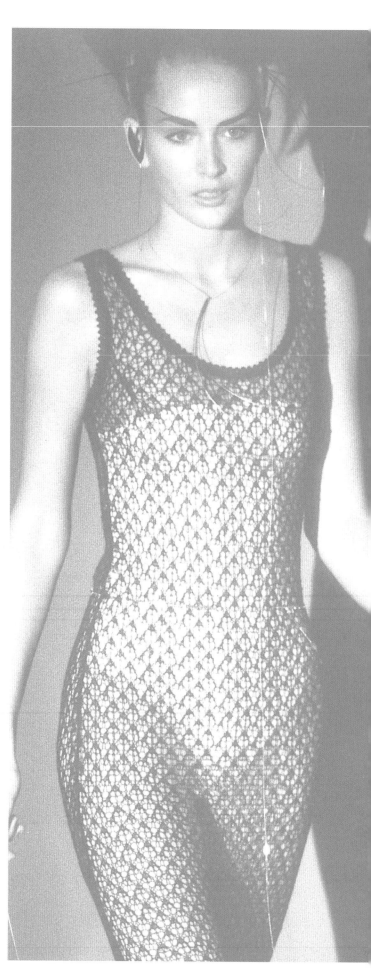

Above Lainey Keogh, autumn/winter 1997/98. Keogh's creations are sensual evocations of the 'goddess' in woman. Keogh knits, crochets or weaves garments which are both alluring and empowering. Textured yarns such as chenilles are favoured for their irresistible touch. Sophie Dahl made her catwalk debut on Keogh's runway in openwork knits and corsets.

Background Karl Lagerfeld, spring/summer 1997. A simple knitted lace structure creates the visual paradox of covering and transparency. The stitches are clearly defined and the quality must be perfection in order for such cobwebs to succeed. Julien Macdonald designed this lace knitwear for Lagerfeld and, exceptionally, was asked to join him for the final catwalk bow.

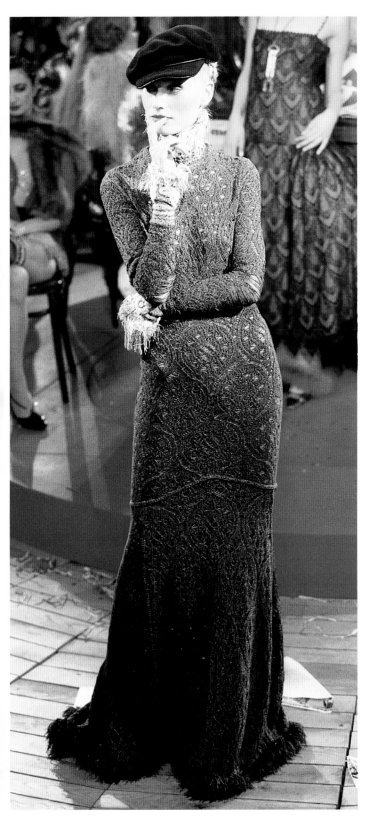

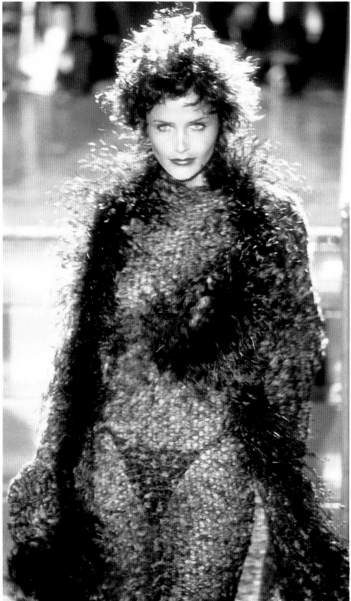

Above Lainey Keogh, autumn/winter 1997/98. A feathery textured yarn is used to create a knitted lace mesh which reveals all but creates an aura of mystery. Other Keogh dresses appear demure in comparison, knitted into dense but voluptuous textures.

Left John Galliano, autumn/winter 1998/99. Galliano approaches his fabric as a couturier, cutting and seaming to create the line he requires. An openwork transfer lace knitted fabric is used here, which can give particular problems of distortion and must be draped on the body so that the movement of the fabric can be predicted.

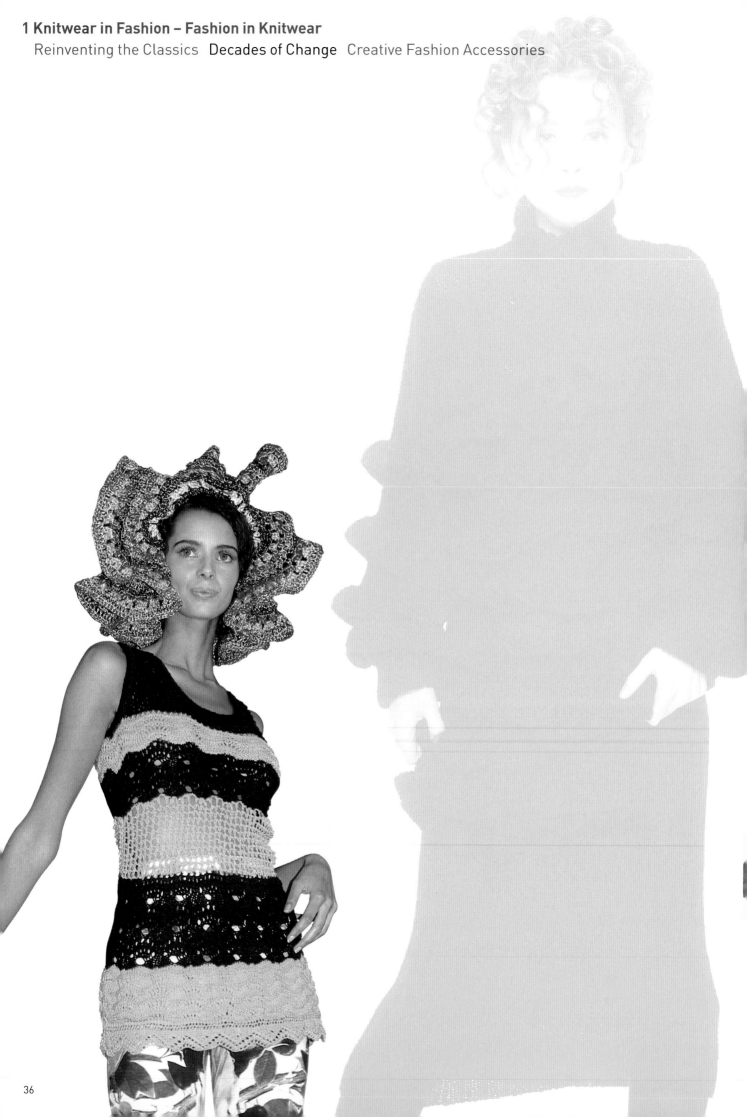

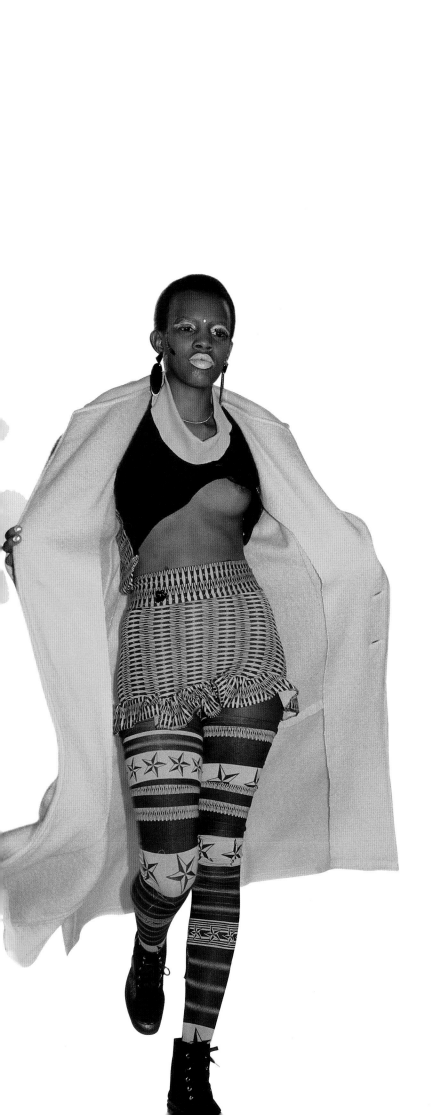

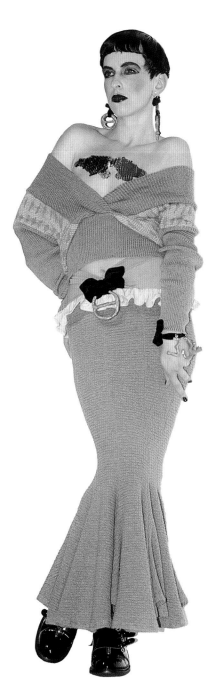

Opposite left Body Map, spring/summer 1990. Eclectic mixes of fabrics and patterns characterized the Body Map image. Here a hand-knitted and crochet top with a stiffened crochet hat and floral print trousers appear in an unusual mix of colours and textures for a quirky look inspired, it seems, by grandmother's dressing-up box.

Background Body Map, autumn/winter 1985/86. At the time of the 'New Romantics', frills were a key element of several Body Map collections. Here viscose and wool frills flow around a hand-knitted wool sweater dress. Knitted diagonally into the dress, using manual short-row knitting, they give a subtle change of texture and a strong silhouette.

Left Body Map, autumn/winter 1984/85. High-contrast prints and jacquard knits in black with white or primary colours create a strong visual impact. The graphic designs by Hilde Smith were integral to Body Map collections. Here they are printed on fine cotton/Lycra blend jersey made up into leggings, which featured the famous portholes, and fun, frilled shorts.

Above Body Map, autumn/winter 1985/86. Body Map were interested in creating a total fashion look, layering heavy knits over fine jersey, or creating volume with fabric. Production was achieved by manual knitting machine for larger items, such as the fishtail or 'petal' skirt, knitted sideways using short-row technique. Note the body jewelry which pre-dated the current vogue by nearly twenty years.

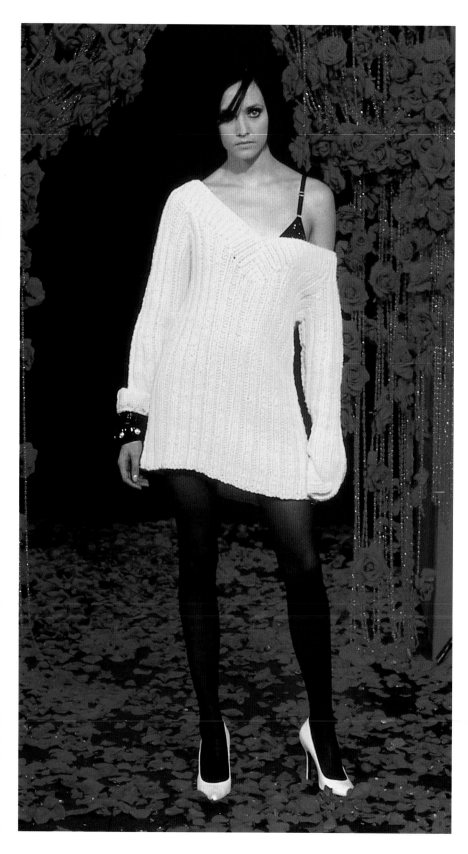

Left Dolce & Gabbana, autumn/winter 2001/02. Knitwear with attitude from the D&G diffusion line, aimed at a younger clientèle. A basic woollen V-neck sweater becomes a sexy dress when oversized and allowed to drop off the shoulder.

Opposite left Fake London, autumn/winter 2001/02. A post-punk 'street chic' look creates impact with a mix of cut-off denims and evening sandals, co-ordinated with patchwork argyll sleeveless top and Union Jack sweater, both designed with the fabric used in reverse, exhibiting the raw cut and unfinished edges of the knitted wool fabric.

Background Fake London, mid-1990s. This Union Jack patchwork sweater – one of the earliest designs launched by Desirée Mejer – encapsulates her fresh and irreverent approach to British emblems and to the classic cashmere sweater, reinventing it for a young, fashion-conscious clientèle. Other motifs included the Queen's head, the bulldog and football lettering. Note the rosette and label in reverse, with 'fake' royal crest.

Opposite right Fake London, autumn/winter 2001/02. Fake London patchworks were originally made from recycled cashmere sweaters but demand soon increased to outstrip supply and production now requires specially knitted fabric. The Union Jack theme – whether reworked in fine stocking mesh, recycled aran, bright colours, pastel shades or, as here, in a total outfit – seems never to be exhausted.

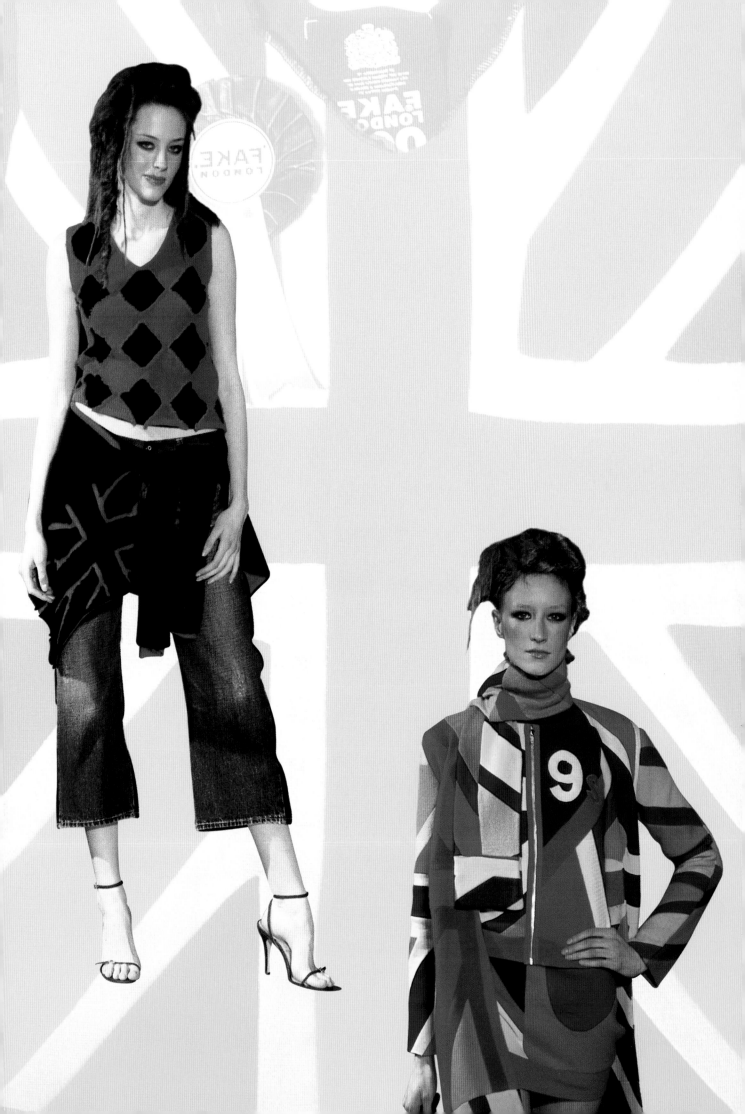

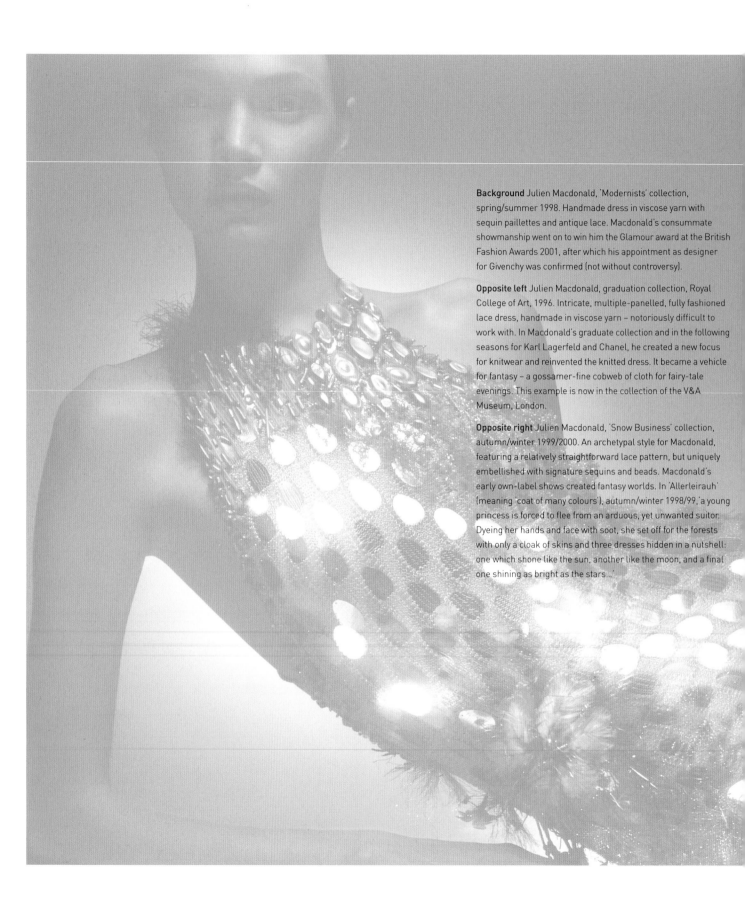

Background Julien Macdonald, 'Modernists' collection, spring/summer 1998. Handmade dress in viscose yarn with sequin paillettes and antique lace. Macdonald's consummate showmanship went on to win him the Glamour award at the British Fashion Awards 2001, after which his appointment as designer for Givenchy was confirmed (not without controversy).

Opposite left Julien Macdonald, graduation collection, Royal College of Art, 1996. Intricate, multiple-panelled, fully fashioned lace dress, handmade in viscose yarn – notoriously difficult to work with. In Macdonald's graduate collection and in the following seasons for Karl Lagerfeld and Chanel, he created a new focus for knitwear and reinvented the knitted dress. It became a vehicle for fantasy – a gossamer-fine cobweb of cloth for fairy-tale evenings. This example is now in the collection of the V&A Museum, London.

Opposite right Julien Macdonald, 'Snow Business' collection, autumn/winter 1999/2000. An archetypal style for Macdonald, featuring a relatively straightforward lace pattern, but uniquely embellished with signature sequins and beads. Macdonald's early own-label shows created fantasy worlds. In 'Allerleirauh' (meaning 'coat of many colours'), autumn/winter 1998/99, a young princess is forced to flee from an arduous, yet unwanted suitor. Dyeing her hands and face with soot, she set off for the forests with only a cloak of skins and three dresses hidden in a nutshell: one which shone like the sun, another like the moon, and a final one shining as bright as the stars...'

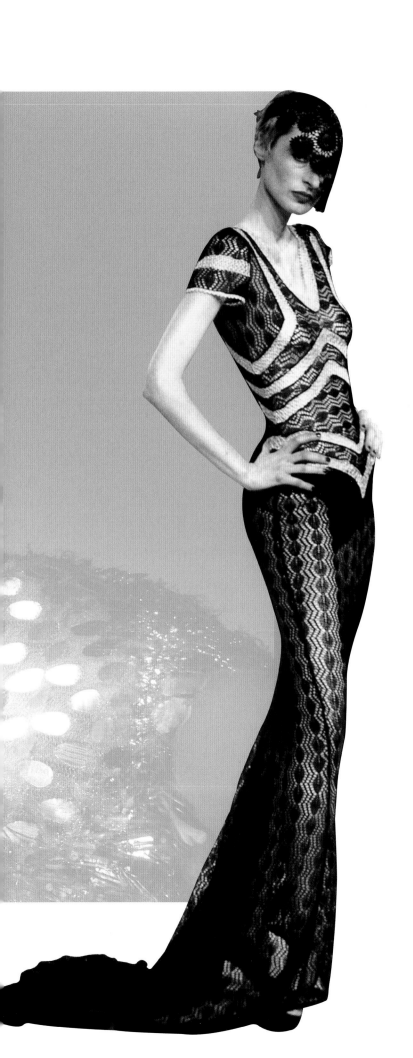
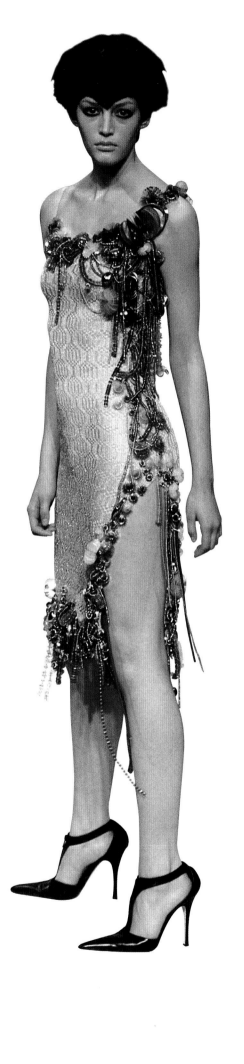

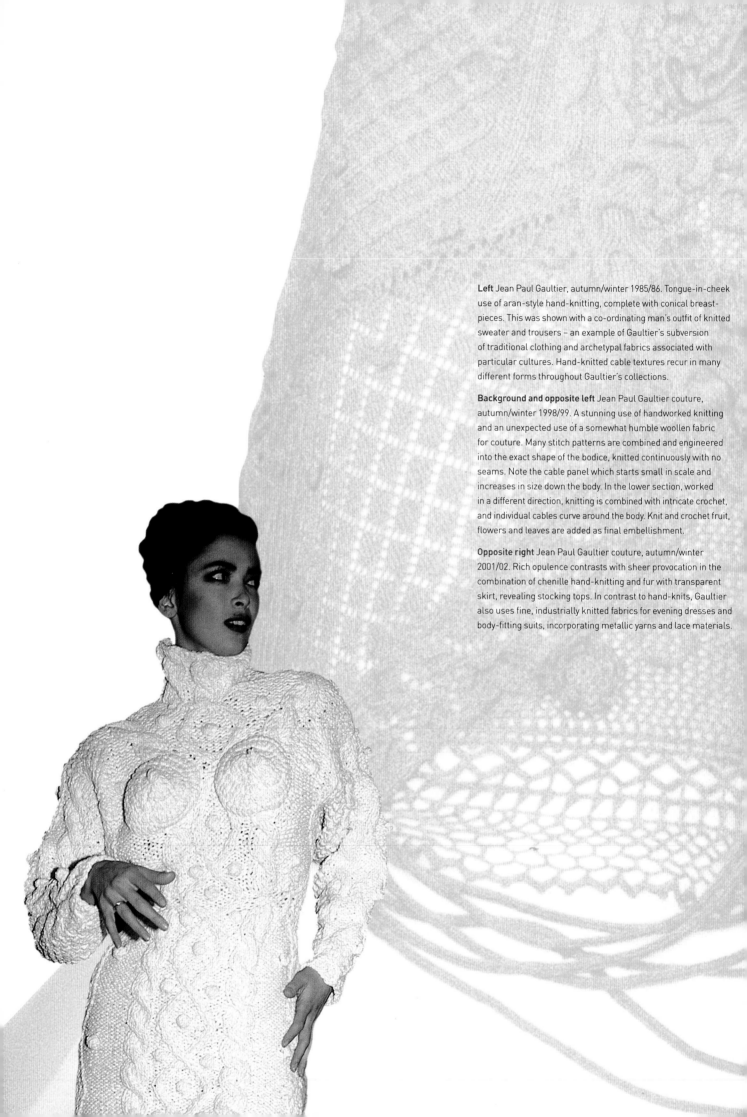

Left Jean Paul Gaultier, autumn/winter 1985/86. Tongue-in-cheek use of aran-style hand-knitting, complete with conical breast-pieces. This was shown with a co-ordinating man's outfit of knitted sweater and trousers – an example of Gaultier's subversion of traditional clothing and archetypal fabrics associated with particular cultures. Hand-knitted cable textures recur in many different forms throughout Gaultier's collections.

Background and opposite left Jean Paul Gaultier couture, autumn/winter 1998/99. A stunning use of handworked knitting and an unexpected use of a somewhat humble woollen fabric for couture. Many stitch patterns are combined and engineered into the exact shape of the bodice, knitted continuously with no seams. Note the cable panel which starts small in scale and increases in size down the body. In the lower section, worked in a different direction, knitting is combined with intricate crochet, and individual cables curve around the body. Knit and crochet fruit, flowers and leaves are added as final embellishment.

Opposite right Jean Paul Gaultier couture, autumn/winter 2001/02. Rich opulence contrasts with sheer provocation in the combination of chenille hand-knitting and fur with transparent skirt, revealing stocking tops. In contrast to hand-knits, Gaultier also uses fine, industrially knitted fabrics for evening dresses and body-fitting suits, incorporating metallic yarns and lace materials.

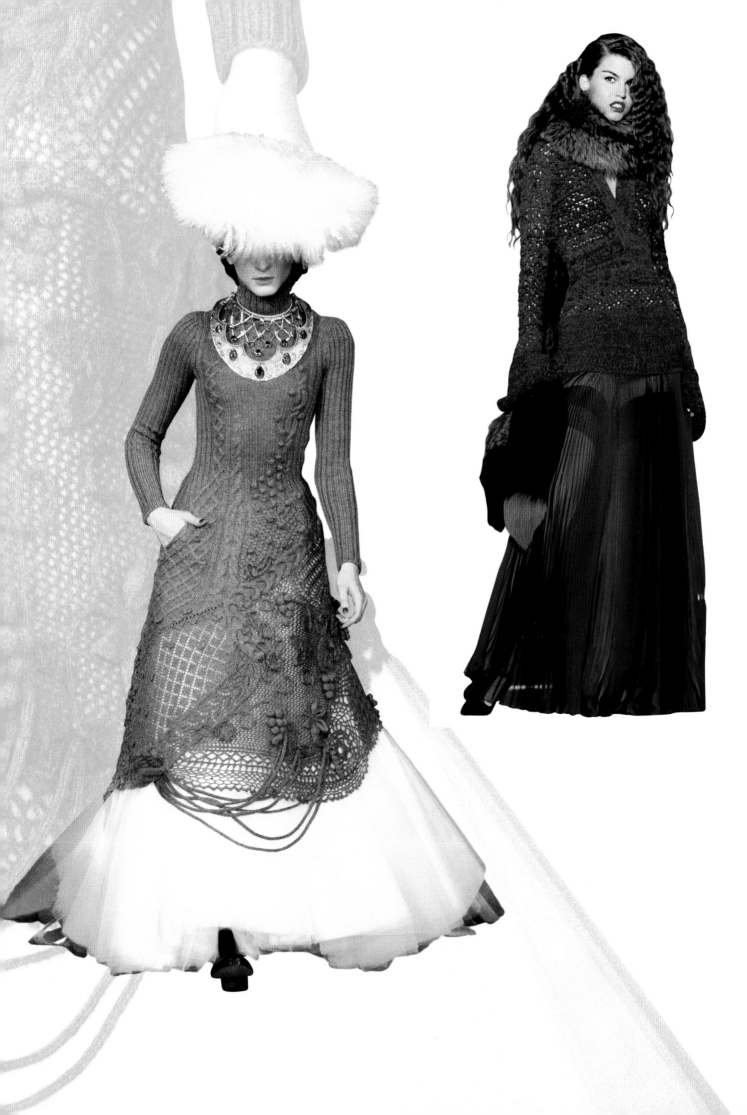

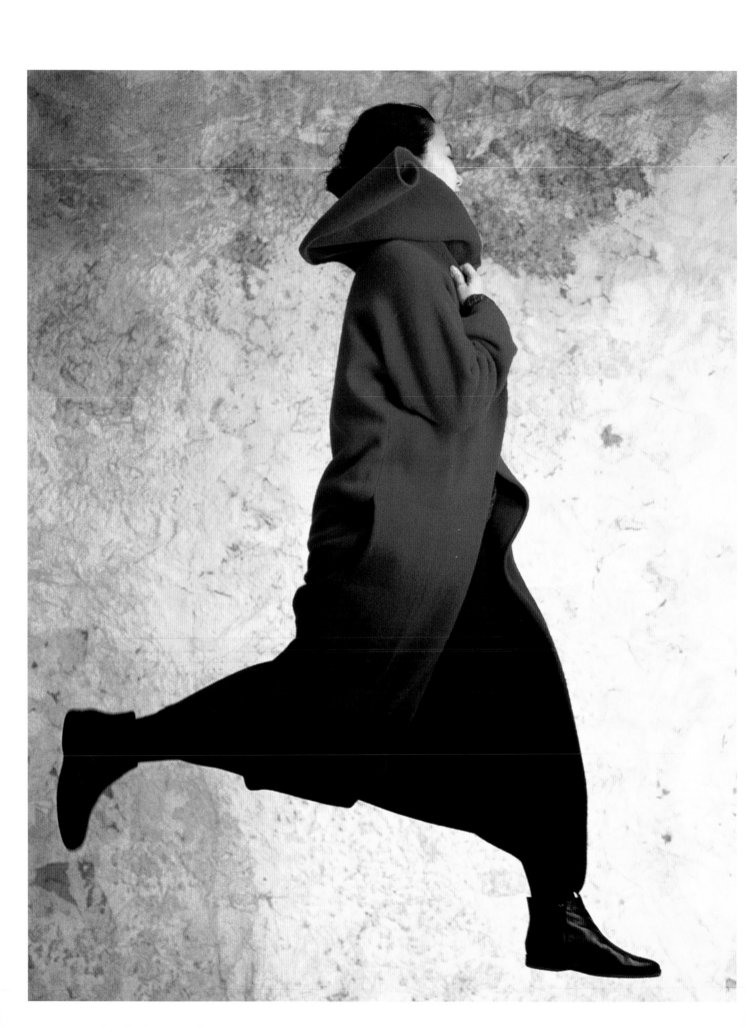

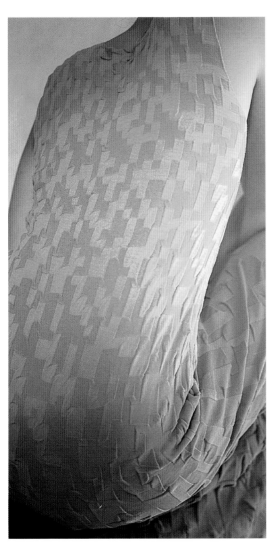

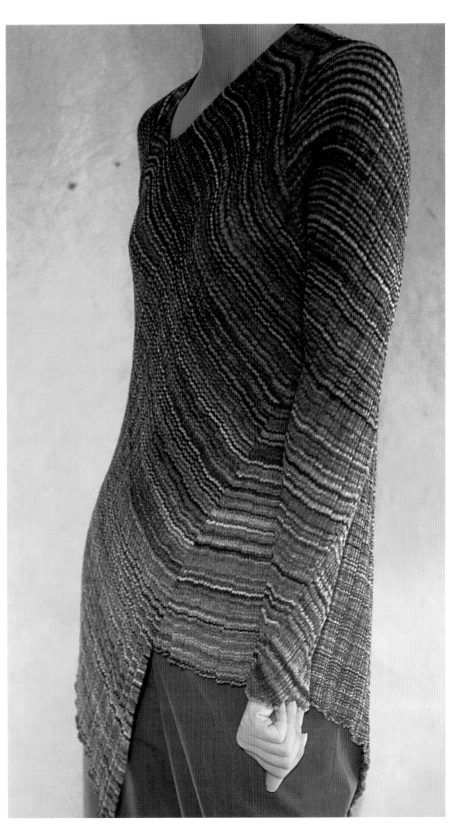

Opposite Jürgen Lehl, winter 2001. The exuberance of colour is conveyed in this knitted and felted wool coat, bokashi-dyed (using a Japanese gradation dyeing technique), with asymmetric collar. Multiple processes are typical of Lehl's complex production, where handworked qualities are imparted to machine-produced fabrics to create depth. Shapes are kept simple and the clothes are therefore both timeless and contemporary, with a universal appeal.

Above Jürgen Lehl, summer 2000. A double gradation is featured in this purl-stitch fabric dress: the geometric pattern grades from small to large down the length of the dress (programmed by CAD system) and the colour grades from yellow to green. The colours are plated to show in distinct areas of knit and purl stitches, enhanced by high-twist cotton yarn.

Right Jürgen Lehl, winter 2001. Six shades of grey high-twist wool used in a random sequence and a fine and unevenly spaced rib create fabric which spirals around the body in minimal and asymmetric form – just fabric (no trims) gives pared down simplicity. The innate characteristics of natural fibres are always preferred in Lehl's collections.

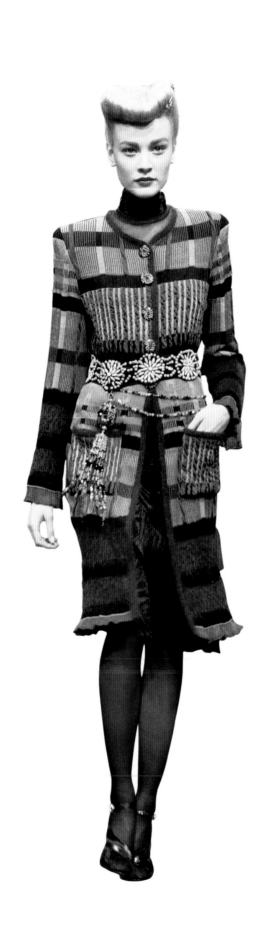

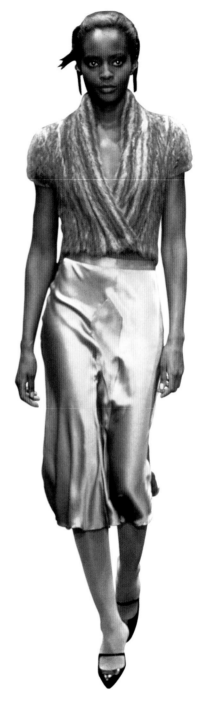

Left Christian Lacroix, prêt-à-porter collection, autumn/winter 1998/99. Lacroix, often inspired by ideas from freelance textile designers, uses ornate and colourful fabrics in rich profusion throughout his couture collections. Here a multicoloured, textured, felted jacquard is striking as an evening coat.

Above Lawrence Steele, autumn/winter 1998/99. In collaboration with his knitwear factory, Steele creates unusual materials for his ready-to-wear collections. This trompe l'oeil fabric, constructed in a quilted jacquard technique using mohair yarn in a cleverly designed graphic, realistically simulates fur when brushed.

Background Marina Spadafora, spring/summer 1999. In keeping with Spadafora's love of openwork and her experimental approach, a fine-gauge mohair lace dress is worn with a jacket from the same lace pattern, but knitted in polyester, permanently pleated and then sprayed with lacquer for a burnished effect.

Opposite right John Rocha, spring/summer 1997. Romantic, whimsical dresses, playing with transparency in both knit and crochet, became a Rocha signature at this time. This fine wool and transparent nylon slip-dress shows one of his early reinventions of traditional lace patterns.

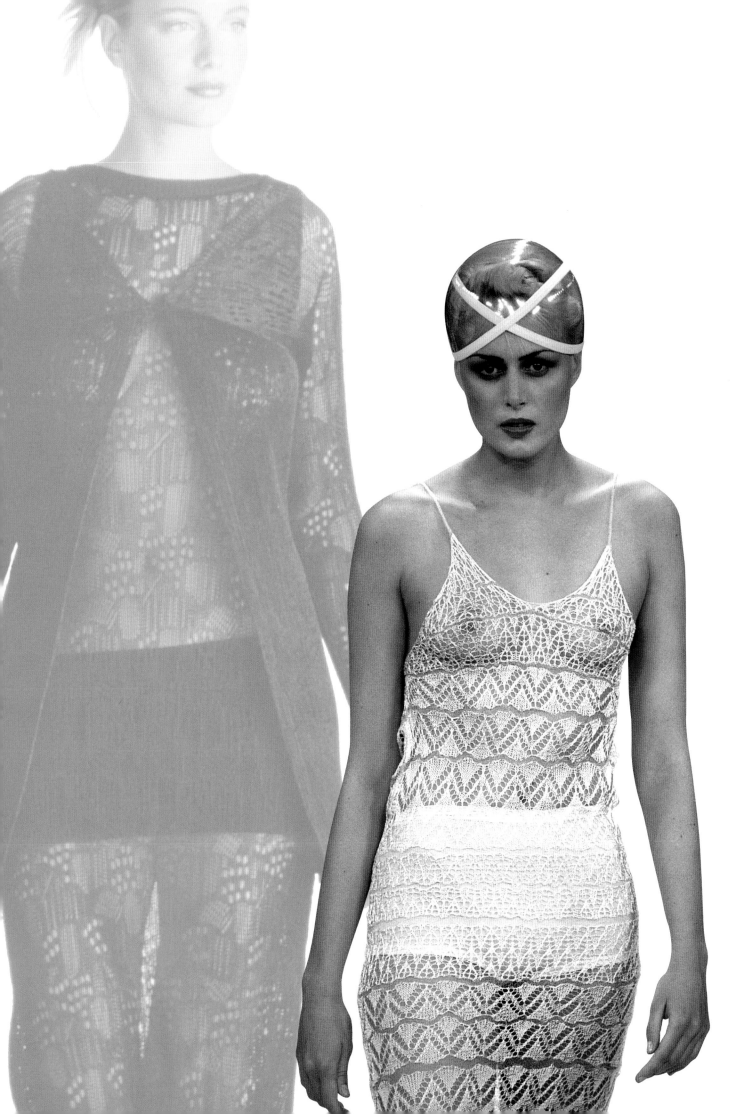

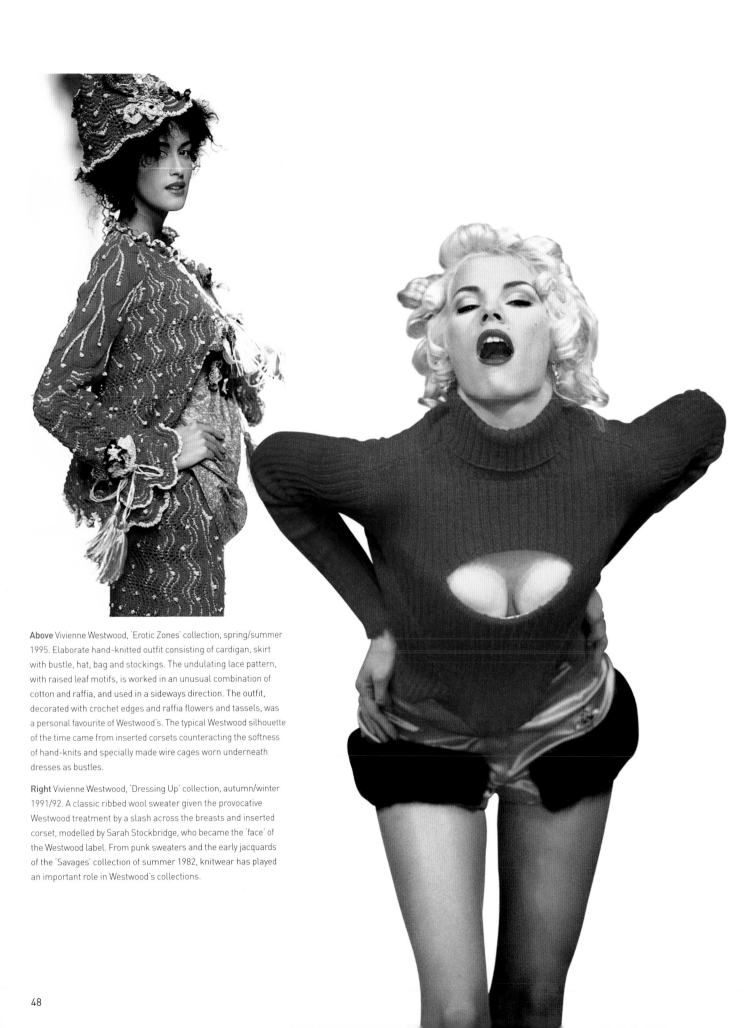

Above Vivienne Westwood, 'Erotic Zones' collection, spring/summer
1995. Elaborate hand-knitted outfit consisting of cardigan, skirt
with bustle, hat, bag and stockings. The undulating lace pattern,
with raised leaf motifs, is worked in an unusual combination of
cotton and raffia, and used in a sideways direction. The outfit,
decorated with crochet edges and raffia flowers and tassels, was
a personal favourite of Westwood's. The typical Westwood silhouette
of the time came from inserted corsets counteracting the softness
of hand-knits and specially made wire cages worn underneath
dresses as bustles.

Right Vivienne Westwood, 'Dressing Up' collection, autumn/winter
1991/92. A classic ribbed wool sweater given the provocative
Westwood treatment by a slash across the breasts and inserted
corset, modelled by Sarah Stockbridge, who became the 'face' of
the Westwood label. From punk sweaters and the early jacquards
of the 'Savages' collection of summer 1982, knitwear has played
an important role in Westwood's collections.

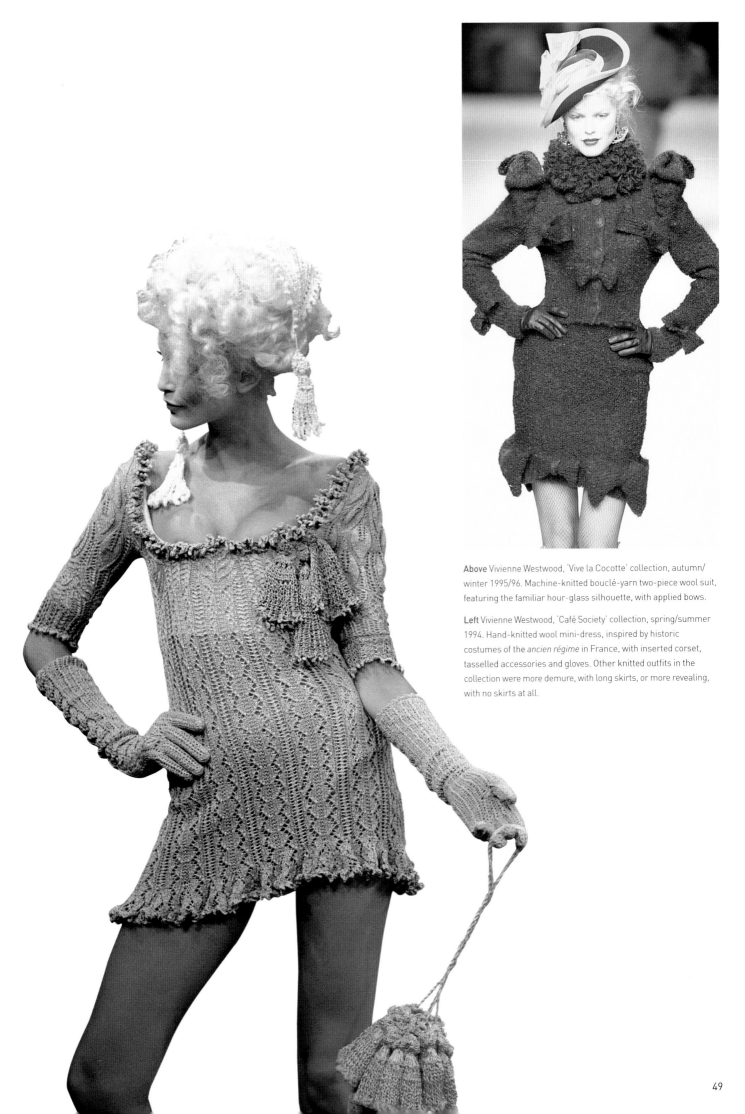

Above Vivienne Westwood, 'Vive la Cocotte' collection, autumn/
winter 1995/96. Machine-knitted bouclé-yarn two-piece wool suit,
featuring the familiar hour-glass silhouette, with applied bows.

Left Vivienne Westwood, 'Café Society' collection, spring/summer
1994. Hand-knitted wool mini-dress, inspired by historic
costumes of the *ancien régime* in France, with inserted corset,
tasselled accessories and gloves. Other knitted outfits in the
collection were more demure, with long skirts, or more revealing,
with no skirts at all.

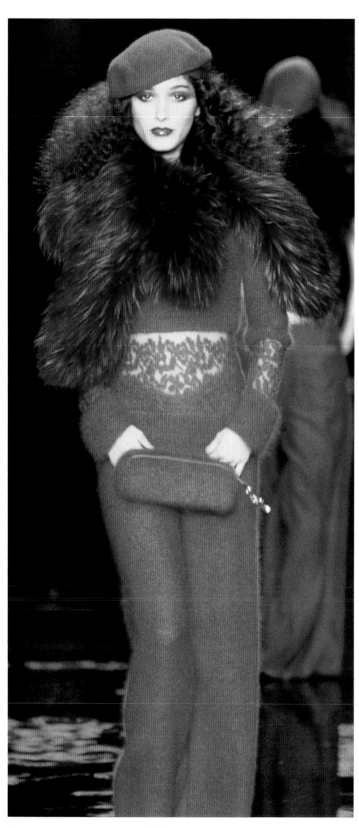

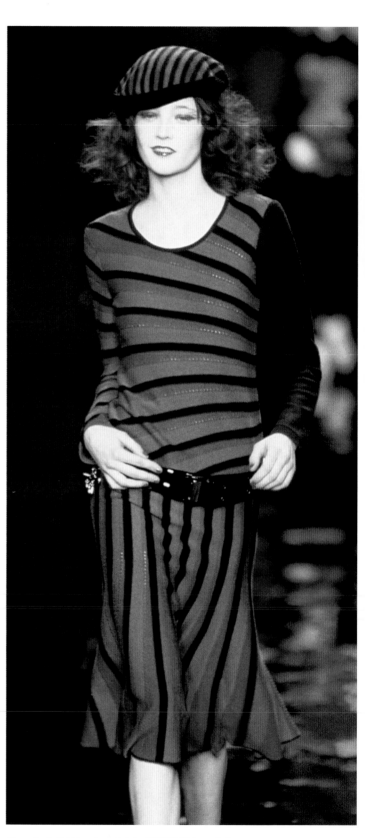

Above Sonia Rykiel, autumn/winter 2000/01. Rykiel is the legendary *grande dame* of Paris fashion, still the owner of her own family-run company after almost forty years. Whilst maintaining a steady presence in designer fashion, the label has recently undergone a renaissance of interest from a wider public and younger clientèle. This complete knitwear look signalled a return to the opulence of luxury angora yarns and fur.

Above Sonia Rykiel, autumn/winter 2001/02. Stripes of all proportions are a permanent feature of Sonia Rykiel knitwear, with regular variations to update the look each season. Here the use of short-row knitting creates a sunray effect, engineered to continue across one sleeve. A change of fabric direction results in a flared shape for the skirt.

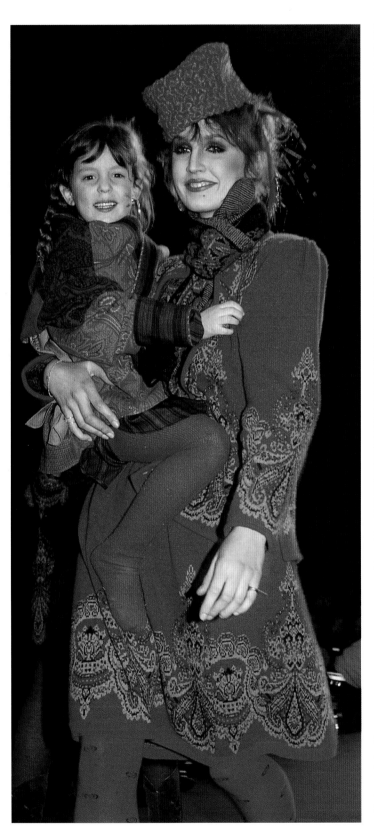

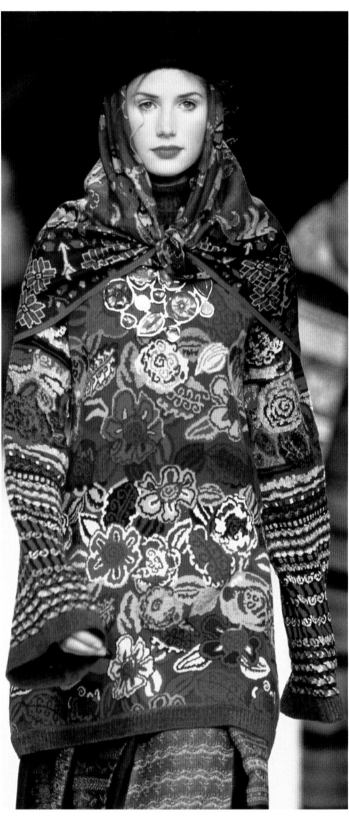

Above Kenzo, autumn/winter 1981/82. Bright colour and intricate patterning, reminiscent of Oriental carpet designs, decorate a layered outfit given a total look by co-ordinated accessories. The pattern is achieved through a four-colour jacquard construction, but in a fine gauge and yarn which allows the fabric to drape. Jacquard and embroidery continue to be strong elements of recent Kenzo collections.

Above Kenzo, autumn/winter 1994/95. Signature mix of patterns, fabrics and Eastern European-influenced styling. The floral, patterned sweater is a cleverly designed four-colour jacquard in which the colours gradually change, giving the impression of many more colours overall. The sleeves change pattern entirely, and a matching necklace blends with the knitted design. Chenille edgings complete the mix.

Background Judit Kárpáti-Rácz, breast-piece, 2000. In 1996 Kárpáti-Rácz began to explore the mythologies of the earth goddesses and the archetypes of femininity – the virgin, the crone and the mother – creating sensual, body-related shapes with timeless qualities. Through exploration of materials, particularly nylon monofilament (familiar as fishing line) in strong colours, she has transformed an ancient knotting technique formerly worked in horsehair for modern accessories.

Opposite Judit Kárpáti-Rácz, hat, 1999. The spiral formation which is fundamental to the construction of most of Kárpáti-Rácz's three-dimensional shapes is a prominent aesthetic characteristic of this hat, which also functions as a veil. Hats which surround or envelop the head are a regular feature. Without the anchorage to the head, the dynamic shape could almost fly away on its feathered spokes.

Accessories have leapt to prominence in fashion during the past ten years and now occupy an important place in the market both in fashion terms and commercially. They can be fun, and follow a proud tradition from Schiaparelli's famous shoe hat of 1937 to Lagerfeld's pastry hats of 1984. Aspirational items, particularly bags – once badges of belonging to a social elite, and the exclusive domain of high-level design houses such as Louis Vuitton, Gucci, Fendi, Dior and Chanel – have spread rapidly from the luxury market to the mass market, stimulated by the increasingly expert and convincing production of fakes. However, the originals seek to keep one step ahead by creating distinctive new designs – for example the Stephen Sprouse graffiti bag and Julie Verhoeven picture bag from Vuitton – and the true fashion cognoscenti will accept no substitute for the genuine item. The Fendi 'Baguette' bag achieved a similar cult status in its many forms, including a version made in grey knitted fabric. Knit has become a fabric which is routinely considered for use in accessories such as shoes and bags but continues to have a surprising visual effect as its context is changed. For the ultimate in total knit dressing, Missoni now make a line of shoes and bags in knit fabrics to match certain outfits, perhaps ironically referring to the 1950s heyday of matching accessories.

Some accessories have become increasingly decorative and impractical – tiny handbags and purses, oversized corsages of raw fabric, shoes which are impossibly flimsy or have highly precarious platform soles – but these are conversation pieces and a relatively small investment for the cachet of the designer label or the attention received. In the mid-1970s Kenzo's Jap label was one of the first to present as fashion a tiny textile pocket bag. This was very influential and is now a commonplace. A market has developed over recent years for items which have been handmade or produced in small batches, satisfying the consumer's desire for individuality and quirky personal expression in a pervasively minimal and hard-edged designed environment. Knitted and crochet bags, once the province of the hippy or the non-fashionable shopper, are now produced in a riot of colourful and not-so-practical but visually appealing bags which echo Victorian beaded bags and knitted purses once used by ladies of leisure.

Young entrepreneurs have discovered a creative niche by setting up micro-businesses making handmade accessories in a way very reminiscent of the craft renaissance of the 1970s. In tandem, small shops-cum-galleries have sprung up in which to display these products, crossing the boundary between craftwork and fashion. Cutting-edge boutiques often include a range of handcrafted accessories, perhaps felt or crochet jewelry and bags. At the opposite end of the spectrum, the British chainstore Accessorize

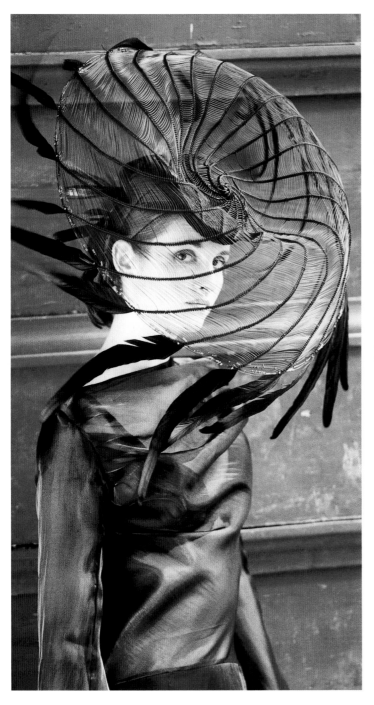

combines commerciality with the craft skills of its producers in India to create colourful interpretations of such trends as embroidered and crochet bags.

Knitted items often feature as one part of a company's range, to give a folksy, cosy, rather bohemian aspect to the collection. Hikaru Noguchi produces a broad and eclectic range of quirky accessories and clothes; Orla Keily makes felted, striped knit bags and co-ordinating sweaters; The Sak create a regular range of hand-crocheted bags. The small scale of accessories allows the designer's imagination to roam, creating the opportunity to experiment with shape, form and materials without too much risk attached. The most exciting work challenges established ideas. Judit Kárpáti-Rácz has developed ancient hand-knotting techniques similar to knitting but using modern materials, notably monofilament nylon yarn and copper, silver and steel wire to sculpt around forms into shapes which symbolize the feminine. The same nylon material is fundamental to Nora Fok's jewelry, its mutability being crucial in creating her sculptural forms, which are often inspired by close observation of natural phenomena.

Textiles and soft materials have begun to be used more frequently as textile designers such as Mie Iwatsubo and Lynsey Walters have turned their attention to manipulating materials into wearable forms of decorative accessories and jewelry. The search for a saleable product has opened up many new avenues for exploration, felted wool fibres and knitted wool fabrics being a favourite for manipulation. The best pieces reflect the ideal combination of craftsmanship and innovation.

Since Mary Quant and Biba first popularized the fashion for opaque coloured hosiery in the 1960s, the development of fashionable tights and stockings has shown no bounds. (In 1998 the holy grail of 'panty hose' or tights construction – a complete, one-piece product devoid of seams – was achieved.) What is worn on the legs is now considered integral to the fashion statement, either as part of the total story, for example in the work of Bernhard Willhelm, or as an echo of the main fashion themes, such as fishnet and heavy lace. Hosiery

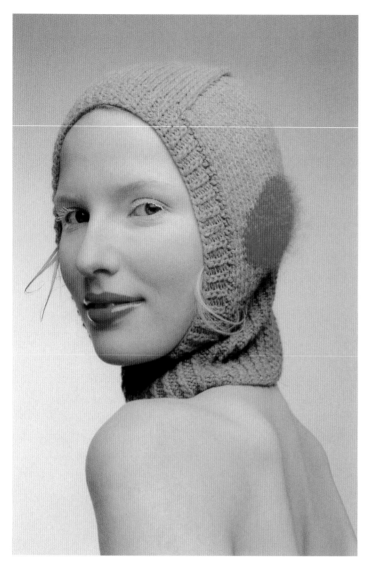

manufacturers have to co-ordinate their products with the prevailing trends. Even at couture level, deconstruction has had its impact. Destroyed fashion needs destroyed accessories: Dior's pre-laddered tights complete an ironic full circle beginning with ripped jeans and punk and ending with Galliano's collaged 'tramp' collections for Dior in 2000/01. Vivienne Westwood proudly displayed a photograph of herself wearing laddered tights in the aftermath of a sexual encounter, so the legend goes. A young French artist Stephanie Piogé has created tights as artwork loaded with meaning by carefully dissecting them and creating precarious assemblages from the parts, expressive of painful emotions.

The humble sock, the most mundane of accessories, has also been reinvented. Colour and pattern have been applied and several designers, including Issey Miyake and Comme des Garçons, now produce co-ordinating socks as a matter of course to accessorize their collections, thereby also providing a relatively affordable buy-in to the range. Jacquard techniques in the very fine gauge used for socks produce myriad visual images which have found their way onto the ankle, including licensed character merchandising from major commercial films. Imagination runs riot and there is less concern for finish than with clothing – threads hang free inside a patterned sock. Anything goes when children's socks are designed. The technical potential for three-dimensionality can be exploited to the full, for example in the ranges produced by Sock Shop, originally inspired by Japanese socks. These are a riot of sock heels forming animal shapes, the heel being a wonderful feat of engineering in which a tube turns a corner due to a special formation of the knit structure.

Women's shoes, meanwhile, occupy a very special position in fashion, with the potential to become fetishized objects both on and off the feet. The sexual connotations of the stiletto-heeled shoe cannot be ignored: many extreme designs and hard shiny materials conjure up the dominatrix and the expression of power. When soft materials such as knitted or felted fabrics are used, the styling changes to comfortable or practical to match the message. The shoe can be a powerful medium for communication of concepts, as demonstrated in the Surrealist art of Magritte and his contradictory feet-shoes, subsequently realized by Pierre Cardin. Dutch maker Simone Memel experiments with shoes that tread the line between art object and practical shoe. She has used knitted fabrics of opposing qualities such as fluffy mohair and hard rope to express conflicts and personalities in semi-wearable pieces, which have been exhibited widely. In some cases it is difficult to distinguish between art-object shoes and the extremes of fashionability. Accessories of all types are an exciting growth area, which, in the most creative hands, merge the boundaries between art, clothing and sculpture.

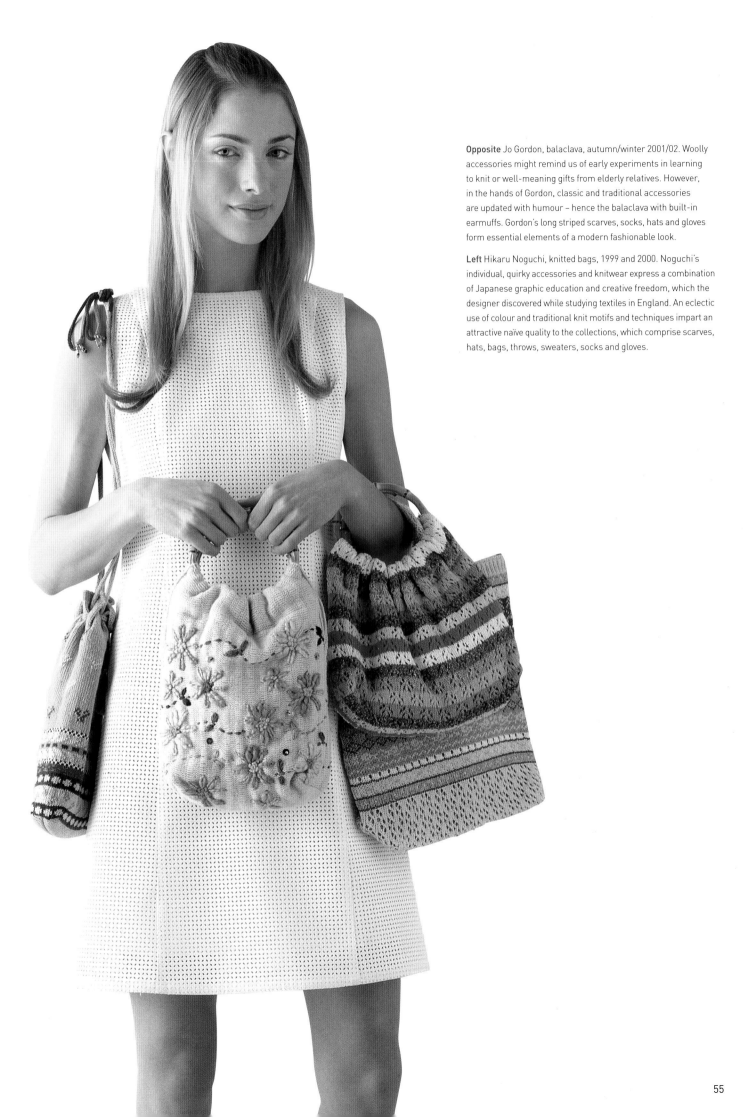

Opposite Jo Gordon, balaclava, autumn/winter 2001/02. Woolly accessories might remind us of early experiments in learning to knit or well-meaning gifts from elderly relatives. However, in the hands of Gordon, classic and traditional accessories are updated with humour – hence the balaclava with built-in earmuffs. Gordon's long striped scarves, socks, hats and gloves form essential elements of a modern fashionable look.

Left Hikaru Noguchi, knitted bags, 1999 and 2000. Noguchi's individual, quirky accessories and knitwear express a combination of Japanese graphic education and creative freedom, which the designer discovered while studying textiles in England. An eclectic use of colour and traditional knit motifs and techniques impart an attractive naïve quality to the collections, which comprise scarves, hats, bags, throws, sweaters, socks and gloves.

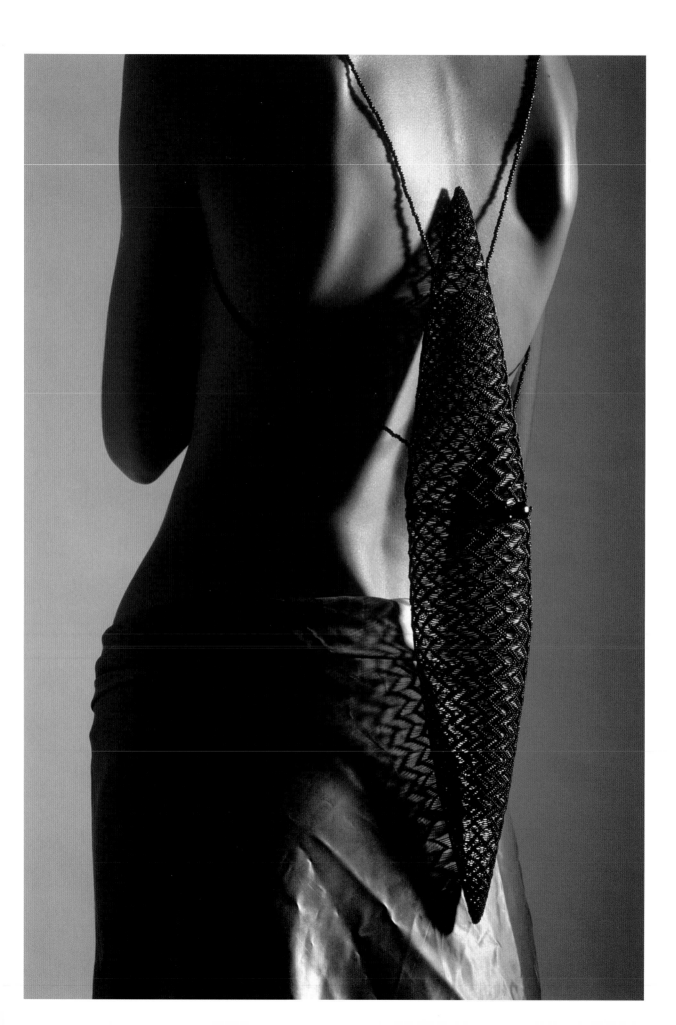

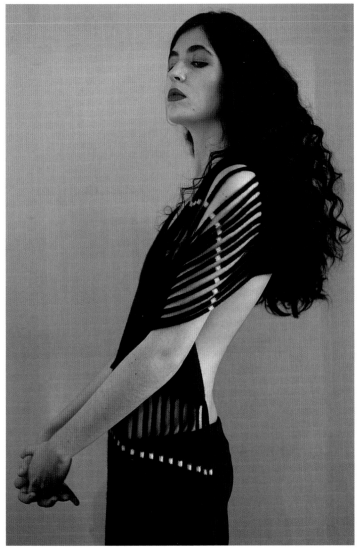

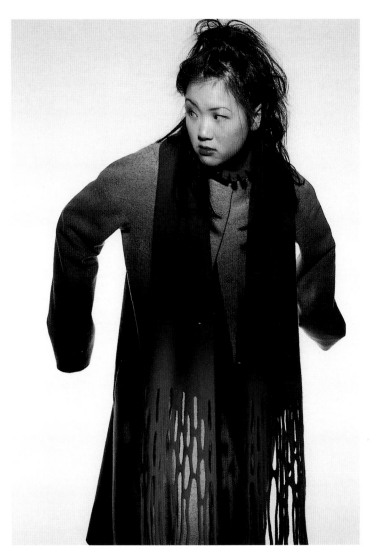

Opposite Judit Kárpáti-Rácz, rucksack, 1996. A beautifully proportioned shape, relating strongly to the curve of the back. Kárpáti-Rácz creates an individual wooden form for each piece – in a similar manner to the shoemaker's last or the milliner's block – around which she creates knotted shapes. The rigidity resulting from the nylon yarn gives practicality to the finished item, which is both lightweight and sturdy.

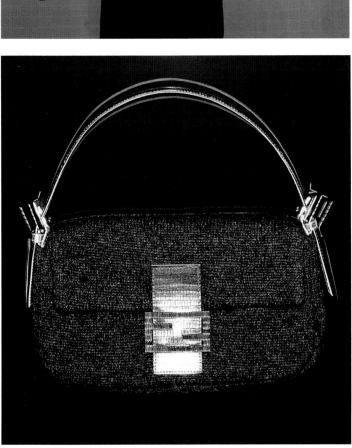

Above left Alan Gallacher, fringed scarf, autumn/winter 2001/02. Gallacher has developed a process for creating knitted and felted fringed scarves with either subtle or bold colour effects, which create a focal point for movement. The range includes large and small scarves and shawls made from merino wool or cashmere. One small scarf with points of colour framing the face is reminiscent of the magnified splash effect created by a water drop; others invoke the hair braids or beads of African tribes.

Above Alan Gallacher, shawl with fringe in the form of a net, autumn/winter 1999/2000.

Left Fendi, 'Baguette' bag in grey metallic knitted fabric, autumn/winter 1998/99. Note the double F logo which is almost as covetable as the double C of Chanel and the double G of Gucci. The Baguette phenomenon was typical of the aspirational status that has been accorded to particular luxury bags since the late 1990s, deliberately heightened by their unavailability.

Right Simone Memel, 'Hard Rope', 1994/95. Memel branched out from her fine arts and three-dimensional studies into the craft of shoemaking in order to express dichotomies and perceptions associated with male and female roles. Her first shoe project was a sock boot, combining sock and shoe, and she has since created many versions of one-off shoes using a range of knitted and other materials. Here hand-knitted string is used to simulate the toughness of rope in a classic wearable style outlined by the knit and purl stitches and the plaited edging.

Below Ann-Louise Roswald, autumn/winter 1998/99. Capitalizing on her father's traditional clog-making business, Roswald was inspired to create matching clogs for her stylized floral printed knitwear. These were quickly taken up by Italian fashion house Marni for their winter 1999 collection, patterned to look like cowskin, and are now manufactured on a larger scale in Sweden.

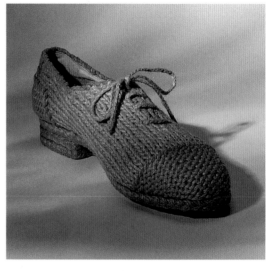

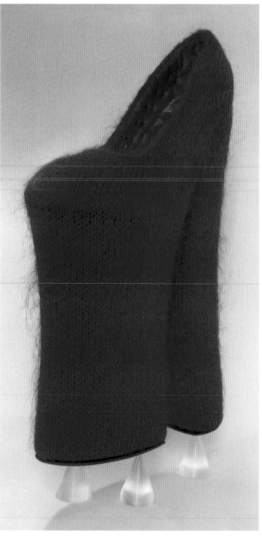

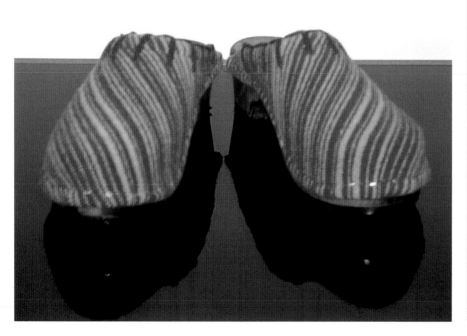

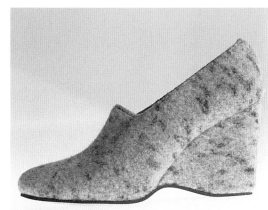

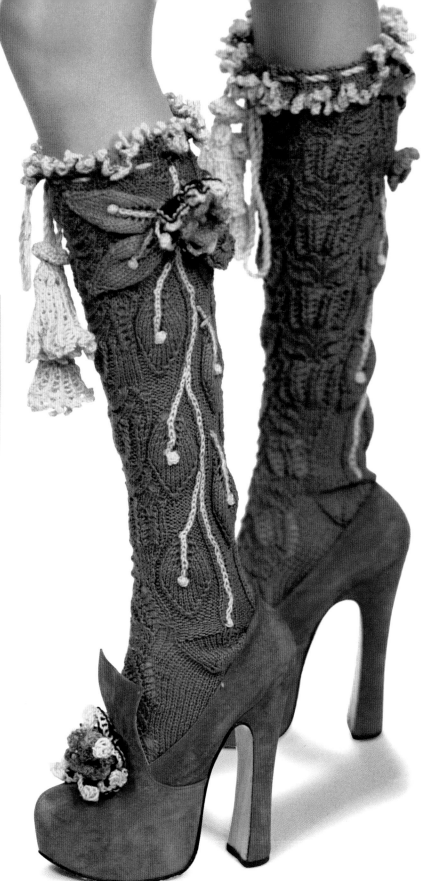

Above Shelley Fox, summer 1996. Felted wool, which was also embossed and used for co-ordinated shoes, formed the fabric for Fox's graduation collection, showing her attention to detail and the importance of unique fabrics to her work. Each outfit had matching fabric shoes – a total-look theme that Fox has pursued through the use of co-ordinated knitted, printed and felted fabrics.

Right Vivienne Westwood, 'On Liberty' collection, autumn/winter 1994/95. Hand-knitted wool stockings with intricate lace and embossed leaf design and appliquéd flowers, finished with knitted tassels, were made to accessorize elaborate corseted and bustled hand-knitted outfits based on historical costume. Note how the knitted decoration extends to the shoes. Bags and jewelry were also created to accessorize.

Opposite Simone Memel, 'Homage à Monroe', 1995. The material defines the shoe in Memel's work – in this case a statuesque homage to womanhood, symbolized by an unwearable shoe in fluffy mohair with a quilted satin lining. In Memel's world Monroe and women stand precariously on their pedestal. Another creation – 'On the Road' – also used a mohair fabric, contrasted with tyre tread-patterned rubber for the sole and heel.

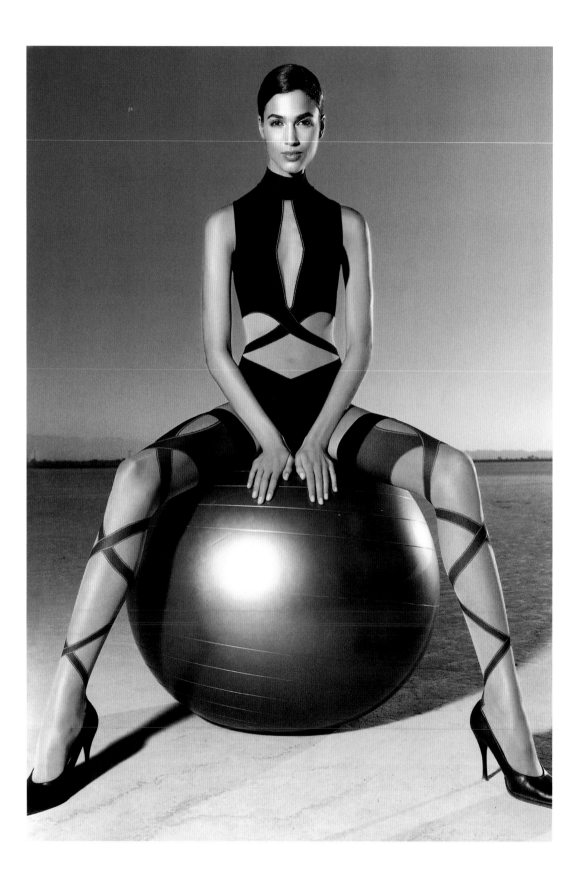

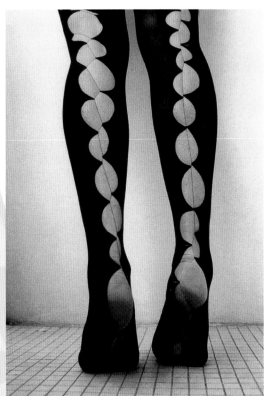

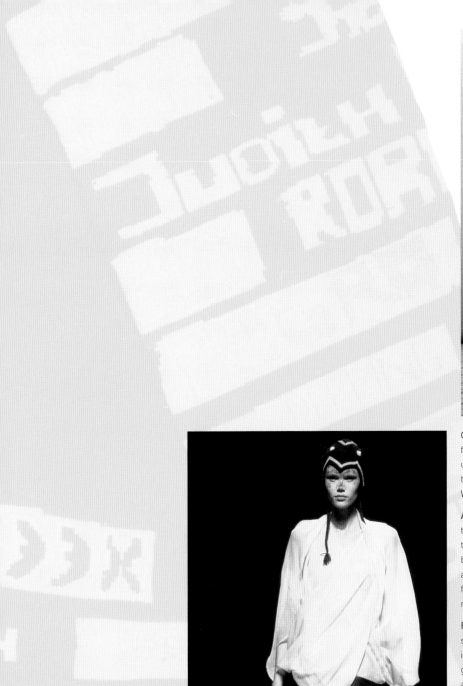

Opposite Wolford, spring/summer 2001. Meshes of all sizes – from fine and heavy fishnets to this bold, ribbon-patterned, hold-up stocking – co-ordinated the designer catwalk collections of the season, from Anna Sui, Guerriero and Jun Ashida to Vivienne Westwood and Helmut Lang.

Above Stephanie Piogé, summer 1999. Piogé's graduation project took tights as a means of expression to convey women's pain: the emotions inside are bursting through the tights, which have been disassembled and now can only function to display anxiety and a precarious position in the world. The appropriation of a familiar item of clothing creates a powerful and disturbing medium of communication.

Background Bernhard Willhelm, autumn/winter 2001/02. Long socks formed a major accessory to the season's collection, knitted industrially with a jacquard pattern of girls' and boys' names. The graphic design takes on an abstract quality when worn, the names appearing as a surprise. The names also featured as an all-over pattern in jersey jacquard fabric for jackets and sweatshirts.

Left Bernhard Willhelm, autumn/winter 2001/02. Outfit accessorized with jacquard socks plus a hand-knitted chevron hat imparting a naïve quality. This collection ranged broadly from Arabic-, Turkish- and Afghan-inspired striped fabric ruffles and tailoring to folkloric hand-knitted sweaters and skirts in 'old fashioned' colours, like patchwork-knitted bedspreads, plus cut and sewn pieces made from the 'names' fabric (see background picture) in jersey.

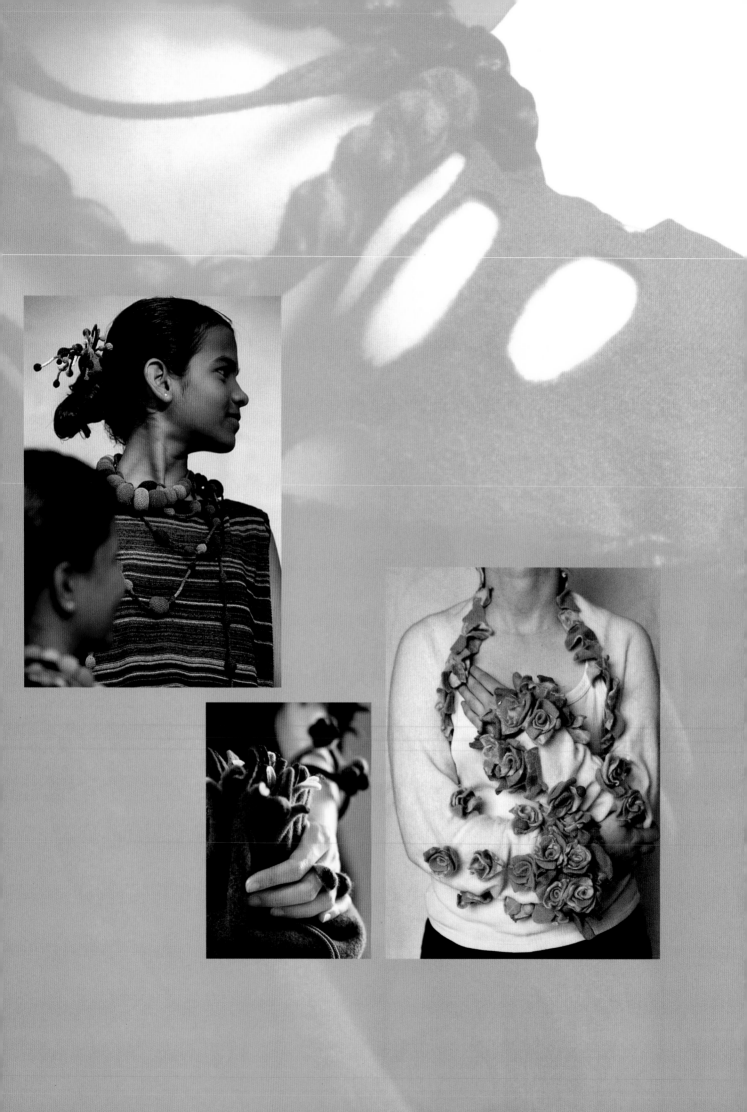

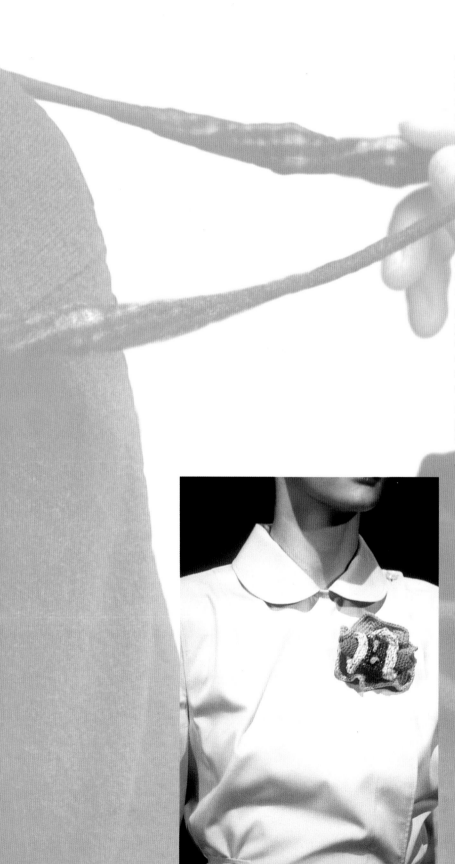

Opposite left Jürgen Lehl, summer 2001. Hand-crocheted cotton necklaces and hair decorations, co-ordinated with linen striped knitwear. Lehl had these made in India. He uses production from many craftspeople throughout Asia, travelling to oversee design and production personally.

Opposite centre Jürgen Lehl, winter 1999. Knitted and felted wool drawstring bag fastened with pebbles. The felt jewelry range included rings, necklaces, hair ornaments and armbands. Felting is a versatile technique, and felt can be made from knitted wool fabric or directly from woollen fibres; many designers favour the knitted fabric method for ease of production.

Opposite right Lynsey Walters, winter 2000. Knitted lambswool shrug decorated with felted flowers. The profusion of flowers are individually made from felted petals which curl realistically. Walters's range of accessories includes quirky aprons and knitted necklaces, handbags and scarves.

Background Jürgen Lehl, autumn 2000. The knitted and felted jewelry created by Mie Iwatsubo, using shibori resist-dyeing technique, co-ordinates here with a knitted lambswool felted sweater with slashed holes over the shoulders. Lehl combines commercial production with handcrafted processes, giving a handmade quality to his collections.

Left Bernhard Willhelm, summer 2001. Handcrafted accessories in knit and crochet, such as this food-inspired knitted and crocheted brooch, and hats of crochet fried eggs, completed the humorous picture of domestic bliss portrayed in this collection. Willhelm usurps the tradition of domestic knitting, with its toys and comforts, and displaces it into avant-garde fashion.

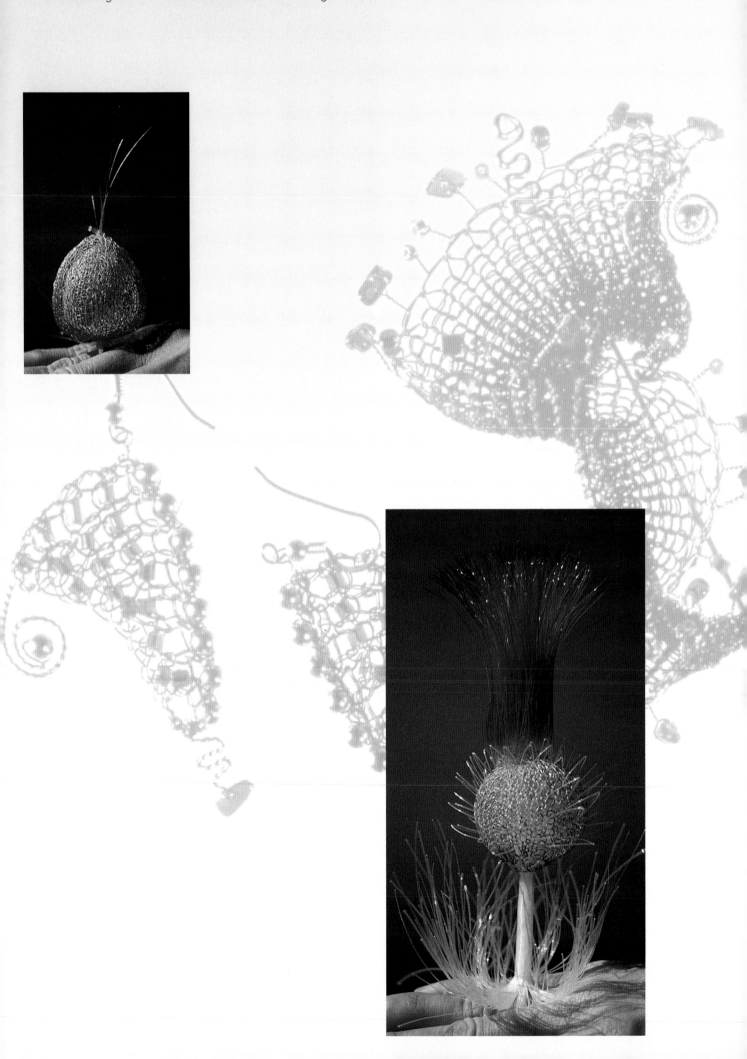

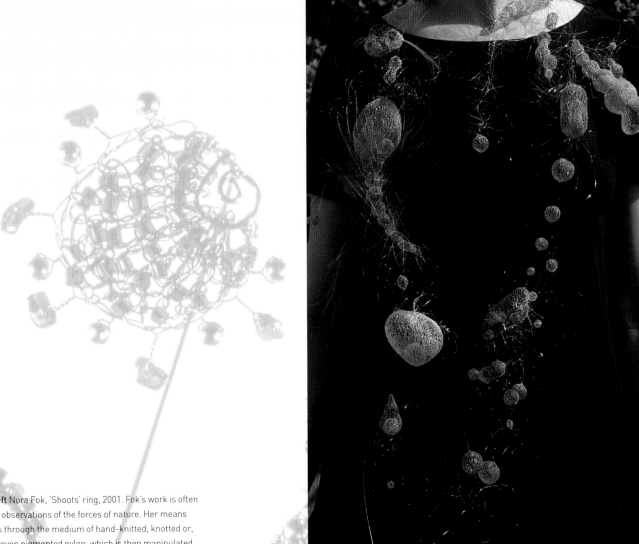

Opposite top left Nora Fok, 'Shoots' ring, 2001. Fok's work is often inspired by her observations of the forces of nature. Her means of expression is through the medium of hand-knitted, knotted or, occasionally, woven pigmented nylon, which is then manipulated through heat to create sculptural forms – a technique that Fok has mastered and made her own over many years of development. The jewelry sculptures have a strong presence, which is enhanced when worn on the body. A series of extraordinary rings express the life-force awakening, including this seed within its protective outer casing, and 'Seedling' (not pictured) which has small, delicate leaves and stands 30 cm high.

Opposite right Nora Fok, 'Thistle' ring, 2001. A further dramatic example of Fok's three-dimensional expression of natural form, standing proudly on the hand.

Background Jan Truman, earrings and brooches, 1997. Truman creates characterful jewelry from knitted copper wire, incorporating into the knitting process multicoloured glass beads and semi-precious gemstones (garnets, amethyst, carnelian, iolite) to create a dance of light and colour. Pieces are made by hand-knitting or by specially adapted machine.

Right Nora Fok, 'Food Chain' neckpiece, 1999. Looking at nature at a microscopic level, this piece depicts the possible beginning of the food chain and the amoeba which exist beyond our normal vision. Each element of the chain is individually formed, sometimes one part inside another.

Opposite Lawrence Steele, autumn/winter 2000/01. By challenging the accepted norms, textiles and fashion move forward, seeking new ideas and experimental processes. Here Steele has combined two unlikely materials, resulting in strong visual impact. Camel hair knitted fur fabric has been overprinted with gold foil, creating a deeply cracked effect – a process which took some persuasion for the factory to produce. (Incidentally, the gold foil was less successful with mink, as commissioned by Anna Wintour, editor of US *Vogue*.)

Innovation is the lifeblood of fashion and for some time textile developments have provided new inspiration for fashion designers. To support the commercial industry in developing new concepts for fabric structures and fibre types, an important part has also been played by knitwear, textile and fashion students at all levels of operation.

In addition to the traditional yarns, designers constantly experiment with new and unconventional materials, breaking down barriers between craft, art and fashion. Experimental 'yarns' have included wire, paper and plastics, and knitted fabrics have been printed, laminated, rubberized, felted, heat-formed and subjected to many other processes. Some experiments perversely seek to combine the inherent structure and form of knitted fabric with opposing effects, such as heat-fixing to make the flexible structure rigid, or coating to fill up the inevitable holes. The newest synthetic fibres are being explored to their limits with surface treatments and combinations of effects which may result in destruction if the correct balance is not achieved. Awareness of all that has gone before means that more and more extremes must be investigated in order to create originality.

Crucial to many experiments are nylon monofilament or polyester materials, which can be heat-set, dyed and transformed in many ways. They have their own inherent behaviour characteristics, such as rigidity, which provide a counter-reaction to the forces found within the knitted structure itself. Many of the processes are, by virtue of their investigative nature, craft-based, manual production methods, giving special qualities to the resulting one-off fabrics, which in turn catch the attention of innovative fashion designers. An artisan-made fabric gives a truly unique selling point to the resulting clothes, and adds value and creates attention when the clothes are used as showpieces on the catwalk.

Many experimental techniques, such as bleaching, dip-dyeing and felting, often practised by students in art colleges, have gradually been adopted by more mainstream production units and therefore have a commercial viability within a specialist, designer-level market. Eventually these techniques appear in mass production (usually utilizing handcraft skills still found in India and Asian countries) and new cycles of experiments are set up. The result has been an increase in the range of textile processes available to the general public.

Student placements are often arranged with established fashion houses, textile design studios and manufacturers, and in this way an endless source of fresh ideas are brought into a company – an exchange of inspiration for experience. For the spring/summer 1994 season, Japanese émigré designer Koji Tatsuno took on a young knitwear

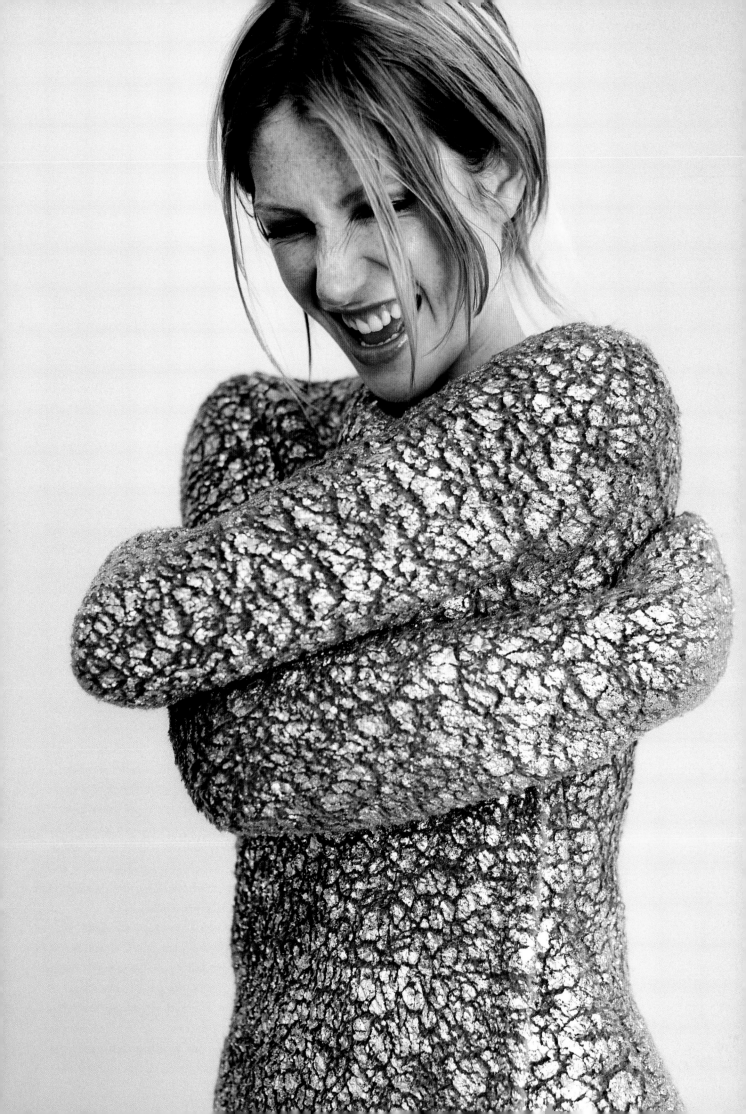

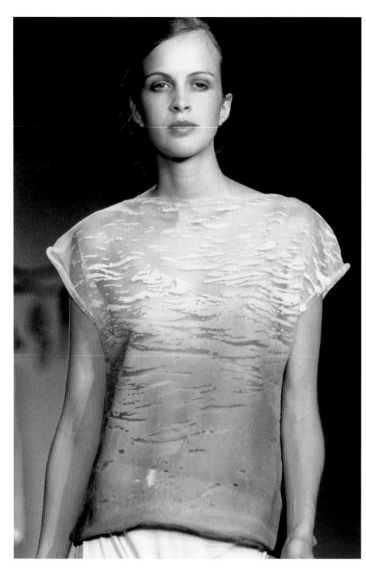

Above Iben Høj, printed knitting, 1997. Machine-knitted fabric combining nylon monofilament and viscose yarns, printed using the devoré technique, in which the viscose is 'eaten' away in the printed parts, creating the image in relief and resulting progression to transparency. The design was inspired by seascapes, and the garment was dip-dyed after knitting. Note the naturally curled edges of the single-bed fabric and trimless styling.

student named Julien Macdonald. Tatsuno had been fêted by the fashion press in the early 1990s for the astonishing bravado and intricacy of his one-off theatrical creations and his sculpting of unusual materials, such as millinery scrim used for an entire dress. Under his visionary but protective eye, Macdonald created some exciting knitted pieces focused on transparency, texture and mix of materials to create chaotic cobwebs of yarn. Macdonald was already experimenting with transparency in nylon monofilament yarns and went on to create his own eclectic showpieces, including dresses festooned with beads and sequins, fluorescent tubes or ironmongers' nuts and bolts suspended from the stitches. Other notable names who cut some of their fashion teeth with Tatsuno are Alexander McQueen and Sharon Wauchob.

Handcrafted processes are feasible only at the exclusive end of the fashion spectrum, its pinnacle being couture, in which each item is individually created and therefore unique. Avant-garde designers utilize craft skills in a range of ways within limited production runs. Martin Margiela has developed a continuing section of his collection which is called 'artisanal production', for which items are processed by hand. His autumn/winter 1998/99 collection, for example, included knitwear and jersey items which were flattened and heat-pressed to plastic, which could be partially removed for wearing, according to preference. Other collections have featured knitwear which has been crumpled and heat-pressed, or distorted and moulded, or reassembled from recycled clothing.

Printing on knitted fabric has long been established: take, for example, the ubiquitous printed T-shirt. In the 1950s, especially in America, there was a vogue for floral printed cardigans which recently inspired designers such as Valentino. Animal-printed knits have also recurred regularly in Italian and French design. British designer Ann-Louise Roswald has taken the technique further in bold, graphic, floral designs that create a head-to-toe statement and are produced in her own studio to retain the designer 'edge'. Printed imagery applied to heavier-weight knitwear is less common and was given a fashion profile by Artwork in the 1980s when they pioneered their quirky 1950s-inspired intarsia knitwear overprinted with cherubs and motifs of Greek and Roman antiquity. For autumn/winter 2000/01, Italian-based designer Lawrence Steele experimented with extraordinary, gold-printed, fur-effect knitted garments, together with lightweight fabric printed to glisten at every movement like liquid gold.

The 'look' of knitting itself is a powerful visual symbol and has been employed in print techniques using offset or directly transferred imagery to create veritable simulacra of knitted garments. Designers apply this idea in a number of ways. Issey Miyake playfully uses the image of textural aran knitting as part of his evolving Pleats Please ranges which have, since 1997, become a site for artistic expression, with artists invited to create designs. In addition to the garments being constructed in oversize and pleated to shrink, the imagery is enlarged to take the pleats into account.

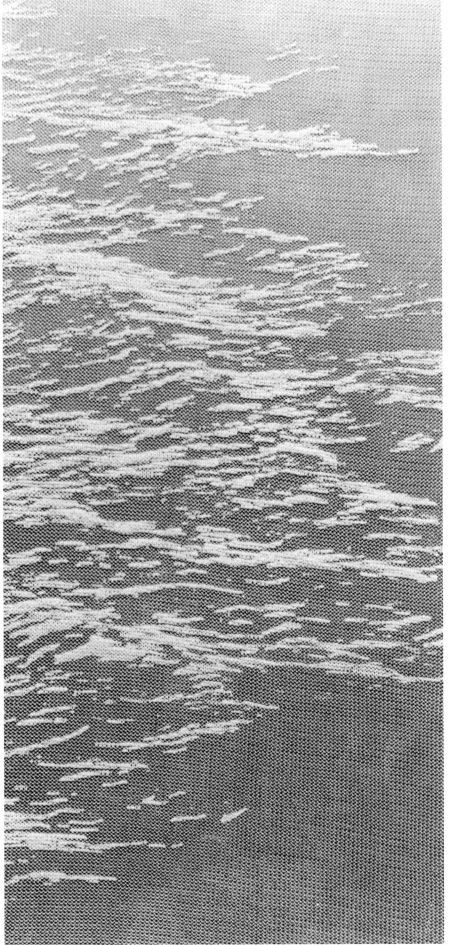

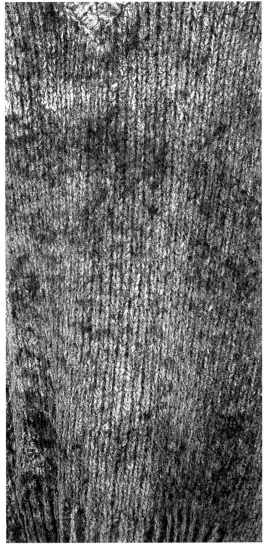

Above Sharon Wauchob, printed knitting, autumn/winter 2001/02. A coarsely knitted classic woollen sweater is overprinted in white pigment through an open screen, without a design, to create a surface effect that enhances the stitch structure. The white print stops short of the side seams of the sweater, resulting in a striking, distressed image, as if the wearer has accidentally encountered wet paint.

Left Iben Høj, printed knitting, 1997. Machine-knitted viscose fabric, using the technical back (purl side) of the single jersey structure, overprinted with Expandtex (also known as 'puff binder') – a chemical which expands when heat is applied, creating a raised image. The effect can be gentle or dramatic, according to the base fabric and the design that is applied.

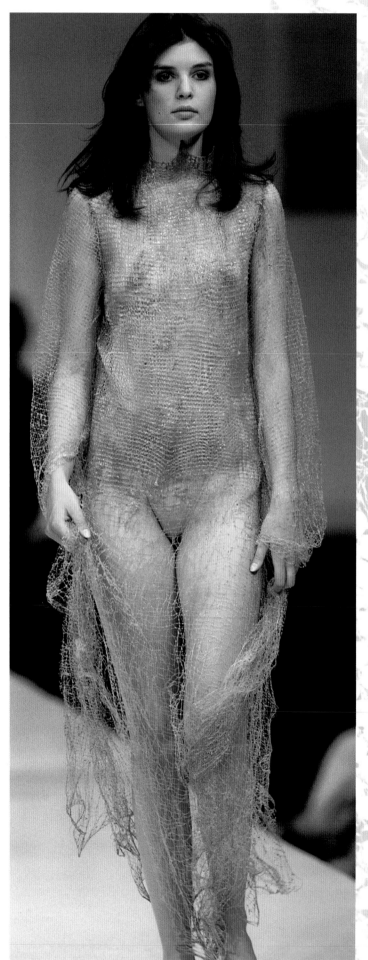

Left Leonie Branston, coated knitting, summer 1994. The net of knitting creates a thin veil to clothe the body in transparency – an experiment which gradually moved from the avant-garde creations of graduate fashion collections to the main fashion runways of the world. Here openwork manipulated lace knitting in shimmering yarns is coated in silicone, giving an otherworldly, slightly reptilian quality to the piece. The flimsy fabric is given weight by the silicone, bringing vision and touch into contradiction.

Background Gina Conquest, decorated knitting, 1999. Precious-looking golden metallic yarn is knitted in a purl fabric with basketweave pattern structure. Silicone is then painstakingly applied by hand in liquid form, drop by drop and stitch by stitch, to create a sumptuous beaded effect. The final fabric has the richness and draping qualities associated with couture fabrics but without the weight of actual beads.

Opposite Koji Tatsuno, coated knitting, autumn/winter 1996/97. Tatsuno was an early exponent of experiments with latex-coating of fabrics. This seemingly simple sweater is given a modern twist by the application of latex onto the raised parts of the knitting, reflecting light in movement. The underlying structure of the sweater is carefully engineered rib transfer – a relatively time-consuming process, even by industrial machine. The resulting chevron patterns are carefully placed to enhance the curves of the body.

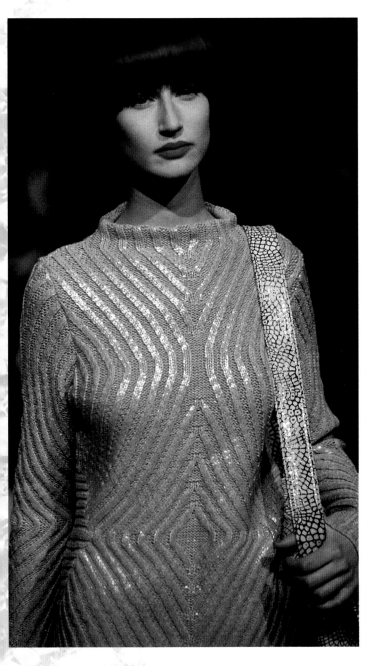

Using a process of heat photogram printing, Rebecca Earley applies the image of knitted clothing, such as a child's jacket or a cardigan, to clothes and accessories, creating visual puns by printing, for instance, the image of a knitted scarf onto a fabric scarf. Her base material is recycled polyester fleece and, as the transfer process exhausts the image, the whole has sound ecological credentials.

In her autumn/winter 1998/99 collection Julie Skarland combined actual heavy knitted fabric with the printed image of the same knitted fabric, produced through the use of digital imaging and digital printing, creating a visual interplay of real and virtual. She also applies knit fabric onto woven fabrics or combines knit with weave to create unusual patched skirts, trousers and dresses.

Martin Margiela presented a collection in summer 1996 (and featured it again in summer 1999) based on the printed image of floral and striped dresses, knitwear, coats and blouses applied to simple shapes in fluid white jersey fabric. The displacement created between image and reality had the effect of democratizing the collection in a manner consistent with the reduction to basic forms evident in Margiela's women's clothing range '6'.

Further inventiveness can be seen in Karl Pinfold's use of the technical image of knit structure in unusual painstaking cut-out form in leather and plastic materials.

Maya Bramwell, meanwhile, bonds oversized hand-knitted fabrics to interlining to create a stiffened fabric with all the visual effect but without the usual qualities of a knitted textile.

The major revolution in stretch fabrics, made possible by the increasing availability and use of elastomeric fibres such as Lycra, has opened the way for major new advances and experimentation and has created a new genre of textile design. Rosemary Moore, a British designer, was the first to recognize and exploit its potential, and in 1985 she secured a patent for her Maxxam ruched jersey. It was also taken up for swimwear and dancewear by American designer Liza Bruce, amongst others. Many designers, including, famously, Azzedine Alaïa and Hervé Leger, have invented new combinations of yarns and structures to create three-dimensional surfaces or supportive, comfortable and sexy second-skin clothes.

One result of experimenting with new processes is the serendipity of mistakes – a situation to which designer Shelley Fox is highly responsive. Many of her signature creased and frilled felted knit fabrics were originally the result of a happy accident, as were the burning and scarring effects which came from an overlooked heat-press.

The Japanese draw less of a distinction between crafts and fine arts, as is evident in museum collections. As the constant textile innovations carried out by companies such as Miyake Design Studio and the Nuno Corporation show, the ability to combine craft skills with an understanding of both old and new technologies can provide the ideas which can influence fashion for a long time ahead.

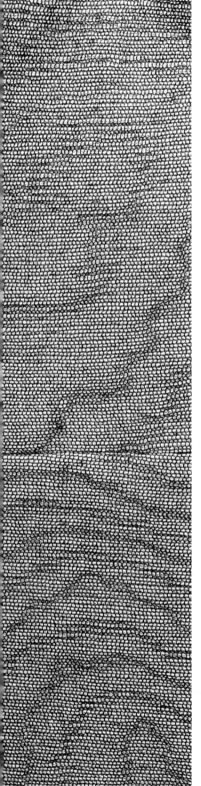

Left and below Alice Lee, autumn/winter 1998/99. Contrasting hard outer surface with soft interior, copper/viscose metallic yarn is knitted, then heat-bonded to cashmere knitted fabric, resulting in an unusual moiré-patterned effect. The fabric has been produced in lengths and made up into a jacket and hat (below) by traditional cut-and-sew methods of semi-structured tailoring.

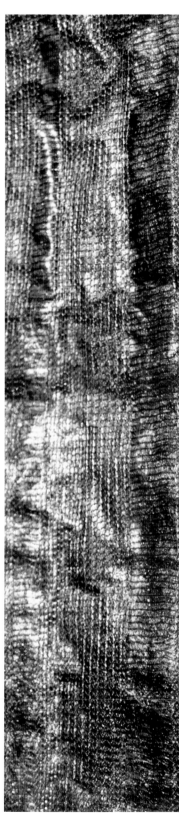

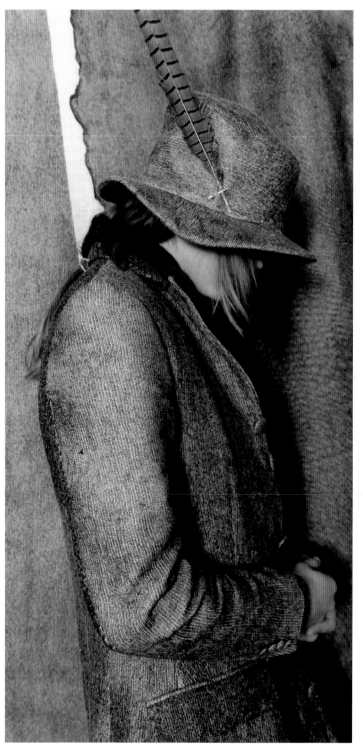

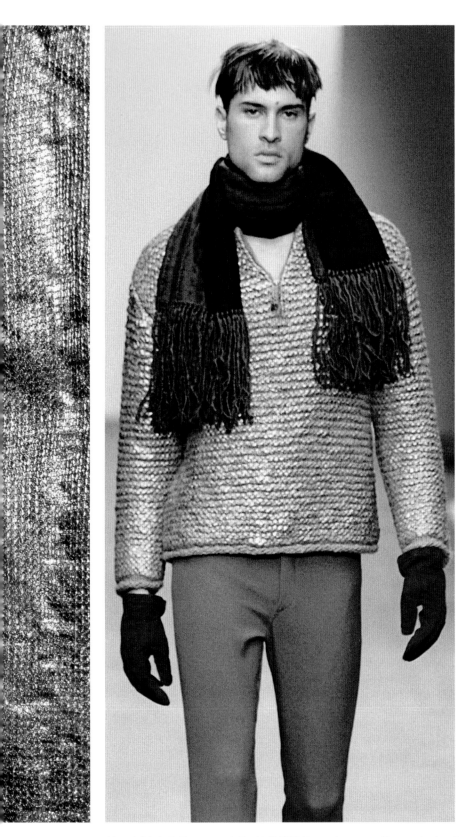

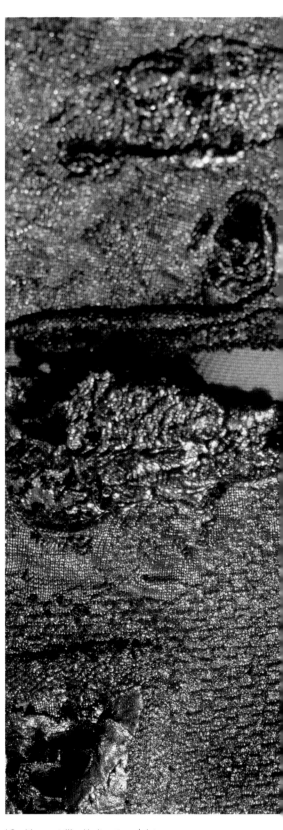

Above left Isabelle Harman, metallized knit, 2000. Harman's metal-coated knitted fabrics have intriguing silver or verdigris surfaces. The fabrics remain flexible and may be distressed or cut away, their knitted origins surviving as surface texture. The underlying knits are usually created with fine viscose yarns in simple tuck-stitch or rib patterns. Harman has designed fabrics for exclusive couture collections by Christian Lacroix and Emanuel Ungaro.

Above centre Jean Paul Gaultier, metallized knit, autumn/winter 2000/01. This heavy-gauge, hand-knitted wool sweater in garter stitch, is given an unreal quality by its sprayed metallic coating.

Above right Frances Geesin, metallized knit, 1994. By applying technologies from metalwork and car manufacture to high-tech yarns, Geesin transforms knitted fabric into metal, which is then adapted to different end products for design or artworks.

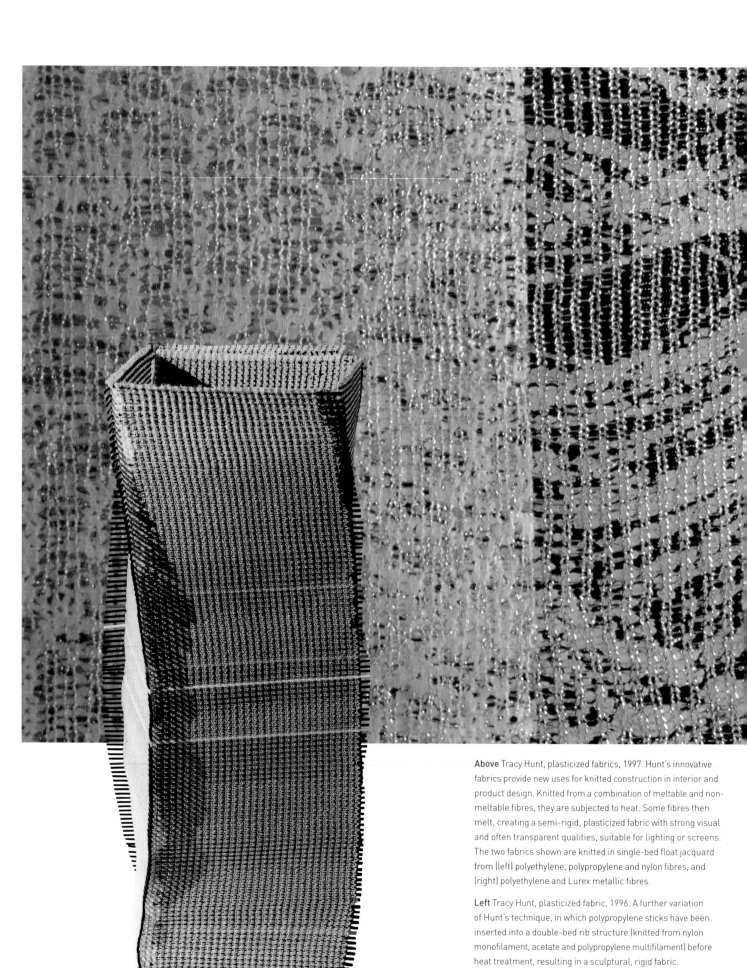

Above Tracy Hunt, plasticized fabrics, 1997. Hunt's innovative fabrics provide new uses for knitted construction in interior and product design. Knitted from a combination of meltable and non-meltable fibres, they are subjected to heat. Some fibres then melt, creating a semi-rigid, plasticized fabric with strong visual and often transparent qualities, suitable for lighting or screens. The two fabrics shown are knitted in single-bed float jacquard from (left) polyethylene, polypropylene and nylon fibres, and (right) polyethylene and Lurex metallic fibres.

Left Tracy Hunt, plasticized fabric, 1996. A further variation of Hunt's technique, in which polypropylene sticks have been inserted into a double-bed rib structure (knitted from nylon monofilament, acetate and polypropylene multifilament) before heat treatment, resulting in a sculptural, rigid fabric.

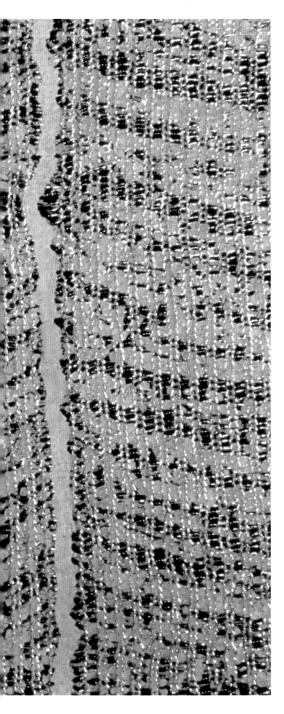

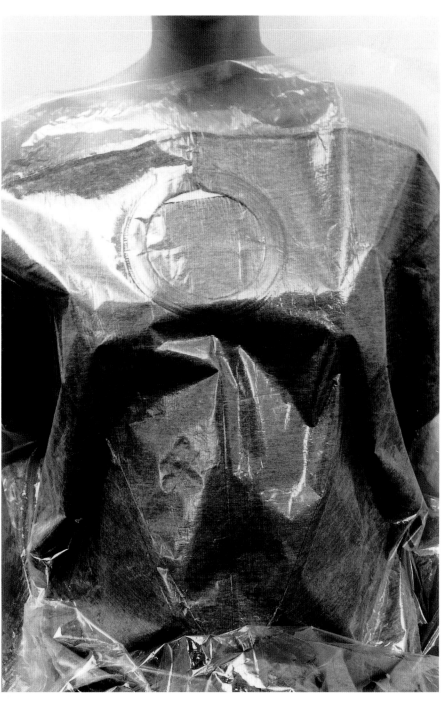

Above Maison Martin Margiela, plasticized sweatshirt, autumn/
winter 1998/99. This sweatshirt was part of a collection in which
the pieces were designed to lie flat when not worn and featured
displaced necklines. Many knitwear items, as well as jersey fabric
T-shirts and dresses, were heat-bonded to plastic, which could
be removed wholly or partially when worn.

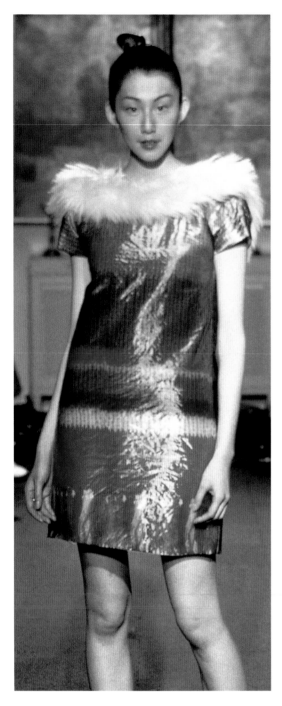

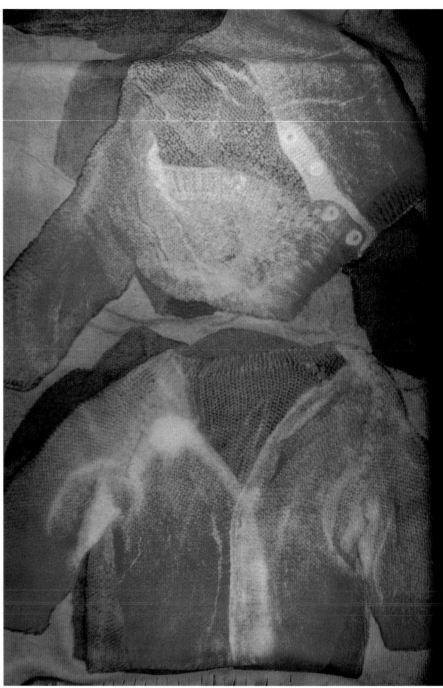

Above Julie Skarland, printed image of knitting, autumn/winter 1998/99. In 1998 Skarland won a multimedia competition to design fabric for digital printing with this trompe l'oeil print based on a hand-knitted scarf. In several outfits in her next collection, she juxtaposed the actual knitting with the virtual knitted fabric. Here the print is used on a plastic-coated fabric. Note the scarf fringe at the hem.

Above right Rebecca Earley, scarf printed with image of child's knitwear, 2000. Earley produces striking collections of clothes and scarves, which use images of garments and gloves as well as natural objects, such as leaves and plants. Her earliest work showed a sweater with the image of another sweater across the front. Images of actual objects are transferred to the cloth by a direct heat photogram process, using a special photographic paper. Luminosity of image is achieved through printing on both sides of the (recycled) polyester cloth.

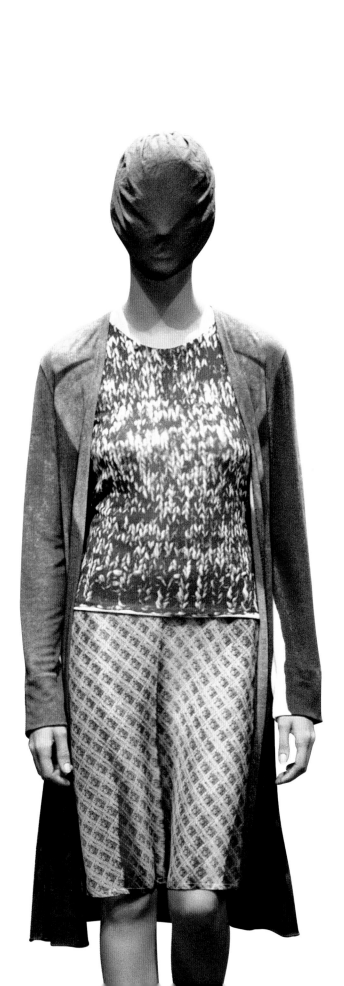

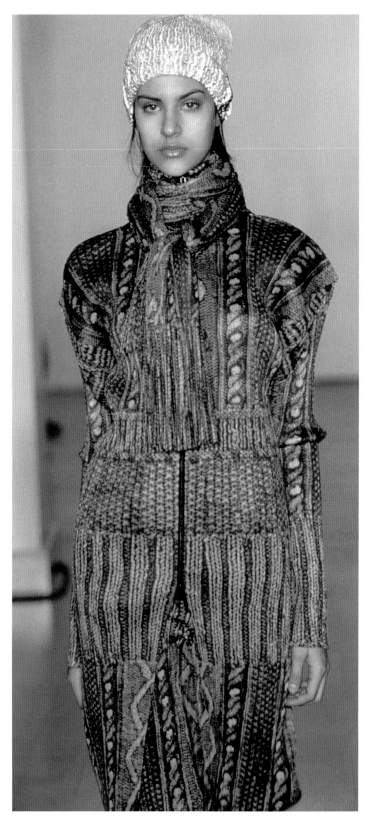

Above Issey Miyake, Pleats Please, autumn/winter 2000/01. Since the Pleats Please range was developed in 1989, in plain colours, Miyake has continually developed variations on the theme: overprinting pieces with guest artists' works, starting in 1996; with flower prints and denim fabric for summer 2000; tartan and diamond prints and this aran knit image for winter 2000; gingham for summer 2001... Instantly recognizable fabrics, such as the aran, create humour, in keeping with the lightness of spirit of the Pleats range.

Left Maison Martin Margiela, spring/summer 1996. This collection consisted of photographs of garments – a sequinned evening dress, a man's overcoat, tweed skirts, print dresses, heavy woollen sweaters – overprinted in grey and sepia tones, evoking old photographs, onto white, fluid fabrics in viscose and cotton, then made up into simple shapes. Knitted fabric again proves to be particularly successful as a print. The anonymity of the veiled faces adds to the contradictory visual impact.

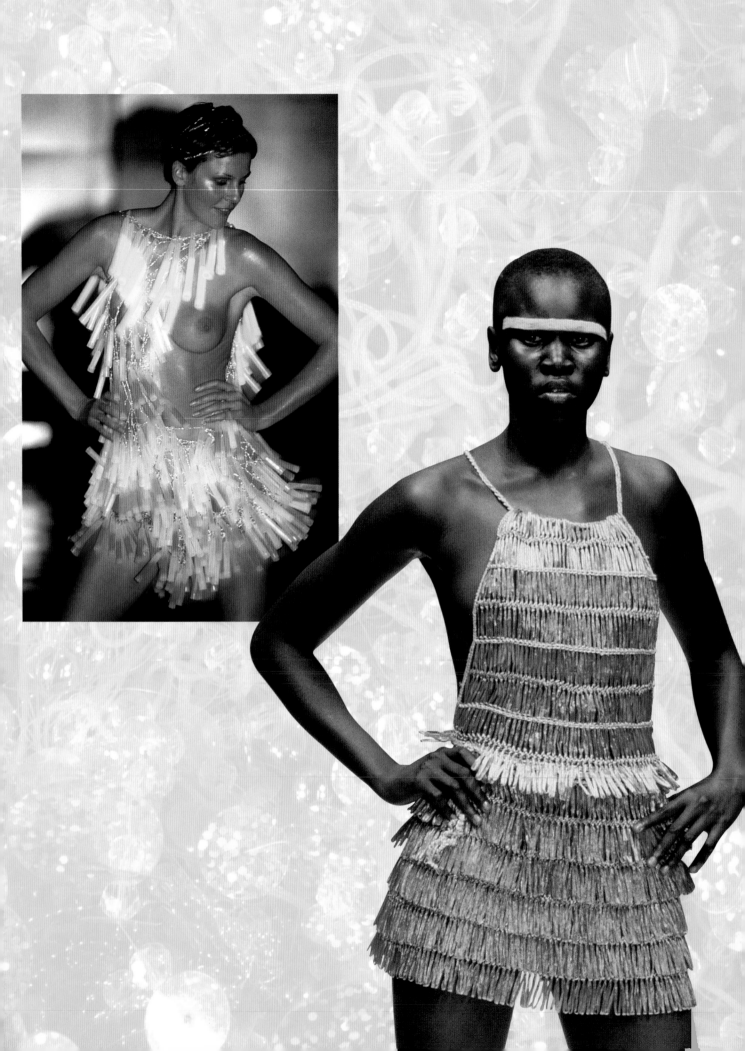

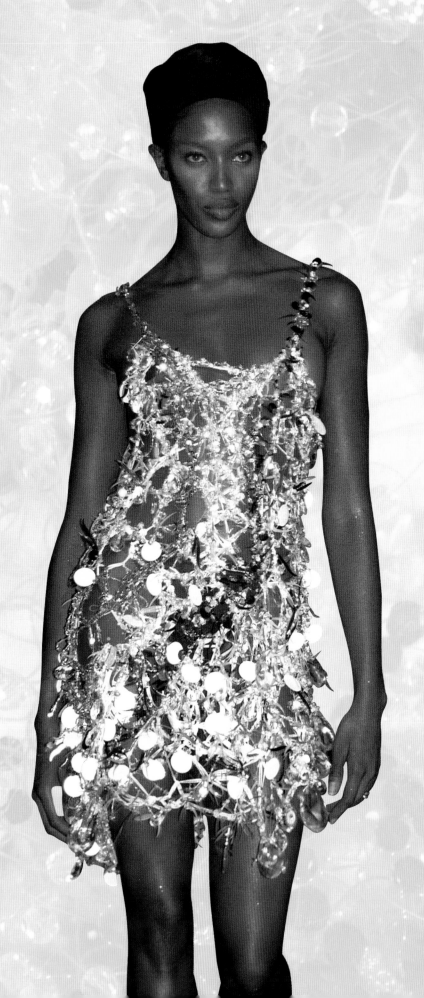

Opposite left Julien Macdonald, 'Metallurgical' collection, spring/summer 1999. Experimental fabrics or unusual processes and materials create visual excitement. This showpiece dress of metallic yarn is hung with fluorescent tubes which glow in the dark for a spectacular catwalk finale.

Background Julien Macdonald, 1996. Detail of beaded and sequinned dress fabric. The hand-knitted base of heavy nylon monofilament yarn is strong enough to take the heavy weight of the decorations. Hand-knitting and crochet techniques allow total freedom to create one-of-a-kind garments – the basis of all couture work.

Right Julien Macdonald, 'Modernists' collection, spring/summer 1998. A signature look: revealing mini-dress of textured metallic yarns and light-reflecting paillettes, perfect for making an entrance. A knitted or crochet mesh base, built up around a body form, can be festooned with beads, sequins or any objects through which the yarn can be threaded during the making of the piece. Further decorations can then be applied by hand-sewing.

Opposite right Marina Spadafora, spring/summer 1998. Dress made to shape from raffia, using a technique of 'floats' between stitches on a coarse-gauge knitting machine to create openwork fabric and fringing. Small-scale production is feasible using semi-manual techniques such as this.

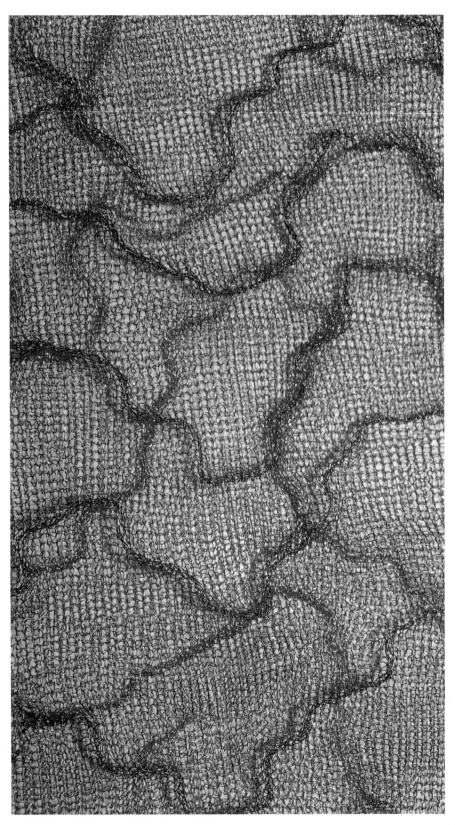

Left Karl Pinfold, copper wire knitting, 1998. Fine metallic wires, as used in electrical products, can be knitted (with some effort) by manual machine. Here a single-bed plain fabric has been shaped by hand into a raised pattern, capitalizing on the qualities of the wire, in a fabric for an experimental bodice. Industrially knitted wire fabrics have many uses in technical textiles for heat and electrical conductivity, reinforcement and filtration.

Opposite left Karl Pinfold, leather cut-out knitting, 2000. For his graduation show, Pinfold produced a unique set of garments based on the technical construction of knitting, but actually created by cutting out strips of leather which simulate the loop formation of a row of knitting. These strips were painstakingly cut and individually linked together, giving the impression of a knitted cardigan. Fringes were incorporated during cutting-out, and the leather was dyed to enhance the effect. Similar experiments were also made in sheets of acetate and corrugated cardboard.

Opposite right Close-up of Karl Pinfold's cut-out leather (see above), showing the interlinking of separate strips.

Background Alice Lee, leather knitting, autumn/winter 2000/01. Large openwork coarse-gauge machine-knitting in fine leather 'yarn' forms a striking mesh for the outer layer of a fully fashioned coat, which has a wool lining knitted integrally. In the same collection, leather sections were knitted into parts of woollen sweaters.

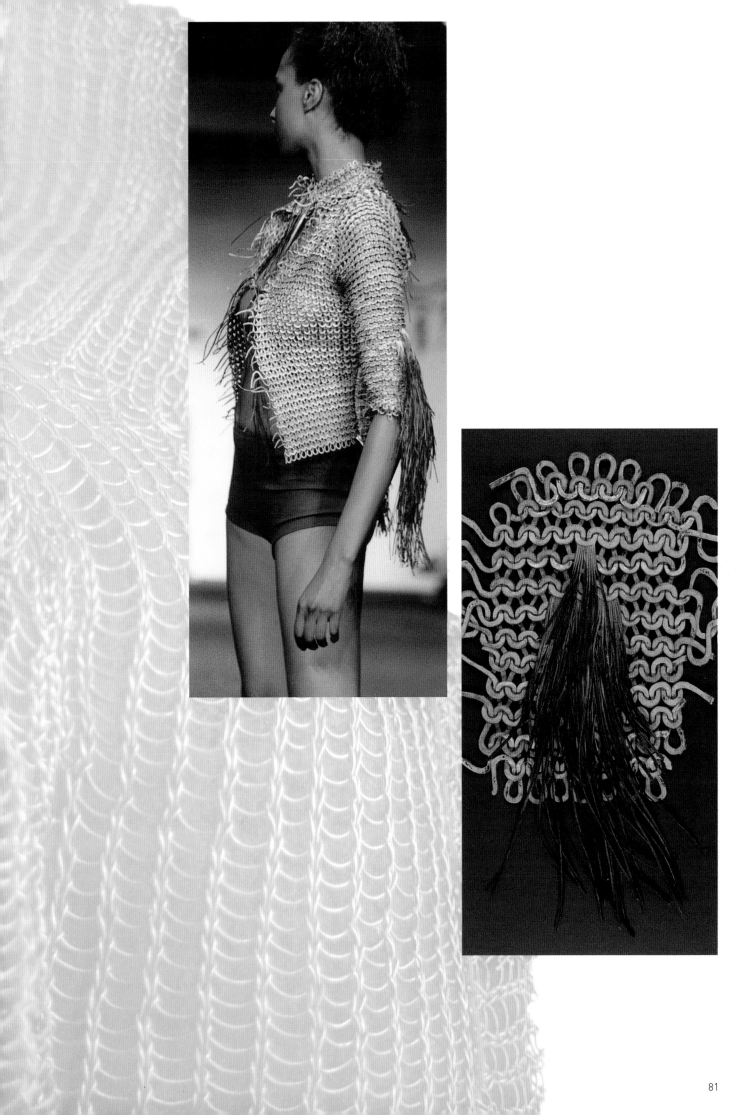

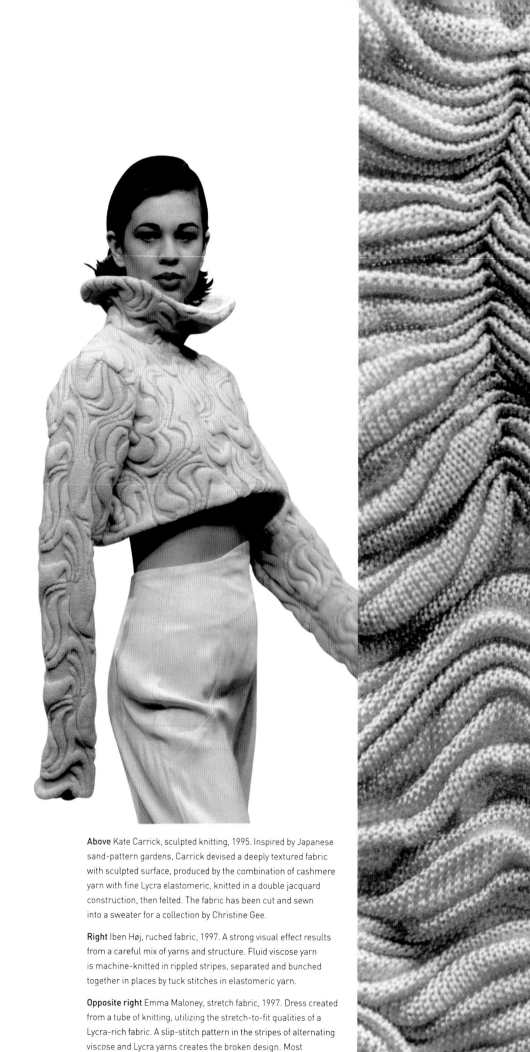

Above Kate Carrick, sculpted knitting, 1995. Inspired by Japanese
sand-pattern gardens, Carrick devised a deeply textured fabric
with sculpted surface, produced by the combination of cashmere
yarn with fine Lycra elastomeric, knitted in a double jacquard
construction, then felted. The fabric has been cut and sewn
into a sweater for a collection by Christine Gee.

Right Iben Høj, ruched fabric, 1997. A strong visual effect results
from a careful mix of yarns and structure. Fluid viscose yarn
is machine-knitted in rippled stripes, separated and bunched
together in places by tuck stitches in elastomeric yarn.

Opposite right Emma Maloney, stretch fabric, 1997. Dress created
from a tube of knitting, utilizing the stretch-to-fit qualities of a
Lycra-rich fabric. A slip-stitch pattern in the stripes of alternating
viscose and Lycra yarns creates the broken design. Most
commercial fabrics contain a very small (less than 5%) amount
of stretch yarn for fit and comfort; garments such as this and
Azzedine Alaïa's famous pieces contain around 30% stretch yarn.

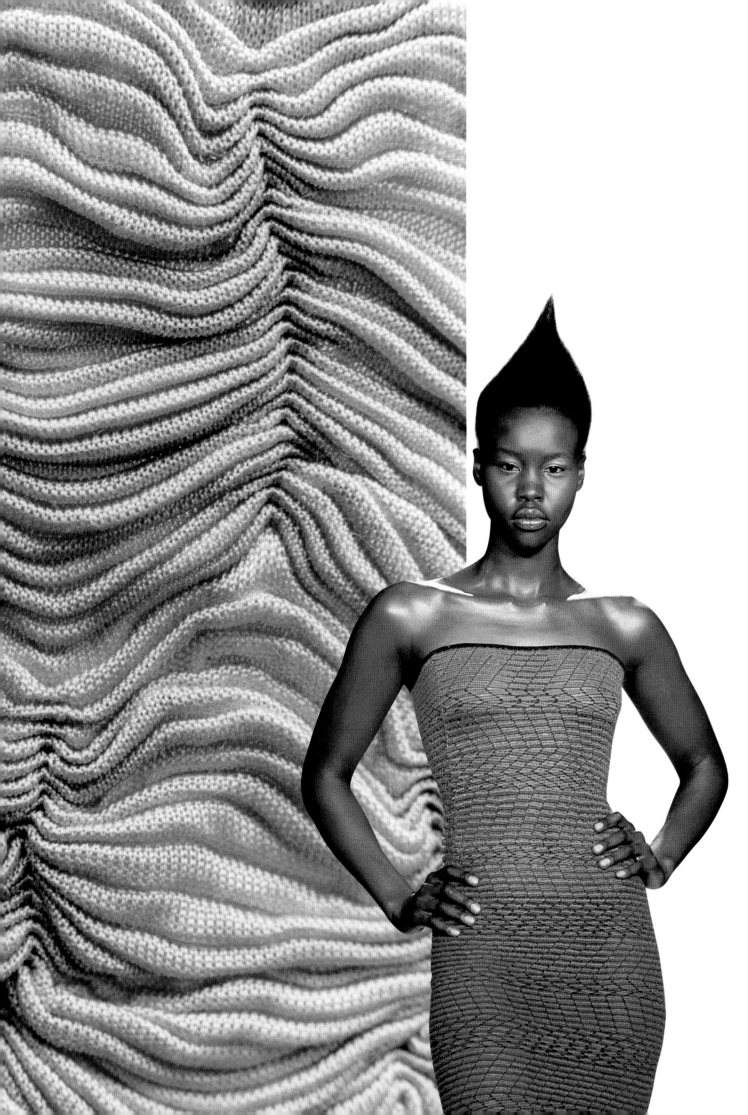

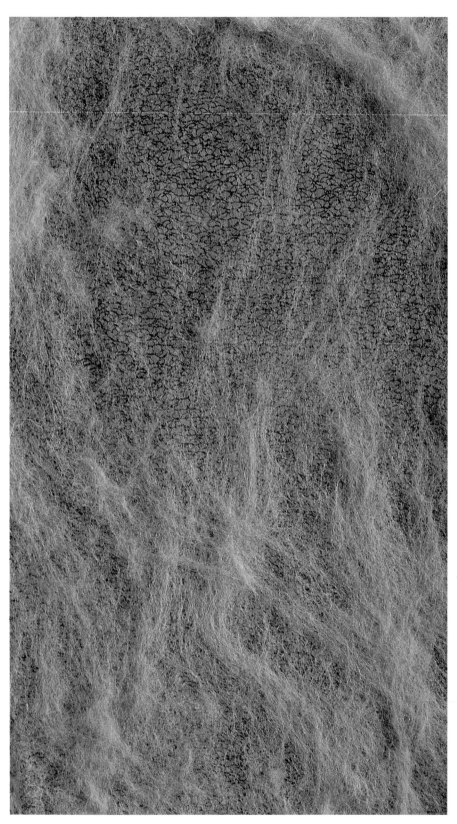

Left Alice Lee, metal and wool felted fabric, autumn/winter 2000/01. A fine tuck-stitch mesh of speciality silk and steel yarn traps felted wool fibres – once again a mix of opposites produces individual fabrics with tactile and visual attraction, used in tops for womenswear.

Below Fatima Saifee, engineered shape (detail of skirt), 2000. Saifee takes an individual approach to garment construction, using the shapes she creates by distortion of knitting to dictate the form. Using the short-row knitting technique on single-bed fabrics, Saifee inserts curves and lines made of Lycra yarn, which shrinks when the piece is felted.

Opposite right Lisa Jansen, felted 'Heavenly' dress, 1998. This ethereal dress appears to float away in the breeze. It is made from knitted silk mesh, inlaid and felted with cashmere and angora fibres and fine chiffon. Jansen's collection explored different ways in which knitted fabrics and fibres could be combined in felts, without processes of sewing, using ties made during the process to fasten the garments.

Opposite left Lisa Jansen, felted dress, 1998. Detail of the back of a dress, showing the merging of the knitted part into the felted fabric.

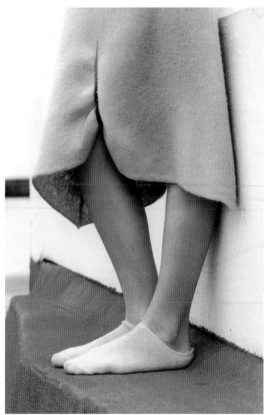

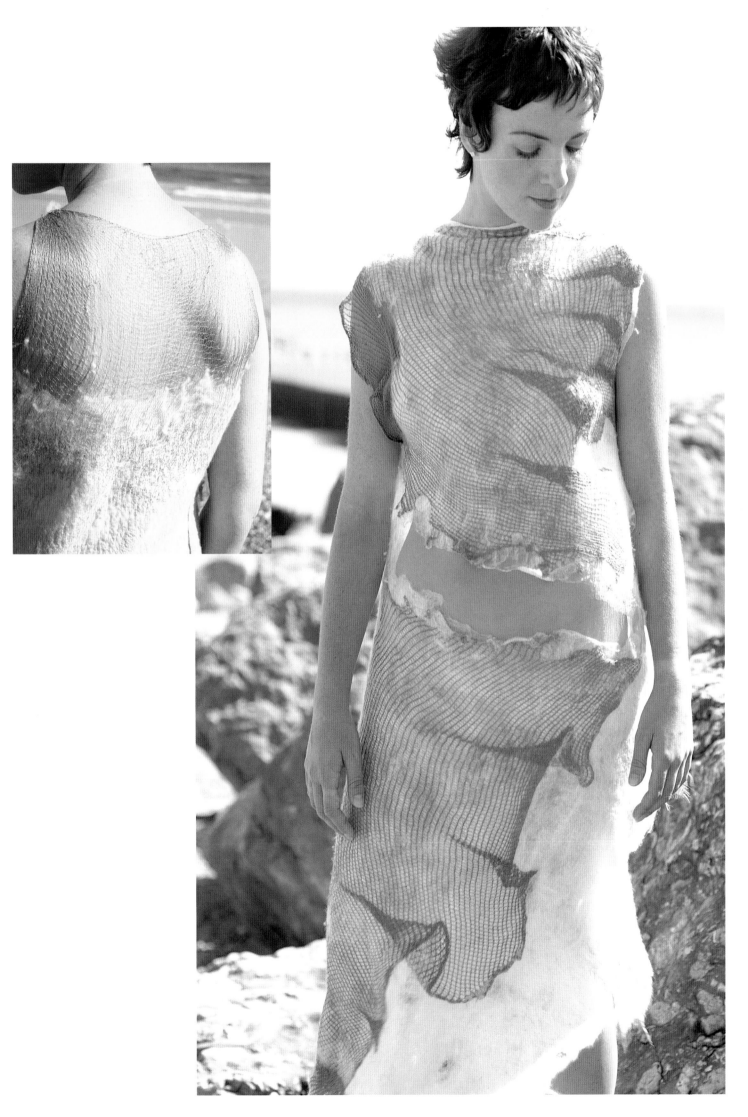

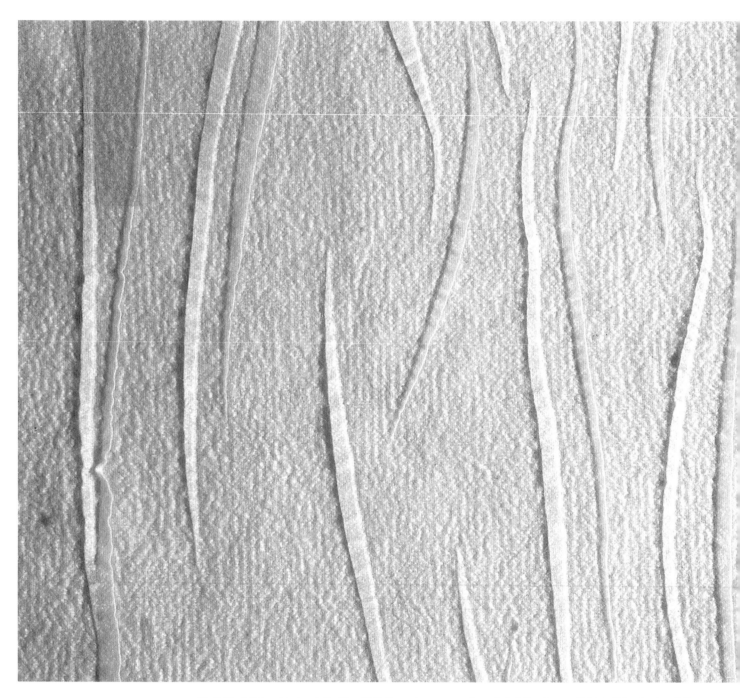

Above Monika Olszynska, bonded knitting, 2000. Olszynska experiments with different ways of manipulating knitted fabrics and surfaces to change the nature and quality of knitting. Techniques such as bonding, printing, cutting, felting, embossing, spraying and dyeing are combined to create innovative and wearable knitted fabrics. Here a cashmere knit is bonded to interfacing, with folds deliberately placed. Bonding effectively eliminates the stretch factor, allowing the production of large knitted garments which will not distort with heavy weight, but retain some characteristics of knit.

Opposite left Maya Bramwell, 'Little Girl' collection, 1999. Bramwell's collection experimented with non-traditional methods of garment construction and the bonding of large-scale hand-knitting to non-woven interlinings to create fabric collages. The underlying motivation for the work is the conflict between maturity and the appearance of innocence, in relation to women's sexuality. Knitting functions as a metaphor for childhood, keying into early memories of learning to knit.

Opposite right Nuala MacCulloch, purl fabric, 1998. An exciting demonstration of the unpredictable forces within some knitted structures, enhanced by choice of yarns. Here a bulky nylon yarn is knitted on an industrial machine to create a stretchy, bouncy piece, which is highly malleable. The basic stitch structure is very simple – blocks of knit and purl loops – but the spiral formation is the surprising result.

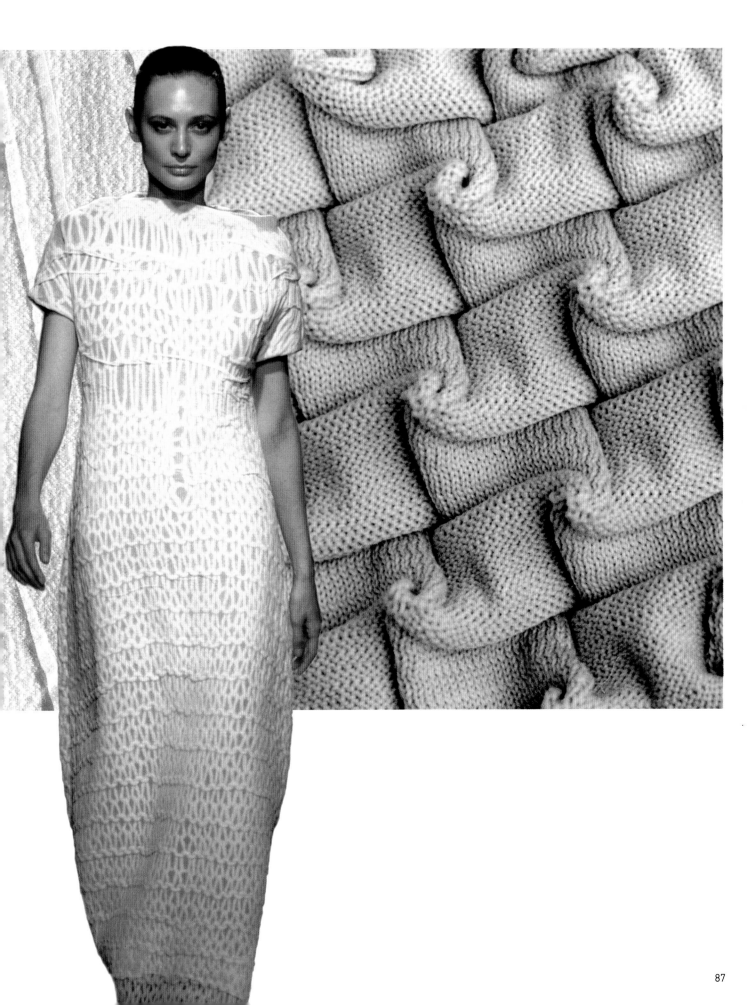

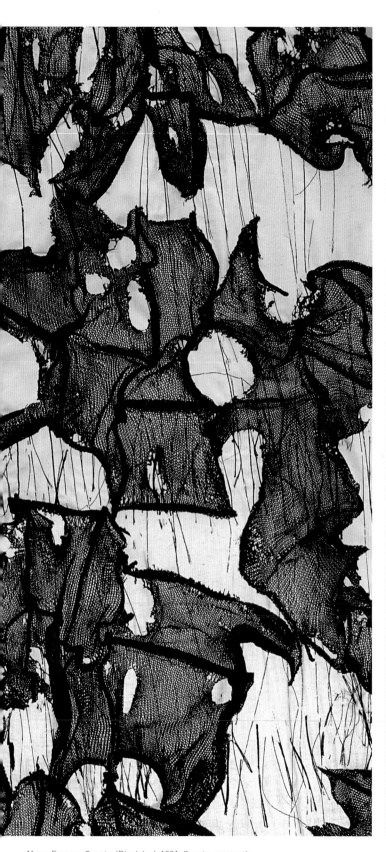

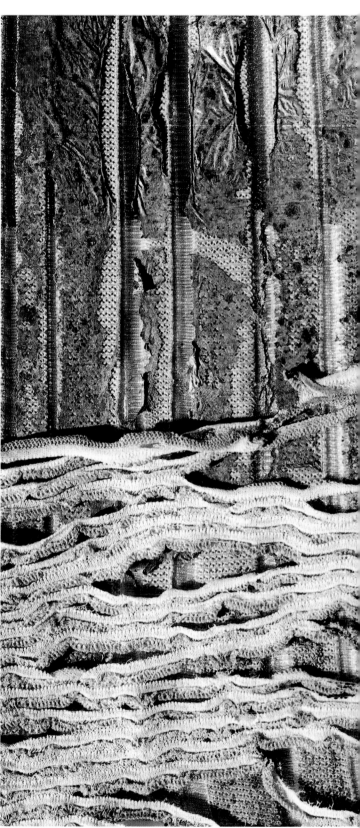

Above Frances Geesin, 'Black Ice', 1981. Geesin constantly researches new fibres and processes. This early experiment was made with synthetic fibres that melt with heat. Polypropylene yarn has been knitted, then fused to calico and heat-distressed using a soldering iron. The abstract result challenges expectations of knitted fabrics. Geesin has continued to investigate the alchemy of fibres and metal in her work with electro-deposition.

Above Rebecca Webber, distressed surface, 2001. Webber is interested in the visual and tactile qualities of distressed surfaces, particularly in synthetic fibres combined with other materials such as plastics, leather and lace. She treats a range of machine-knitted fabrics – ribbed, blister jacquard and stripes of various yarns – to processes of burning, melting, bonding and printing, in order to find an engaging, fragile beauty in deconstruction.

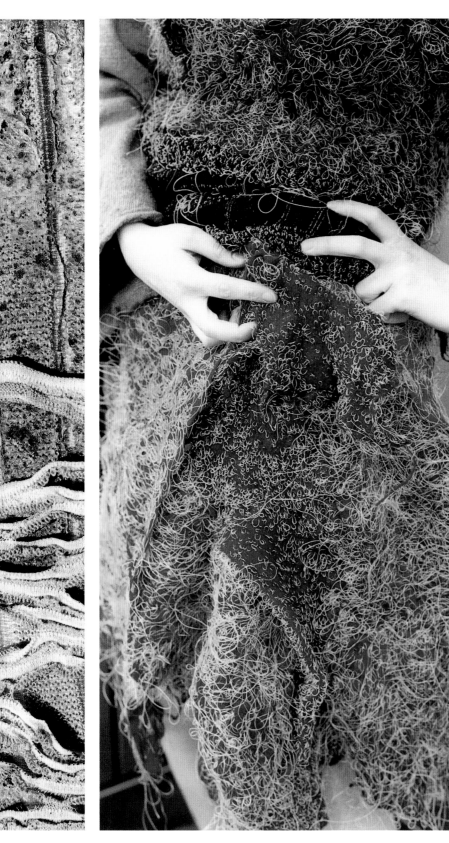

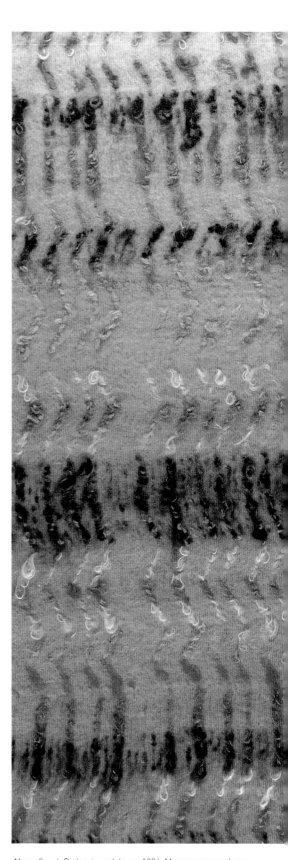

Above Tamara Kemoklidse, surface effects, 2001. Inspired by the intensity of colour found in Persian miniature paintings of medieval times, Kemoklidse mixes natural and synthetic yarns into chaotic, dense surfaces. Her methods include working with yarns inlaid and floated across a machine-knitted fabric containing Lycra, which, when shrunk and relaxed, forms the loops on the surface.

Above Sarah Bigley, tweed dress, 1996. Many processes have been combined to produce the patterns and depth of colour in this 1950s-inspired, tweed-effect fabric. Wool yarn was knitted loosely, dyed in graded colour, unravelled, reknitted with contrast yarns inlaid into a double-bed fabric (trapped between the beds whilst knitting), and finally felted and shrunk into a dense fabric. This was then cut and sewn into a dress.

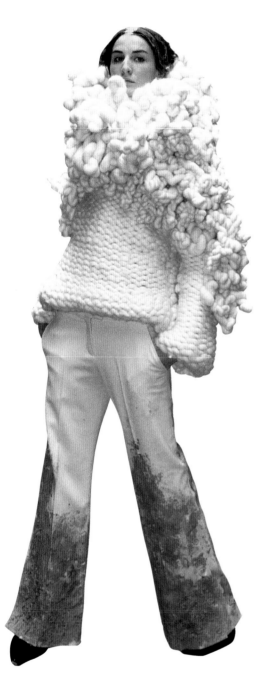

Above Alexander McQueen, autumn/winter 2000/01. McQueen's shows create unforgettable spectacle, each one surpassing the previous for theatre and drama. His outrageous or extreme clothes ensure sensation and press coverage, backed by more commercial lines which still retain the McQueen edge and now-legendary 'neo-couture' tailoring. When McQueen uses knitwear, he does it with the same sense of the extreme, illustrated by the large-scale knitted showpieces shown here.

Opposite left Alexander McQueen, 'The Overlook' collection (named after the hotel in the horror film *The Shining*), autumn/ winter 1999/2000. McQueen mixes the sinister and the surreal – such as the painting of a white strip across the eyes of his models – to challenge perceptions and find beauty in ugliness. This large-scale knitted sweater deliberately evokes body proportions that are the antithesis of the model body shape.

Radical designers and radical ideas appear at intervals in fashion, as in other design disciplines, throwing existing ideas into question, challenging assumptions and the aesthetics of established taste. Shocking as they are at first, we gradually absorb these new ideas until they become less strange to our sensibilities, and slowly there develops a fundamental shift in perceptions and we reach another plateau of acceptance. The radical avant-garde consisting of the Japanese triumvirate of Issey Miyake, Rei Kawakubo and Yohji Yamamoto have been designing for around thirty years, and their impact and influence on international fashion continues to grow. They have launched protégés (Naoki Takizawa, Junya Watanabe and Atsuro Tayama, for example) and inspired countless numbers of design students to follow their lead. Their so-called 'intellectual' canon has now been augmented by younger designers, notably Martin Margiela, Alexander McQueen and Hussein Chalayan, who have become no less influential in their uncompromising approach to clothing and display. Other designers whose approach can be considered radical in terms of knitwear and textile fabrication are Delphine Wilson, Ernestina Cerini, Alice Lee, Koji Tatsuno, Bernhard Willhelm, Shelley Fox and Véronique Branquinho.

A language of the modern avant-garde has now been established and the signs are clearly recognized: asymmetry (left to right side of body, hemlines); the appropriation of fabrics and materials from outside fashion; the juxtaposition of fabrics of contrasting weights and visual qualities; the 'cutting up' of classic, particularly tailored, pieces; reassembled clothing confounding expectations of inside and outside; raw and unfinished edges; folded, twisted and draped fabrics creating a trapped or distorted body silhouette; shrunken or oversized proportions; innovative fabric treatments and constructions often with a chaotic feel. These are some of the elements now stripped of their initial shock value and entering mainstream fashion. The influences of 'la Mode destroy', as Harold Koda called it, or 'deconstruction fashion', as many journalists have called it, are now widespread – witness the mass-produced fashions that incorporate raw and frayed edges, or have frills and fabric attachments applied for somewhat gratuitous decoration at every opportunity. Ripped denim jeans were shocking when first seen, but although they may have coded meanings, they no longer cause the same consternation.

Martin Margiela utilizes the basis of classic knitwear garments and applies one or more radical shifts to subvert expectations of the way they behave or are worn – a perfect knitted wool sweater is carefully cut through the collar and hem; the neckline of a classic merino wool cardigan is uncut and unfinished, left to curl with threads trailing. He plays with proportion by knitting enlarged Barbie doll's garments complete with the distortion of scale and errors that the enlargement calls for, such as oversized press studs. Notable

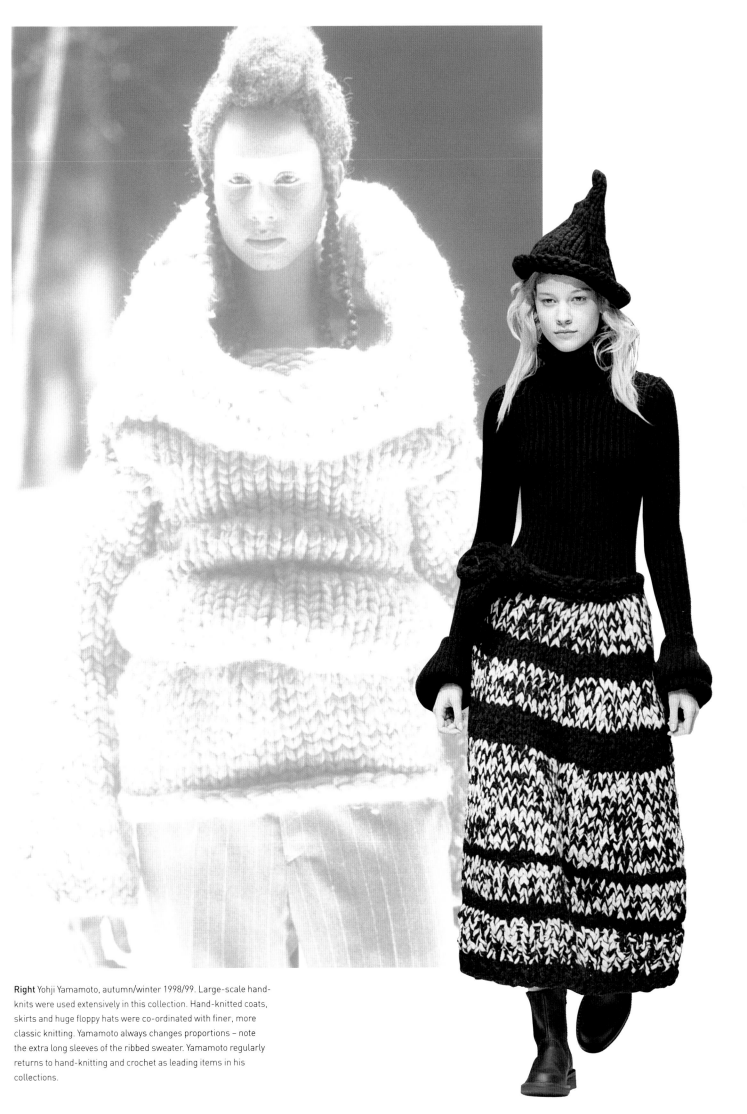

Right Yohji Yamamoto, autumn/winter 1998/99. Large-scale hand-knits were used extensively in this collection. Hand-knitted coats, skirts and huge floppy hats were co-ordinated with finer, more classic knitting. Yamamoto always changes proportions – note the extra long sleeves of the ribbed sweater. Yamamoto regularly returns to hand-knitting and crochet as leading items in his collections.

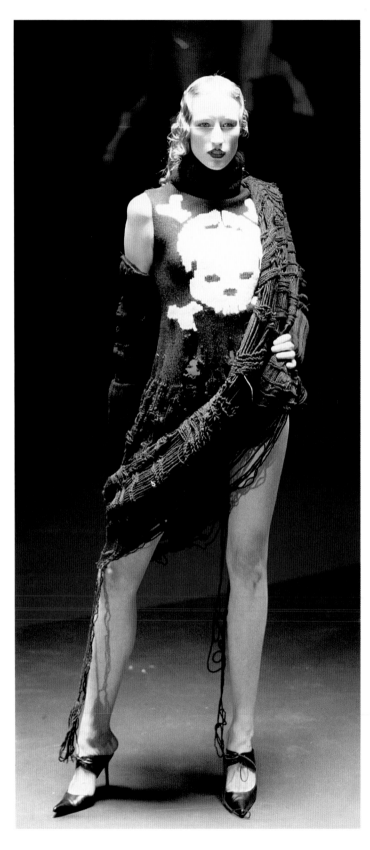

are the oversized sweaters and 'grandad' cardigans for winter 2001 womenswear, knitted from a mix of heavy wool and polyester, making them responsive to heat treatment to mould and fix the size and shape away from the body. Some incorporate distressing of the fabric, including torn and incomplete edgings. The summer and winter 2001 collections were made entirely in a notional Italian size 78, then folded back and sewn to create the appropriate fit. A cardigan appears unwearable with its sleeves folded and stitched half inside the arm-holes – the less brave unstitch it to become a 'normal' cardigan (albeit with underarm opening). In comparing the oversized knitwear of, for example, Shirin Guild with that of Margiela, the difference is that the proportions are not adjusted with Margiela – the sleeves are also size 78, whereas Guild's sleeves are extremely short to compensate for the width of the body when worn.

Knitted fabric can, uniquely, be made in the round (without seams), or it can be manipulated and twisted into sculptural new shapes for clothing. Seams can be displaced and repositioned, as in the work of Delphine Wilson. Pieces can be reconfigured with internal darts, and lines of relief stitches can be contoured around the body. At its simplest level of single jersey fabric, knitting is particularly malleable. Individual garment pieces can be shaped at will and, according to choice of yarn and finish, can either result in something perfect and balanced or something distorted and untamed – qualities which are exploited in Yohji Yamamoto's Y's knitwear. When his pieces are worn on the body, edges curl, straight lines distort, inside becomes outside, pockets and sleeves appear or disappear in playfully designed but intricately thought-out configurations of cardigans, sweaters, jackets and skirts, many of which are reversible. In a notable extension of ideas from the signature range for winter 2001, Y's included a cardigan which incorporated its own shoulder bag.

The net of knitting recurs as a visual icon in fashion (punk first introduced the concept of web-like coverings; see p. 14), reducing the function of the sweater to an absurdity. Both avant-garde and more mainstream designers have used the large open loop and mesh structure of knitting to bold effect – ironically not expected to be perfect, thus creating a visual dislocation. In 1981 Rei Kawakubo famously designed a sweater full of holes which cleverly gave the illusion of destruction, but each hole had been carefully executed with a casting-on and casting-off process in order to maintain the fabric stability, without which the garment would gradually unravel. In contrast, Martin Margiela's recent knitwear is physically distressed by simply cutting and fraying the fabric, or by a separately knitted ribbed edging which has partially 'fallen off' the machine (in fact this is intricately engineered). Margiela earlier produced a version of the distressed sweater full of holes created by random lace knitting. A younger designer, Winni Lok, has made her signature knitwear by ignoring all the construction rules of classic knitwear and roughly piecing together sections of knit and meshes, leaving raw and frayed edges.

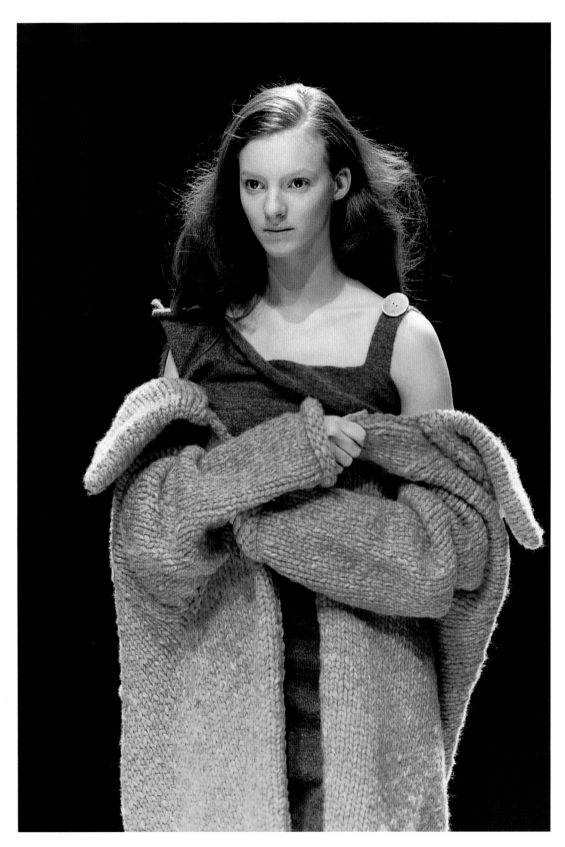

Opposite Alexander McQueen, autumn/winter 2001/02. For a collection performed around a carousel but with dark and gothic overtones, McQueen created distressed knitting, including this dress with skull and crossbones in the process of unravelling itself. This is not the first time McQueen has played with imagery evocative of violent undercurrents. In a 1997 collection, a model appeared to have been lashed into a dress knitted from heavy rope.

Above Yohji Yamamoto, autumn/winter 1998/99. In contrast to McQueen, the simplicity of hand-knitting and the basic construction of Yamamoto's pieces conjured a romantic innocence and naïveté, as the models hugged the comforting knitting around themselves. The shapes of the coat and dress are simple rectangles, the edges left to curl. The accompanying advertising campaign showed the clothes in strange, magical settings in the forest in full moonlight.

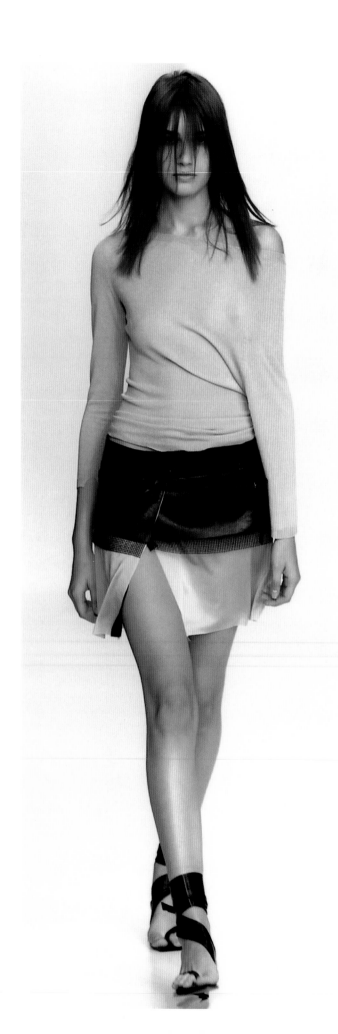

Cut-up is a favoured technique of several designers, from Comme des Garçons' bifurcated garments of winter 1993/94, which combined cut-up knitwear with fine chiffons, to the half-garments of Gaultier and the couture collage creations of John Galliano's summer 2000 Dior collection. The grunge impact of recycled sweaters overlocked together in Xuly Bet's 1993 designs shown in Paris also created a strong reaction at the time, just as Desirée Mejer's Fake London label began the recycling and patchworking of old cashmere sweaters into fashionable and irreverent designs.

In the late 1980s and early '90s Ernestina Cerini was creating her distinctive labyrinthine, braided and manipulated knitwear which occasionally appeared to unravel into chaos. Her unconventional approach came from being self-taught and from having the ability and means to experiment. Together with designer Marina Spadafora, the two labels dominated the Italian knitwear press for several seasons.

Alice Lee (a partnership between Alice Smith and Lee Farmer) have developed a unique series of knitted viscose dresses which utilize a particular feature of knitted construction called 'short row' or 'partial' knitting, resulting in linear patterns and fluid shapes around the body. The conceptual aim of the work is to create a one-piece dress without the need for sewing: Alice Lee have almost succeeded. The mental and mathematical agility required to design and execute these pieces – made by hand-frame knitting – is considerable.

Shelley Fox has a background in both textiles and fashion, and creates textures and shapes through a process of experimentation with materials and a geometric approach to pattern-cutting which she has evolved into her own 'circle cutting' technique.

Recent graduate Fatima Saifee has created distorted and graphic knitted fabrics through combinations of wool and Lycra, which she has developed for avant-garde designer Kei Kagami.

Bernhard Willhelm presents strongly themed and visually powerful collections that combine a child-like vision with inventive construction, fabrication, embellishment, colour and styling. The naïve charm of some of his collections is derived from the techniques and imagery used, as, for instance, in his reworking of the late 1970s landscape sweater in his winter 2000 collection, and in the homely hand-knits of winter 2001 contrasted with darkly patterned fabrics. Fine jersey jacquard knits always echo the imagery at a smaller scale, as in spring/ summer 2002's Venetian mask-inspired collection.

The Comme des Garçons Homme Plus menswear line includes patterned, pieced, overprinted, intarsia, textured and plain fine sweaters, all co-ordinated to the season's main themes by the details of their design.

Knitwear can be as radical as the imagination and expertise of the design team creating it, but without the creative vision of one designer it would be unlikely to come to fruition.

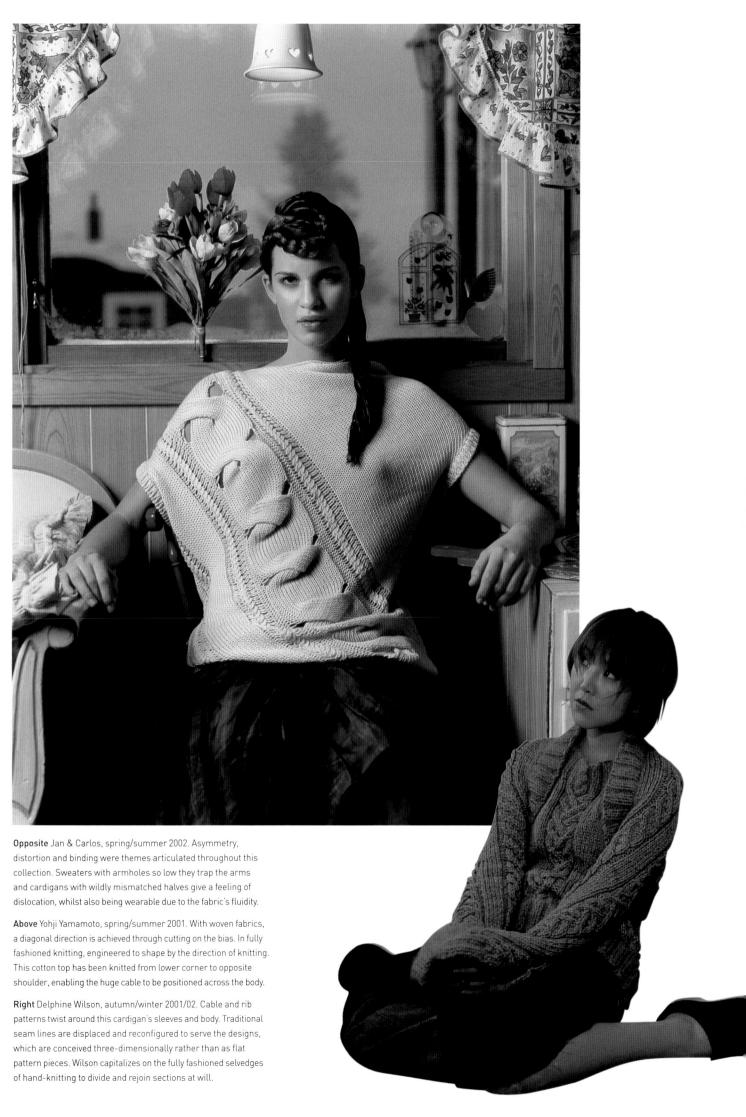

Opposite Jan & Carlos, spring/summer 2002. Asymmetry, distortion and binding were themes articulated throughout this collection. Sweaters with armholes so low they trap the arms and cardigans with wildly mismatched halves give a feeling of dislocation, whilst also being wearable due to the fabric's fluidity.

Above Yohji Yamamoto, spring/summer 2001. With woven fabrics, a diagonal direction is achieved through cutting on the bias. In fully fashioned knitting, engineered to shape by the direction of knitting. This cotton top has been knitted from lower corner to opposite shoulder, enabling the huge cable to be positioned across the body.

Right Delphine Wilson, autumn/winter 2001/02. Cable and rib patterns twist around this cardigan's sleeves and body. Traditional seam lines are displaced and reconfigured to serve the designs, which are conceived three-dimensionally rather than as flat pattern pieces. Wilson capitalizes on the fully fashioned selvedges of hand-knitting to divide and rejoin sections at will.

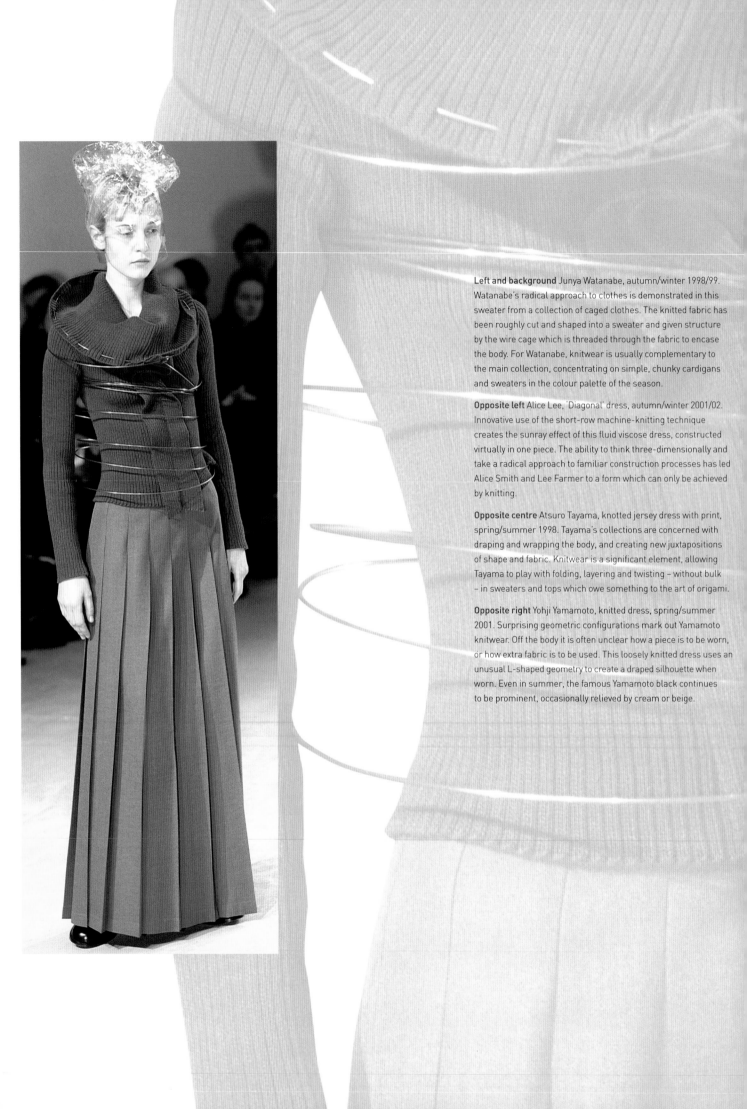

Left and background Junya Watanabe, autumn/winter 1998/99. Watanabe's radical approach to clothes is demonstrated in this sweater from a collection of caged clothes. The knitted fabric has been roughly cut and shaped into a sweater and given structure by the wire cage which is threaded through the fabric to encase the body. For Watanabe, knitwear is usually complementary to the main collection, concentrating on simple, chunky cardigans and sweaters in the colour palette of the season.

Opposite left Alice Lee, 'Diagonal' dress, autumn/winter 2001/02. Innovative use of the short-row machine-knitting technique creates the sunray effect of this fluid viscose dress, constructed virtually in one piece. The ability to think three-dimensionally and take a radical approach to familiar construction processes has led Alice Smith and Lee Farmer to a form which can only be achieved by knitting.

Opposite centre Atsuro Tayama, knotted jersey dress with print, spring/summer 1998. Tayama's collections are concerned with draping and wrapping the body, and creating new juxtapositions of shape and fabric. Knitwear is a significant element, allowing Tayama to play with folding, layering and twisting – without bulk – in sweaters and tops which owe something to the art of origami.

Opposite right Yohji Yamamoto, knitted dress, spring/summer 2001. Surprising geometric configurations mark out Yamamoto knitwear. Off the body it is often unclear how a piece is to be worn, or how extra fabric is to be used. This loosely knitted dress uses an unusual L-shaped geometry to create a draped silhouette when worn. Even in summer, the famous Yamamoto black continues to be prominent, occasionally relieved by cream or beige.

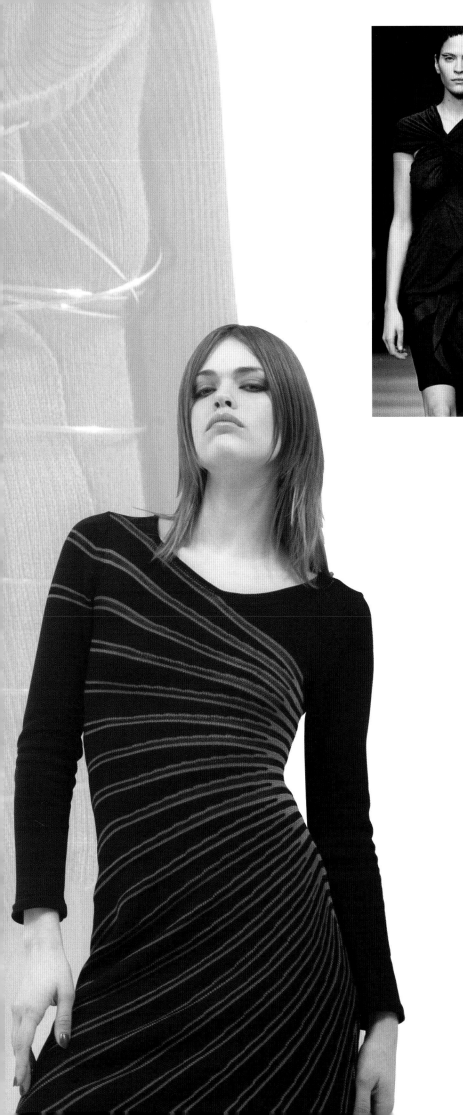

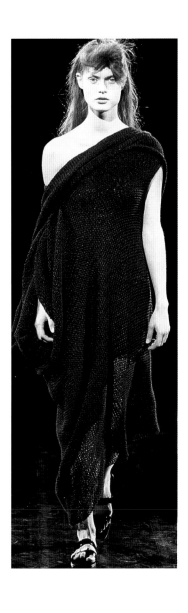

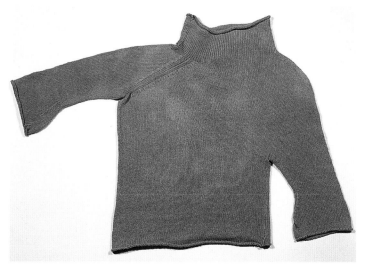

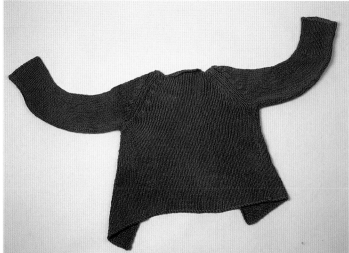

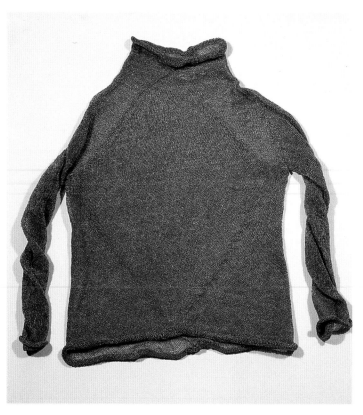

Above Yohji Yamamoto, Y's collection, spring/summer 2001.
The Y's range is Yamamoto's original Japanese label, started
as menswear for women. It includes a wide range of knitwear
not shown on the catwalk. This asymmetric cotton sweater has
one sleeve knitted integrally with the body, and the other knitted
separately with a fully fashioned raglan seam. When worn, the
stretch of the fabric creates fit, and the obvious effect is in
mismatched armhole seams.

Above right Yohji Yamamoto, Y's collection, spring/summer 2001.
Unusual garment shapes are common in the Y's collection. When
viewed two-dimensionally, garments may have an asymmetrical
silhouette, extra fabric or loops. This fully fashioned, heavy cotton,
trimless cardigan features curved arms created by short-row
knitting. A matching sweater has arms which curve inwards
to the body, each subtly affecting the fit.

Right Yohji Yamamoto, Y's collection, spring/summer 2001.
Several Y's designs have a twisted look, with seams in the 'wrong'
place. The single-bed structure of this distorted trimless sweater
in high-twist metallic yarn results in the dramatic displacement
of the side seams, although the shape remains standard.

Opposite above Maison Martin Margiela, autumn/winter 1994/95
and spring/summer 1999. Cardigan based on Barbie doll's
wardrobe, with authentic 'details and disproportions reproduced
in the enlargement' as stated on the label. Margiela returns
increasingly to the theme of scale and sizing, as in his 2000
and 2001 collections produced in a notional size 78.

Opposite below Maison Martin Margiela, autumn/winter 1991/92.
Recycled sweater made from military sweaters and socks.
Margiela was an early exponent of recycling, which has remained
a consistent theme of his collections. His reworked, handmade
garments are now produced under the title of 'artisanal
production' and labelled '0' for women and '0/10' for men.
In 1999 Margiela reworked – in grey – ideas from the previous
ten years' collections.

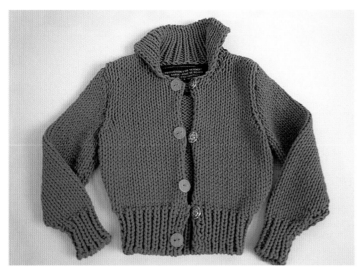

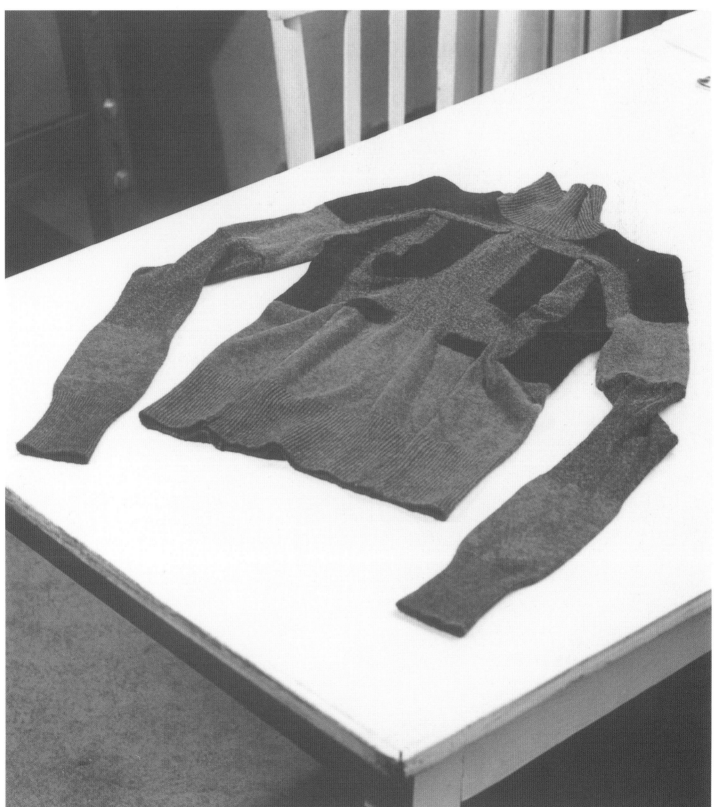

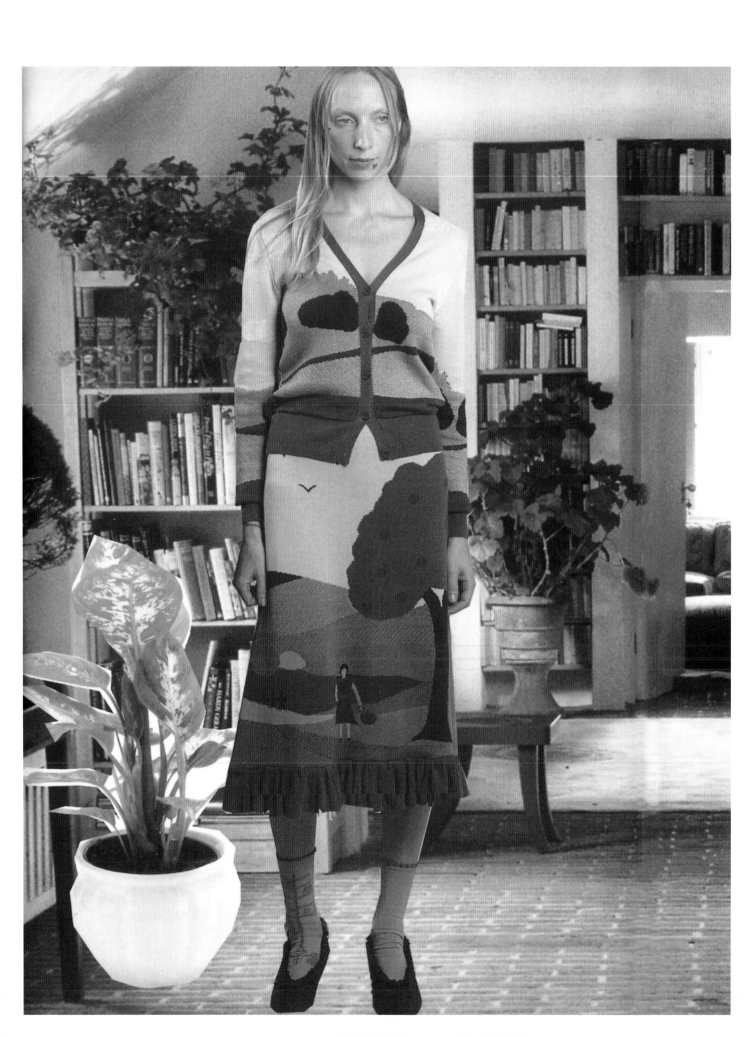

Opposite Bernhard Willhelm, spring/summer 2001. Faux-naïve pictorial knitwear created using jacquard technique, enhanced by embroidery. Pictorial sweater designs were also shown for men. The innovative catalogue for the season placed the models in domestic interiors, some performing chores. Original presentation and storytelling are continuing features of Willhelm's work.

Right Atsuro Tayama, autumn/winter 1998/99. A dress created by wrapping the body in a spiralling length of knitted wool fabric, like a bandage, demonstrating Tayama's love of working on the dress-stand to formulate his designs. Narrow knitted fabric with a selvedge requires no edge finishing, has stretch qualities and is therefore a practical solution to the wrapping concept.

Below Yohji Yamamoto, Y's collection, autumn/winter 2001/02. A shoulder bag is incorporated as an integral part of a shetland wool cardigan, worn either over one shoulder or diagonally across the body. Inside becomes outside as the fabric is used on the 'wrong' (purl) side and seams are external. The only fastening is a kilt pin.

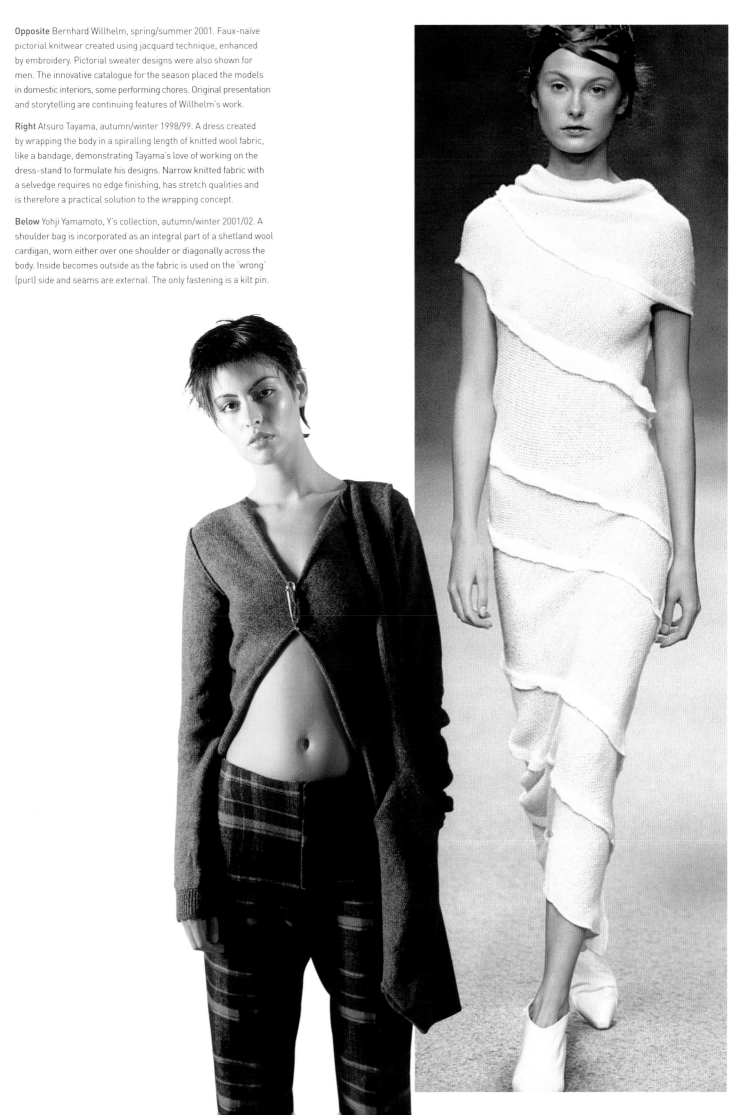

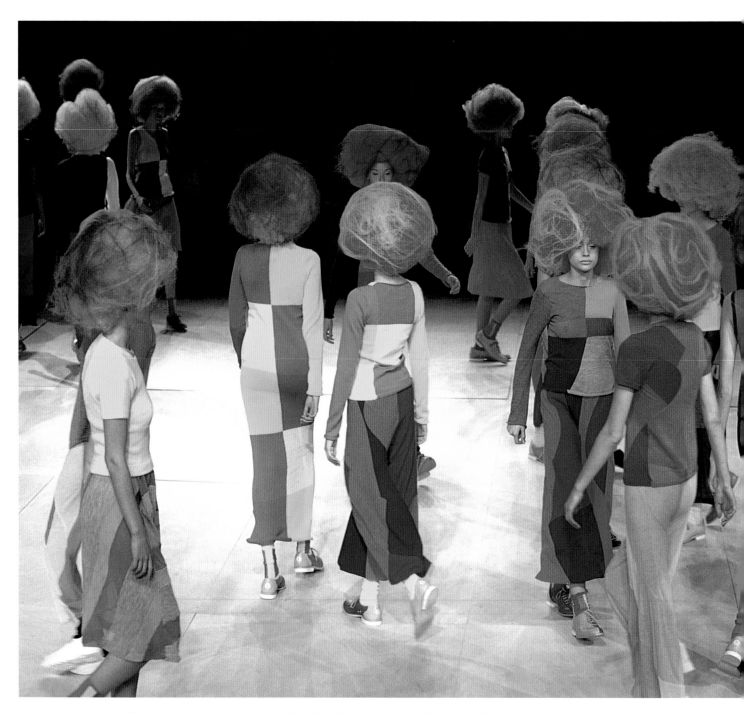

Above Comme des Garçons, 'Kaleidoscope' collection, spring/ summer 1996. Rei Kawakubo's radical designs at first astounded and eventually delighted press, buyers and customers. Knitwear is usually a minor element in the mainline collection – an accessory – but in the collection shown here, it was forefronted. The acid bright patchworks comprised knitted nylon dresses and tops (pieced and intarsia), combined with pieced or overprinted jersey skirts. Note the naturally rolled edges of the knitwear without additional finishes. For winter 2002 Kawakubo has again turned to knitwear featuring twisted and displaced constructions.

Opposite left Comme des Garçons, 'Fusion' collection, autumn/ winter 1998/99. The subtle colour-blocking within the knitwear is achieved through careful mixing of yarns with a neutral base. The knitwear is constructed in traditional fully fashioned manner, with finished edges but external seams, its classic simplicity providing a foil for the elaborate asymmetric drapery of the skirt.

Opposite right Comme des Garçons, 'Sweeter than Sweet' collection, autumn/winter 1995/96. The tight-shouldered silhouette, with deeply inset sleeves which entrap the arms, recurs in several collections. It is here shown in classic cotton jersey manufactured in the style of a sweatshirt with hemmed edges and neckline. Kawakubo works a great deal with jersey fabrics, often twisting, wrapping and distorting the silhouette.

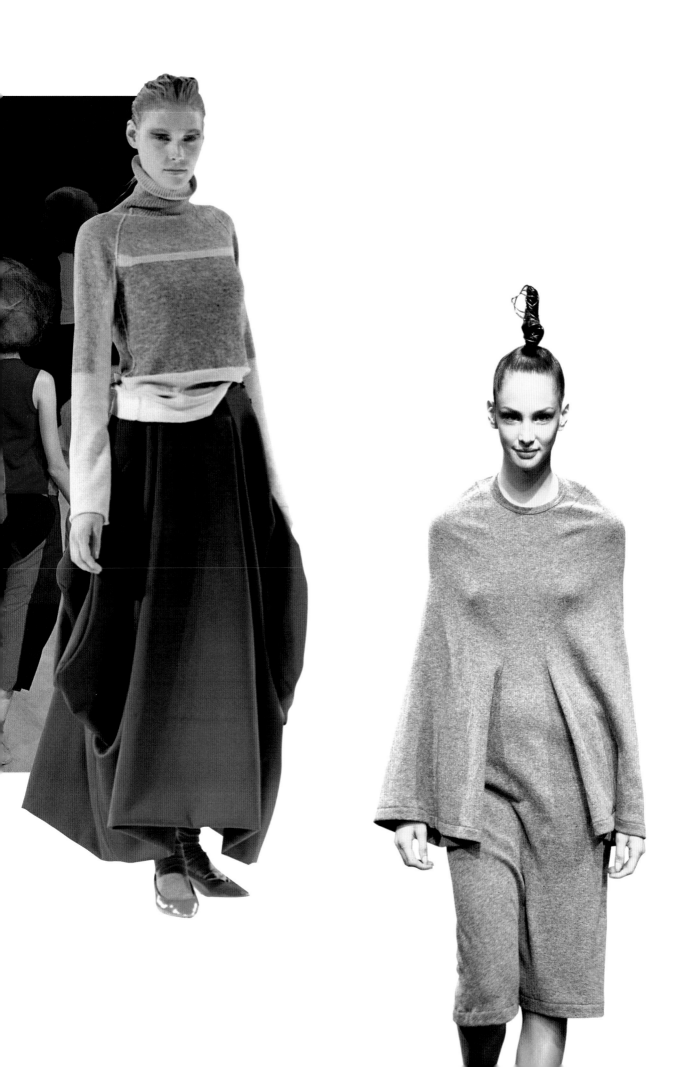

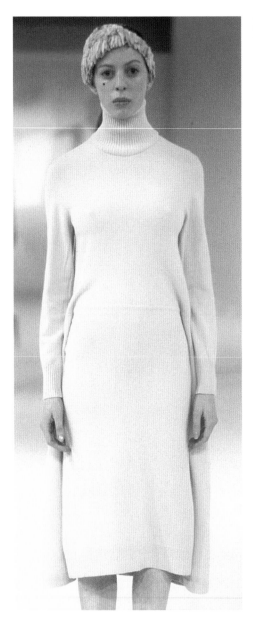

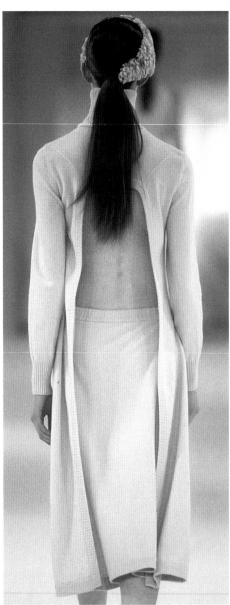

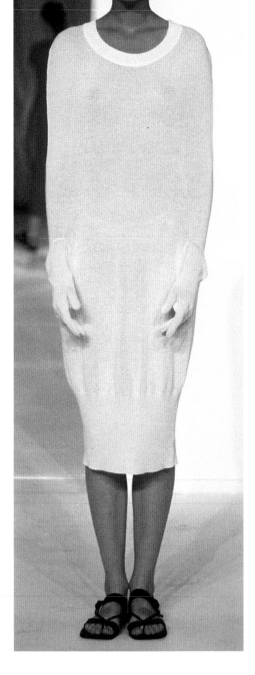

Above left and centre Hussein Chalayan, 'Echoform' collection, autumn/winter 1999/2000. Chalayan developed ranges of knitwear in the late 1990s (with the assistance of Winni Lok) which have become a permanent feature off the catwalk. At first glance, the knitwear appears very traditional, but often there is a twist. An extreme example is this fully fashioned wool/cashmere dress which from the front appears straightforward, but is in fact backless, with an integrated skirt.

Right Hussein Chalayan, 'Between' collection, spring/summer 1998. Bound arms recur as a motif in the collections, indicating restriction, and are sympathetic to the static, meditative style of presentation favoured by Chalayan. Jersey fabrics are either used to bind or are cut away in large sections, as in the printed jersey dresses of winter 1998, with sides cut out in oval shapes. In this 'Cocoon' dress, an amusing concession to practicality is made in the built-in mittens, reminiscent of a space-suit.

Right Hussein Chalayan, 'Scent of Tempests' collection, autumn/ winter 1997/98. Chalayan's work sometimes raises political or religious issues. Commenting on covering up women's bodies, this collection features exposure of a subtle kind, achieved through semi-transparent sections of knitted wool fabric within a dress or sweater.

Below Hussein Chalayan, 'Scent of Tempests' collection, autumn/winter 1997/98. Chalayan's somewhat provocative commentary on the contradiction between Islamic women's dress and modern society was shown a year later in a collection featuring models dressed only in diminishing versions of the chador. This sweater with slit mask was a forerunner, and created some controversy itself.

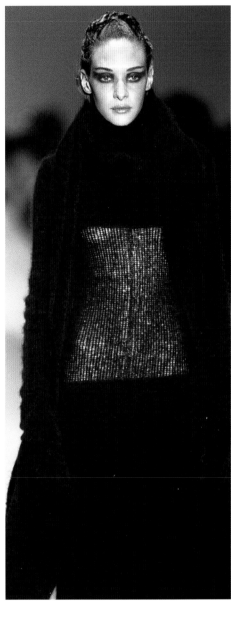

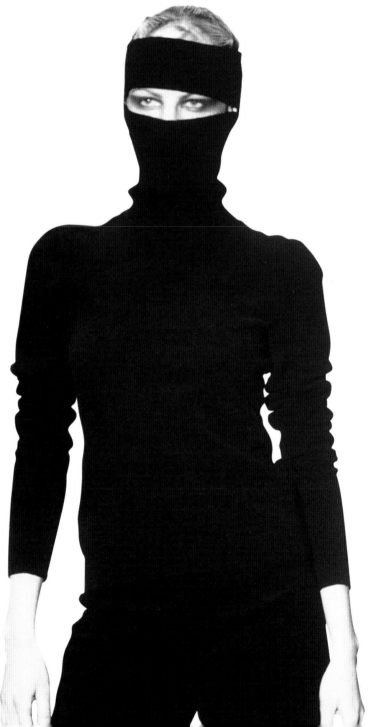

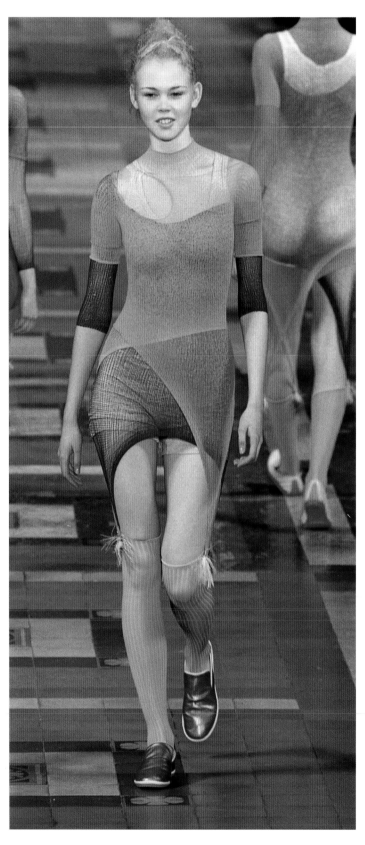

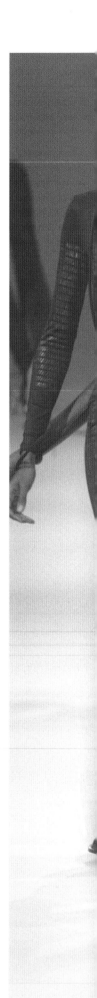

Left Issey Miyake, autumn/winter 2000/01. Two parallel strands can be observed in Miyake's work: the first in which clothing envelops the body, and the second in which the form and silhouette of the body are revealed in second-skin clothing. These can be seen especially in the 'Bodyworks' exhibitions of 1983–5, led, as ever, by investigation into new materials and textiles. Textile designer Makiko Minagawa has worked with Miyake in his Design Studio since its inception. Here experimental ultra-stretchy knitted meshes were layered over each other and tied down in order to form coverings. When relaxed, the pieces are minute in scale. This experiment fed into the development of the one-piece Spider knits that form part of the A-POC range – tiny sweaters knitted in one piece, which stretch greatly to fit.

Opposite left Issey Miyake, 'Tattoo Bodies', spring/summer 1992. Second-skin bodysuits and leggings in stretch jersey with raised print in patterns reflecting the scarification of the skin, as practised by certain African tribes. (The photographs of Leni Riefenstahl made an impact on Miyake.) The tattoo body has appeared in earlier collections, particularly in winter 1989, when graphic-patterned printed stretch bodysuits literally covered the body from neck to toe, mimicking painted skin.

Opposite right Issey Miyake, autumn/winter 1996/97. Striped knitted jersey T-shirts and leggings are shown with radical accessories in rubber-backed jersey fabric, taking the sportswear theme to extremes, whilst remaining essentially practical: the extra padding at the elbows and knees has zipped openings. Miyake revisits and updates ideas first tried out in an early collection of 1971, where the padding was traditional sashiko quilted cotton.

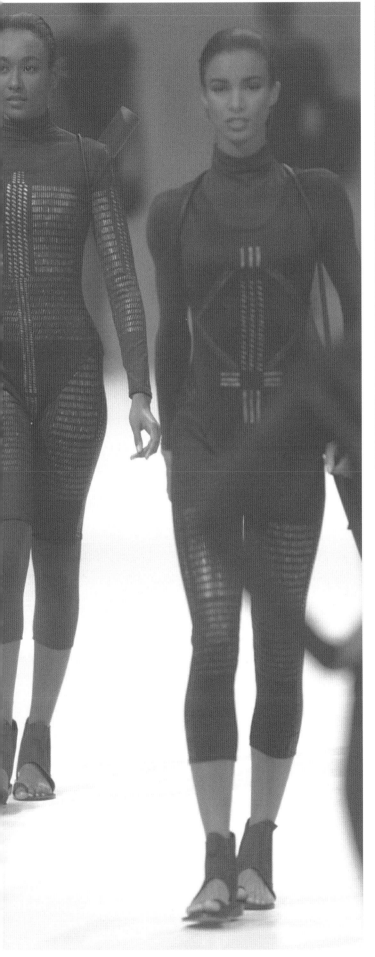

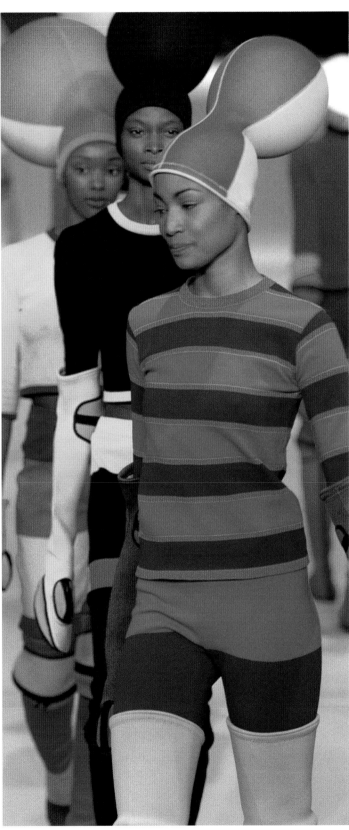

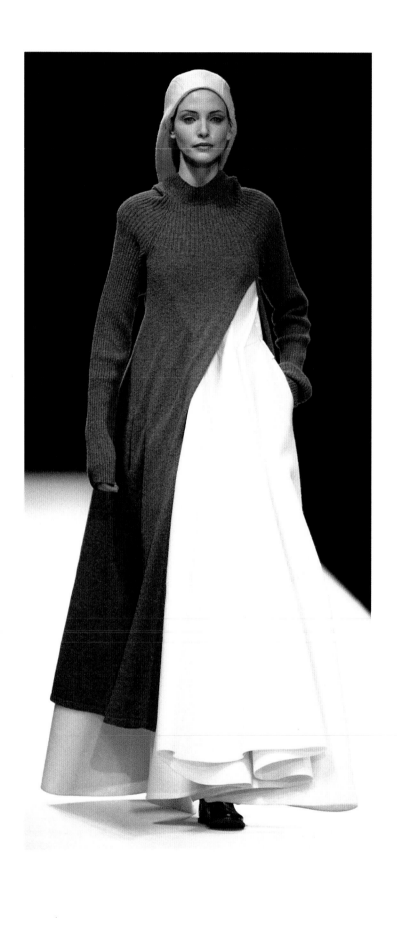

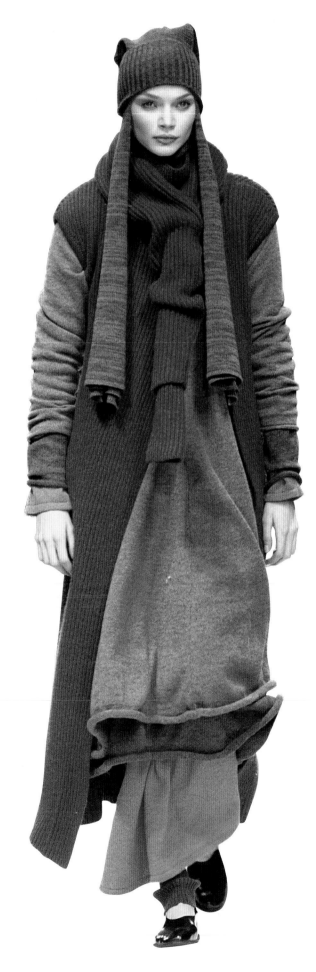

Opposite left Yohji Yamamoto, autumn/winter 1996/97. Knitwear was the major theme in the collection. This silhouette has a flattering, almost nun-like presence – a white dress partially covered by a fully fashioned knitted wool overdress, with shaped rib yoke. The image is refined whilst still featuring asymmetry. Yamamoto has said he does not seek perfection but leaves something to be completed by the wearer.

Opposite right Yohji Yamamoto, autumn/winter 1996/97. Layers of woollen knitting worn under a ribbed outer garment, the single-bed knitting of the underlayers left unfinished and curled, in contrast to the ribbed outer layer which does not curl. Multiple-layered clothing was common at this time but may now appear cumbersome. Relaxed long cardigans replaced the structured jacket as acceptable outerwear.

Right Yohji Yamamoto, hand-crocheted outfit, autumn/winter 1991/92. Although Yamamoto is known for black and dark colours, he does periodically make a statement with bright colours. He is one of the few designers to present crochet in a high-fashion context, using large scale once again for strong visual impact. Crochet reappeared most recently in menswear for autumn/winter 2001/02 in wool suits based on French peasant clothes.

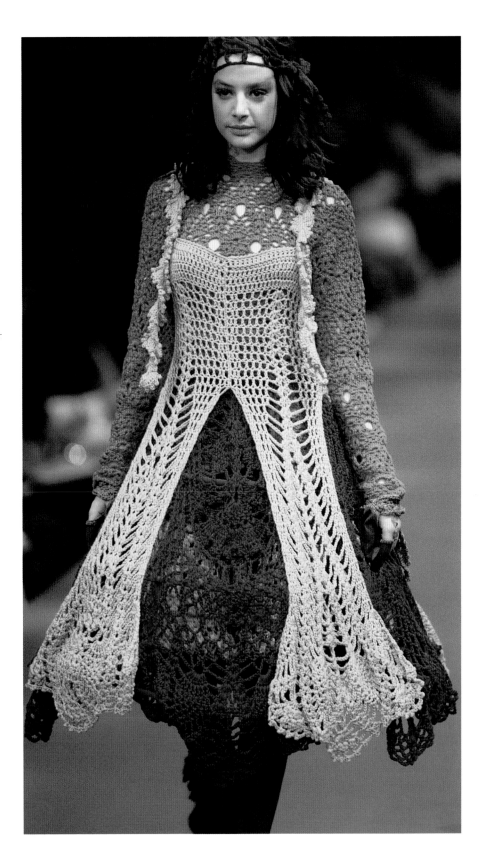

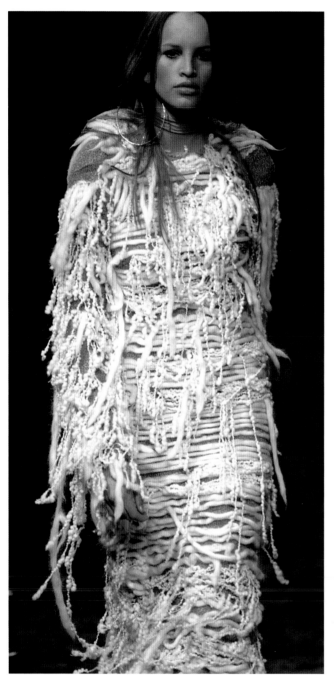

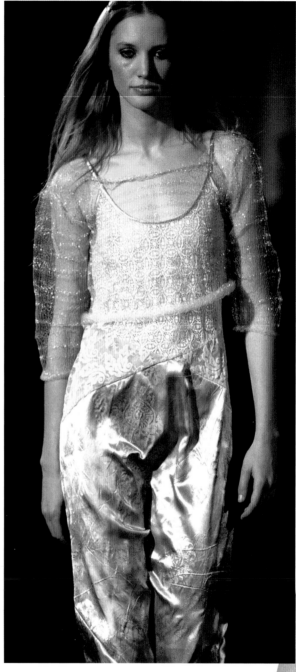

Above left Koji Tatsuno, autumn/winter 1993/94. Tatsuno started his career by tailoring vintage fabric into sumptuous waistcoats and jackets, but he also developed a more experimental approach, working not as a fashion designer but more as an artisan-couturier staging spectacular shows and selling avant-garde pieces to individual clients. In 1993 he became interested in knitwear and knitted construction. Assisted by Julien Macdonald for two seasons, he produced highly innovative, deconstructed knitwear, such as this dress of 'floating' wool strands, created by laying unspun wool into a transparent knitted backing.

Above right Koji Tatsuno, spring/summer 1994. Experiments with transparent nylon monofilament yarns were highly unusual at this time. Transparent fabric shimmering with metallic thread formed illusory garments and almost invisible layers. This theme was developed in sweaters with inlaid mohair yarns which snaked around the body.

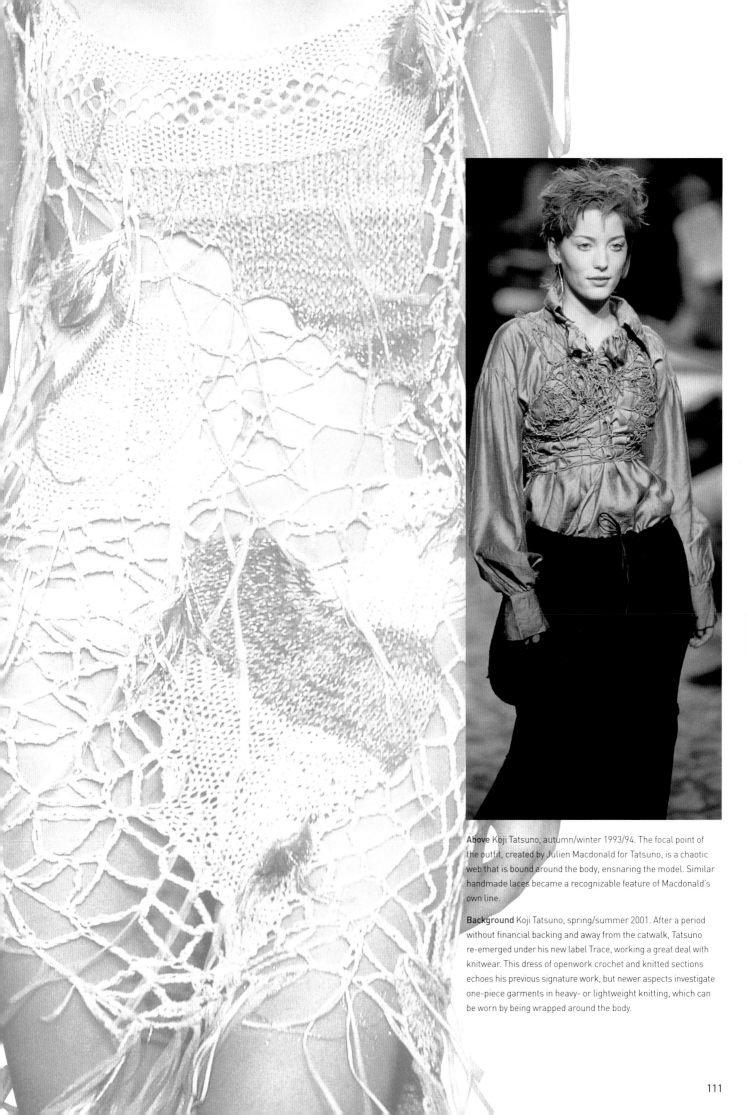

Above Koji Tatsuno, autumn/winter 1993/94. The focal point of the outfit, created by Julien Macdonald for Tatsuno, is a chaotic web that is bound around the body, ensnaring the model. Similar handmade laces became a recognizable feature of Macdonald's own line.

Background Koji Tatsuno, spring/summer 2001. After a period without financial backing and away from the catwalk, Tatsuno re-emerged under his new label Trace, working a great deal with knitwear. This dress of openwork crochet and knitted sections echoes his previous signature work, but newer aspects investigate one-piece garments in heavy- or lightweight knitting, which can be worn by being wrapped around the body.

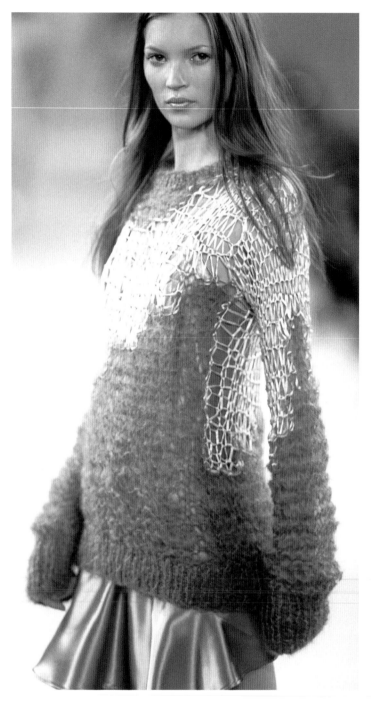

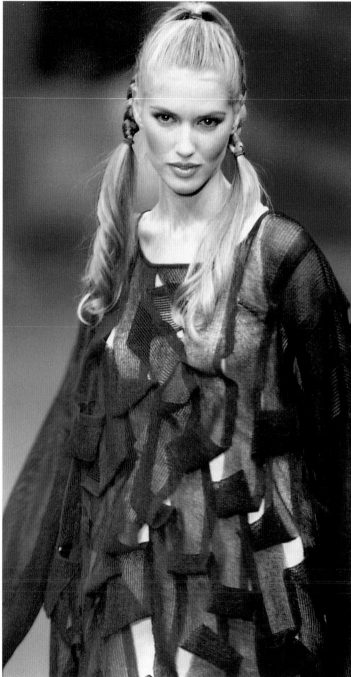

Opposite left Anna Sui, spring/summer 1994. At the height of the 'grunge' fashion phenomenon, with echoes of earlier punk knitwear, the loosely hand-knitted sweater was revived for the catwalk. A combination of contrasting yarns, texture and colour, and the resulting uneven knitting, came to represent this brief anti-fashion fashion, which could not sustain itself at designer level.

Opposite right Ernestina Cerini, spring/summer 1993. Cerini came to prominence in the 1980s with her complex, often hand-manipulated knitwear, inspired by decorative ironwork. In her garments she pieced together knitted braids, created unusual textural patchworks and investigated original silhouettes. This collection comprised pieces made from draped and manipulated knitted fabrics and handmade openwork macramé tunics.

Right Xuly Bet, autumn/winter 1993/94. Lamine Kouyate had launched his recycled collections on to the Paris fashion circuit to great acclaim the previous season. This dress is made from patched, recycled knitwear, overlocked and decoratively stitched. Representing a particular moment in fashion history, this reworked use of old clothing can be seen in several collections, including From Somewhere by Orsola de Castra, and Martin Margiela. Fake London started with recycled cashmere, and the use of vintage clothing in new fashion is now accepted.

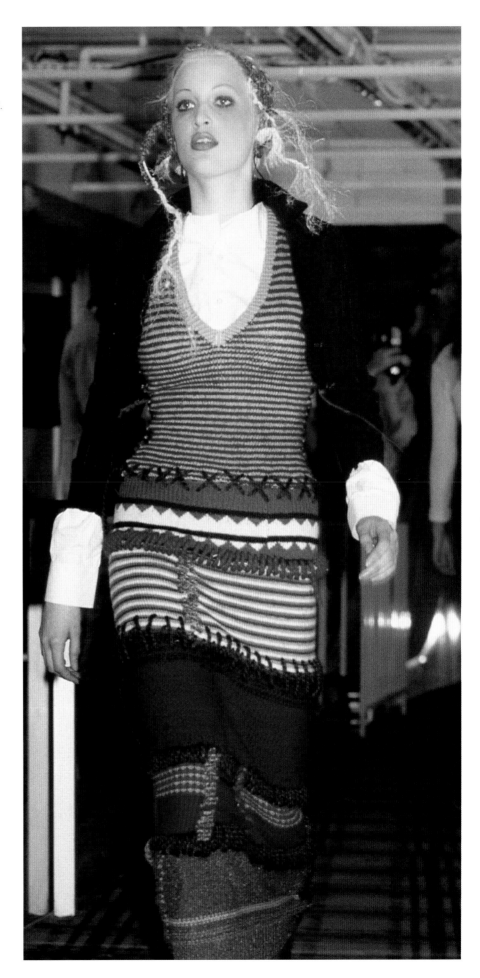

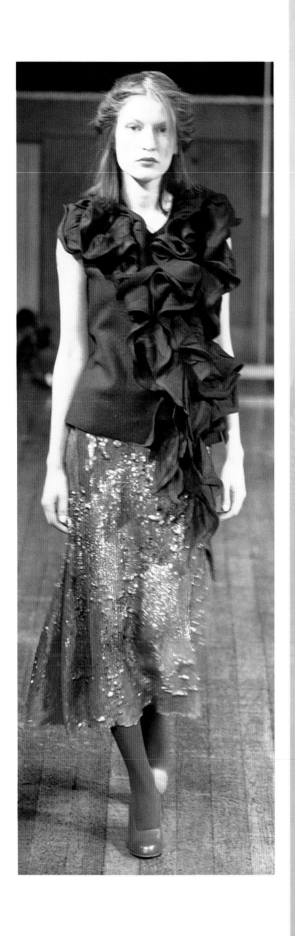

Left Shelley Fox, autumn/winter 2000/01. Fox is an innovator who creates high fashion out of experimentation and serendipity. Manipulating and developing many fabrics herself, she also researches new approaches to construction, and has developed her own geometric 'circle-cutting' technique. This sequinned skirt is made from fabric that has been singed and the frilled top is constructed from knitted and felted wool, with frills applied. Due to the felting process, each piece is unique and unpredictable.

Background Fatima Saifee for Kei Kagami, spring/summer 2002. Kagami creates avant-garde clothes which break away from current fashion trends. Working in the manner of haute couture, he commissions collaborators to achieve his vision. Saifee's use of random insertions (here using fabric) and organic shapes, achieved with the integration of Lycra into knitted fabrics, caught his attention and resulted in a knitwear collection for this and the previous season.

Opposite left Sharon Wauchob, sweater, autumn/winter 2001/02. Wauchob's background in both commercial design (Louis Vuitton) and experimental design (Koji Tatsuno) has led to an individual look. Handmade showpieces are combined with more mainstream designs. This woollen sweater is adorned with grotesque twisted cable (reminiscent of Kawakubo's early knitwear) and pom-poms, which also figured in skirts and accessories.

Opposite right Sharon Wauchob, sweater, autumn/winter 2001/02. Wauchob's concept of luxury designs contains extreme elements and complex layers and silhouettes, with fabrics manipulated, printed or overworked. This fine wool sweater is decorated with metal studs, giving weight and impact.

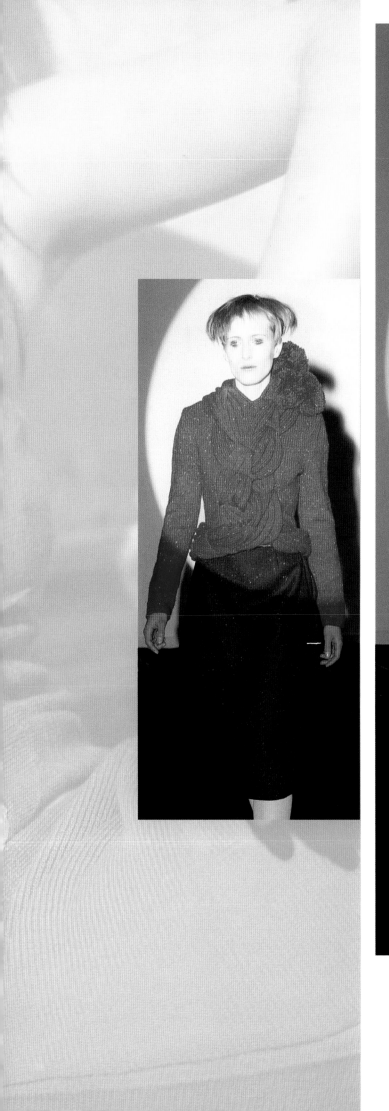
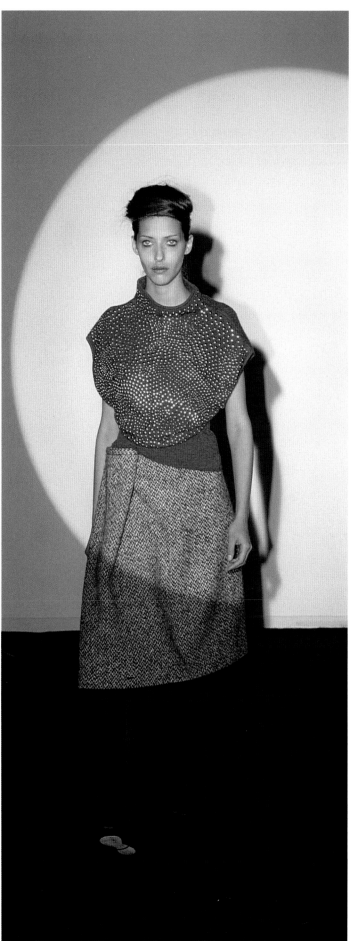

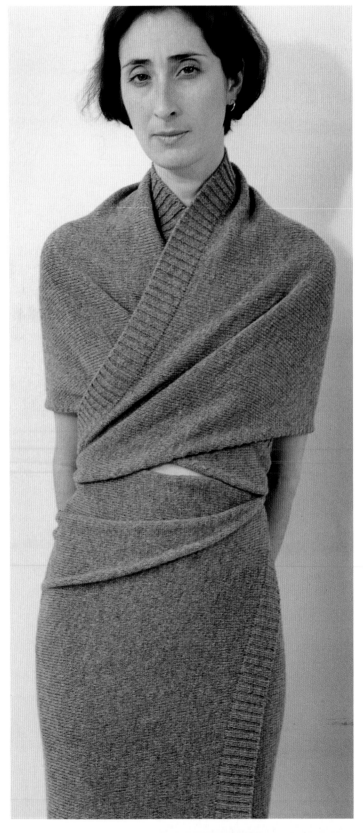

Left Maison Martin Margiela, autumn/winter 1999/2000. Wrapped shetland woollen dress made from two pieces of knitted fabric, one shaped. This concept reflects the simplest form of body-covering used from ancient times. The pieces are knitted 'garment blanks' with a traditional rib for the welt, but used in a direct manner instead of being cut and sewn into a classic shape. Margiela interrupts the knitwear production process at a very early stage.

Opposite above Maison Martin Margiela, spring/summer 2002. The theme of the collection was 'Circles, Folding and Cut'. The circular section included knitwear of several weights, which, when flat, formed circles of several sizes (including a large circular cape) but, when worn, the pieces draped subtly to hint at their construction. Here the circular cardigan sleeves are cut and sewn, but the ribbed edging has been meticulously shaped in a curve.

Opposite below Maison Martin Margiela, spring/summer 2001. A collection in which oversized menswear was worn by women. All the garments were enlarged to an Italian size 78. Woven pieces were folded and stitched back to fit a standard size, whilst knitwear was crumpled and moulded to shape. Here a classic man's cardigan is worn with trousers which are the same back and front. The models' eyes were again obscured (see p. 77), creating anonymity and drawing attention to the clothes.

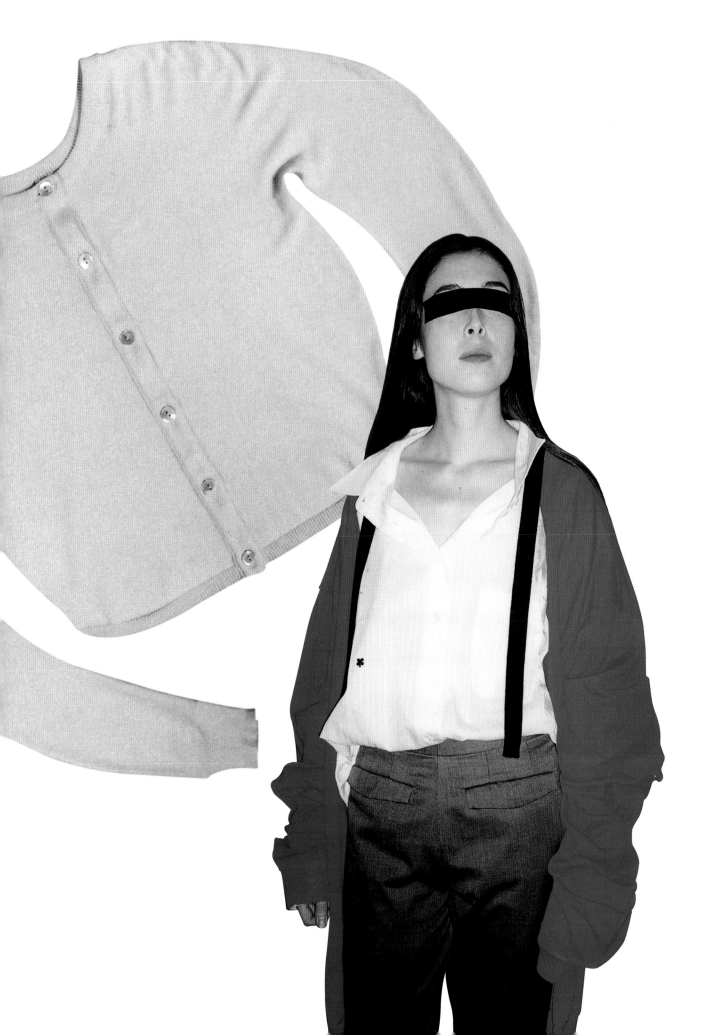

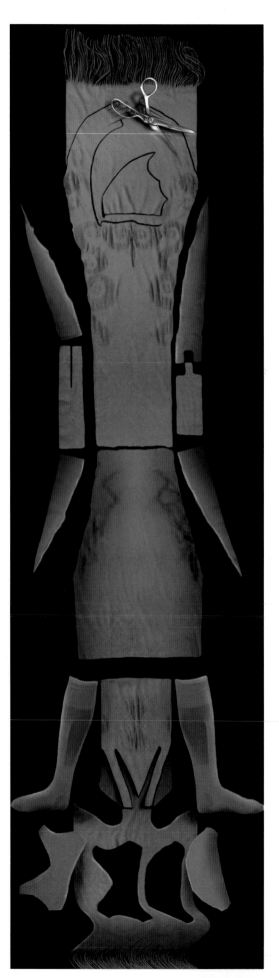

Two of the most significant developments in knitwear manufacturing, which could have a major impact on the fashions we wear and on clothing production, are seamless (or integral) construction – currently seen in socks, gloves, underwear, lingerie and more recently in some sweaters – and the revolutionary clothing concept A-POC from Issey Miyake, in which a knitted tube of patterned cloth ingeniously separates into a whole wardrobe of garments, breaking new ground aesthetically, technologically and in its retail concept. Both developments use totally different technologies – integral knitting is based on weft knitting, A-POC on warp – but each depends on the computer control and design capabilities working at the interface of machine innovations and advanced yarns.

The concept of seamless knitting is as old as knitting itself, as shown by fragments of Egyptian socks dating from the fifth and sixth centuries held in museums. In medieval times, Britain and Spain were two of the foremost producers of hand-knitted seamless stockings. Since the Industrial Revolution, when knitting was mechanized, industrially knitted garments have been produced either in shaped sections on flat-bed machines or cut from fabric produced on flat or circular machines, both of which require a finishing process. The seamless, garment-by-garment, industrial manufacture of knitwear, requiring little or no making up, has long been something of a mission for machine builders. In 1965 the Japanese company Shima Seiki invented the first machine for manufacturing seamless knitted gloves to meet the demand for work gloves used daily by taxi drivers, construction and factory workers throughout Japan. The company has since remained at the forefront of integral knitting technology. Though the ability to knit in the round without seams is the oldest form of knitting by hand, it took until the later twentieth century to replicate by machine the gansey, sock, glove and cap – all perfect examples of seamless, three-dimensional knitting.

The hosiery industry has recently led developments in machinery and adapted their expertise in fine gauge production with synthetic yarns to create new engineered and sculpted lingerie, swimwear and underwear which have quietly infiltrated the mass market via companies such as Wolford, Benetton and Marks & Spencer. Much lingerie is now without side seams and increasingly features differential structures to add support and define shape in one-piece underwear.

Machine builders, such as Santoni, and manufacturers are now turning their attention to outerwear formed from basic body-sized tubes, which have tremendous potential for new forms of clothing. Philippe Starck and Wolford created the versatile

Opposite and right A-POC Queen, from 'King and Queen', spring/summer 1999. Seeing A-POC for the first time we are not quite sure what to make of the vague patterns and occasional gaps discernible in the cloth. Fortunately there is a computer animation to explain it. We are shown the fringed roll of cloth, the application of the scissors and one by one a wardrobe is released: dress, skirt, underwear, hat, gloves, socks and bag. They are put on by an invisible model who walks away delighted.

Below A-POC Alien, autumn/winter 1999/2000. Alien is possibly the most complex design to visualize. It contains the body in double layers of mesh fabric – dress over trousers, and face initially masked. In the fashion show presentation, two assistants cut away and opened up the fabric into a more wearable form, and the model emerged.

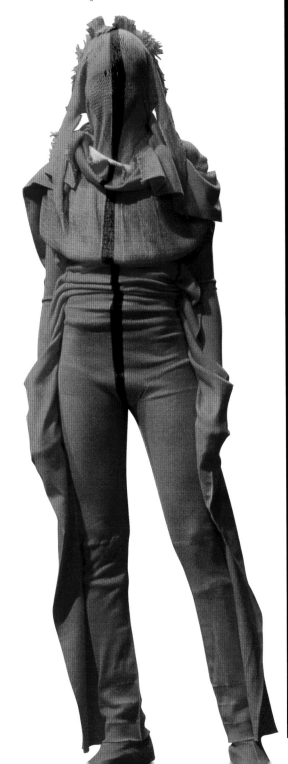

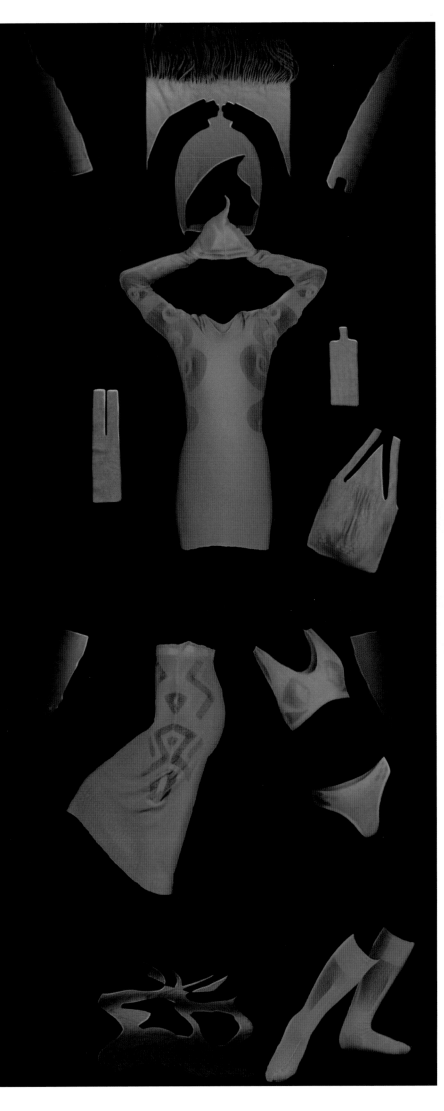

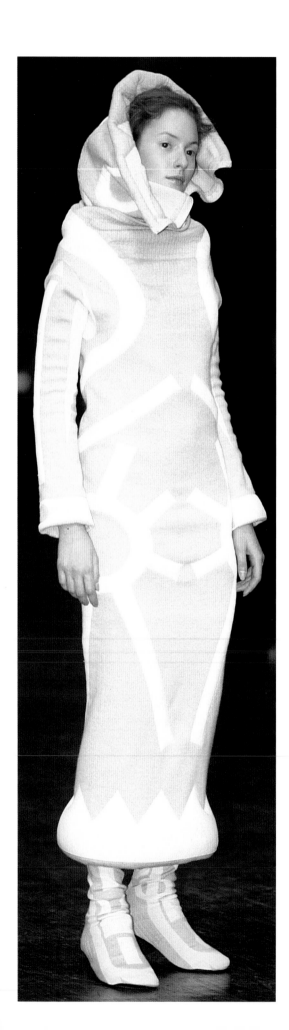

tubular dress 'Starck Naked' in 1998. Testu, a new design company, have created ranges of unisex pieces made from fine knitted tubes but deliberately shaped and distorted in the knitting process to create bizarre, two-dimensional forms which fall into folds when worn on the body. As with most innovations in technology, early use has tended to merely replicate the basic existing knitwear constructions. However, new design research is beginning to take place; for example, the work of Caterina Radvan focuses on unconventional shapes that create volume and drape in seamless garments.

Technological advances in knitting have at present outstripped the market's ability to absorb and utilize it, and the customer has to be educated to recognize the benefits. The role of technicians and designers must inevitably merge closer together to create a dialogue from which design innovation can spring.

Issey Miyake remains unsurpassed in his commitment to the development of new forms of textiles and clothing which cross both international and fashion boundaries to have universal appeal. With his integration of old and new technologies, experimentation with processes and questioning of assumptions whilst resolutely looking to the future, Miyake has revolutionized our perceptions of clothing the body. The A-POC concept represents a simultaneous leap of the imagination and application of technology. A-POC (an acronym for 'A Piece of Cloth' and play on the word 'epoch') was first shown in 1997 and is a collaboration between Issey Miyake and Dai Fujiwara, one of the Miyake Studio design team who originally trained as a weaver. The whole process is an experiment designed in four stages – a continuing work-in-progress – in which the customer also participates. These stages are conjugated like Latin – APOC, APOS, APOM, APOE. As the technology of the cloth is perfected, they will turn their attention to the yarn (A Piece of String), then design the machinery to have complete control, and then hire A Person of Education and Dedication to create a fully integrated company. They see no boundaries or limits to what might be achieved – just technical problems to be overcome and refined. As Fujiwara says, 'Design is functionality and function is beauty.'

The fundamental philosophy is one within which Miyake has operated since he set up his studio in 1970 – to create the maximum with one piece of cloth; no waste, minimum cutting and seaming and, in the case of A-POC, no after-knitting processes at all. This has similarities to the classic construction of the kimono from one long roll of narrow cloth, and Miyake has applied it in many ways, with knitwear, woven garments and also moulded pieces. Indeed the first garment entitled 'A Piece of Cloth' was knitted and shown as early as 1976. The A-POC application may be the concept's most perfect realization as it involves no seaming or finishing processes except the cutting out of the chosen variation from the tubular roll of cloth which is presented to the customer. As such, it also represents a unique mix of customization and mass production.

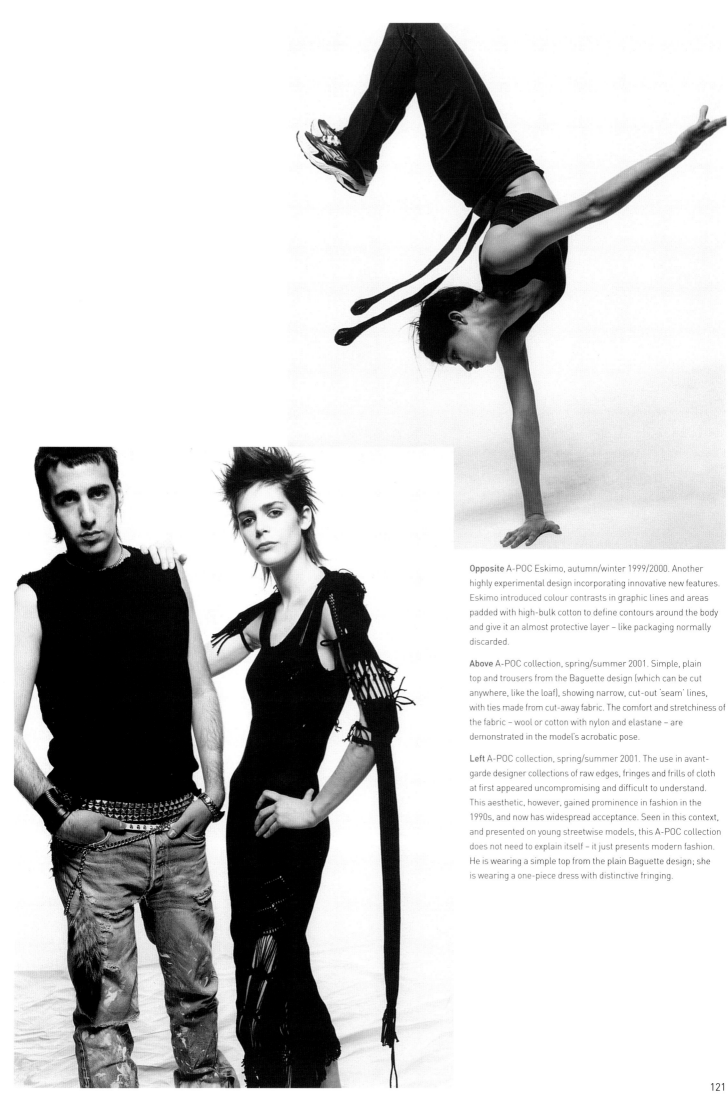

Opposite A-POC Eskimo, autumn/winter 1999/2000. Another highly experimental design incorporating innovative new features. Eskimo introduced colour contrasts in graphic lines and areas padded with high-bulk cotton to define contours around the body and give it an almost protective layer – like packaging normally discarded.

Above A-POC collection, spring/summer 2001. Simple, plain top and trousers from the Baguette design (which can be cut anywhere, like the loaf), showing narrow, cut-out 'seam' lines, with ties made from cut-away fabric. The comfort and stretchiness of the fabric – wool or cotton with nylon and elastane – are demonstrated in the model's acrobatic pose.

Left A-POC collection, spring/summer 2001. The use in avant-garde designer collections of raw edges, fringes and frills of cloth at first appeared uncompromising and difficult to understand. This aesthetic, however, gained prominence in fashion in the 1990s, and now has widespread acceptance. Seen in this context, and presented on young streetwise models, this A-POC collection does not need to explain itself – it just presents modern fashion. He is wearing a simple top from the plain Baguette design; she is wearing a one-piece dress with distinctive fringing.

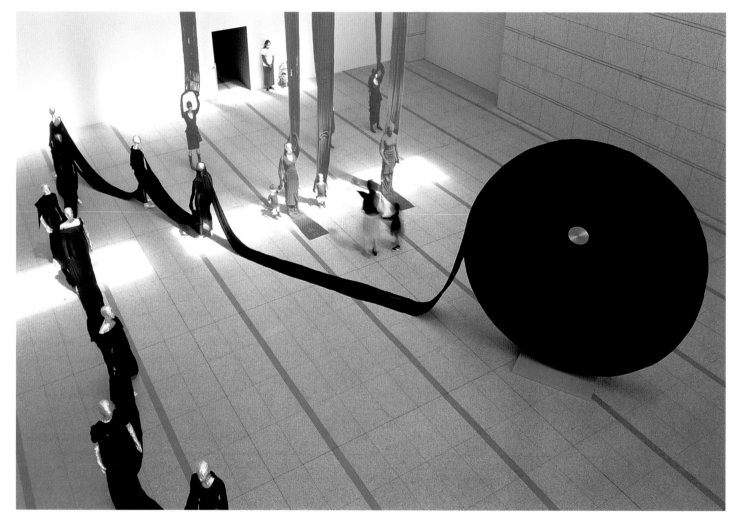

Above Issey Miyake, 'Making Things' exhibition, Tokyo, summer 2000. First presented in Paris in autumn 1998, the exhibition also travelled to New York. The A-POC section received more prominence in Miyake's home country, spectacularly filling the space with continuous lengths of cloth worn on mannequins and making the point of mass production by the presence of the huge roll of knitted fabric.

Opposite above A-POC Le Feu, spring/summer 1999. The A-POC concept was at first shown as part of the Miyake fashion show presentations, before becoming a collection in its own right. This dramatic display demonstrated the revolutionary concept by a series of models wearing a T-shirt and skirt, based on a square shape, each one connected to the next.

Opposite below Close-up of the 'Making Things' installation, showing the warp knit partially cut away, leaving the fringe effect and spaces in the knit, which create larger fringes.

Attention has been given to the technical details, such as creating the right mesh fabric for appropriate stretch, and working out the different diameters of tube required for all the garment parts (the ideal body size was found to be 55 cm). With the right amount of stretch, however, these tubes can fit all sizes.

A-POC is manufactured using computer-controlled, warp-knitting technology, which creates fabric from a fine mesh of individual chain stitches flowing vertically, each linked together. A high level of stretch is derived from the cotton or wool/nylon (polyamide)/polyurethane mix. The innovation was to develop this technology in circular knit form and adapt it from socks to body-sized pieces, and then to design the contours of the garment shapes within the large tube, using graphic patterning on a computer interface and creating a subdivided tubular shape which, when released, opens to form three-dimensional garment pieces with internal patterns of mesh. The cutting lines are subtly delineated by gaps where the individual warp threads are not connected to each other. These create the signature fringing effect which demarcates all the outlines of the pieces within the flat fabric tubes, as well as the major sections such as tubes for arms and legs. As the experiment has developed, the garment shapes, internal designs and fabric patterning have evolved, each developed painstakingly on the computer screen.

One of the intrinsic qualities of A-POC in its first incarnation – 'Just Before' – was the unfinished, raw appearance derived from the fringed edges just released, the extra fabric from the sides of cloth remaining from cutting out (utilized as rough belts), and the raw-edged collars and necklines formed from removing the attached fabric. The effect was arresting and at first a little shocking: like any totally new concept it challenged our assumptions about clothing. The ragged edges have since undergone refinements and developments with each successive design until the simplest 'Baguette' sweater and its companion trousers show only the most discreet external 'seams'.

All the A-POC designs can be varied according to choice – round neck, V-neck or loose collar, short or long sleeves, short or long length, and so on. A computer-generated video shows the process of releasing the wardrobe from the cloth. The innovative retail concept of the A-POC shops is that they are to be seen as a laboratory in which the customer can view many examples of the variations on each theme and can cut their own garments from the piece or the roll, with help from the well-informed sales staff. In Tokyo Dai Fujiwara works with his assistants, all wearing white coats, in a laboratory at the back of the shop, separated from it by glass walls, so that they can feed customer reaction back into the design process. A live experiment indeed.

A-POC Eskimo and A-POC Alien were two designs from 1999, each incorporating new features such as areas padded with bulky yarn to define contours around the body and give it an almost protective layer. Further experiments have incorporated other features: the Millennium Pillow carries portable furnishings with the wearer, and Mobile is an anthropomorphic cross between clothing, furniture and plaything. Although sometimes a little difficult to understand, and not so universally wearable as Pleats Please, the A-POC concept will, according to Dai Fujiwara, eventually realize the merging of woven and knitted textile production to create new clothes for living in the twenty-first century.

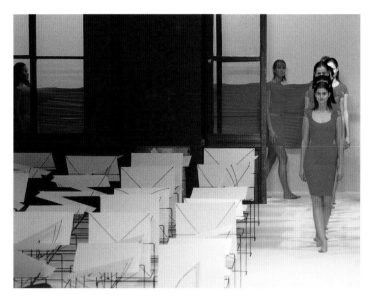

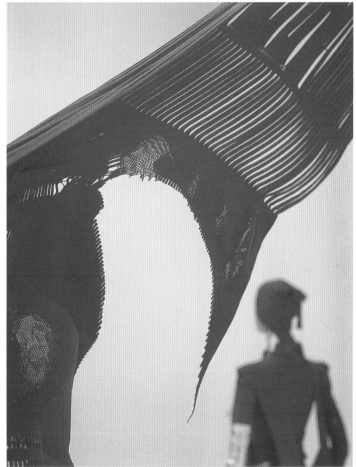

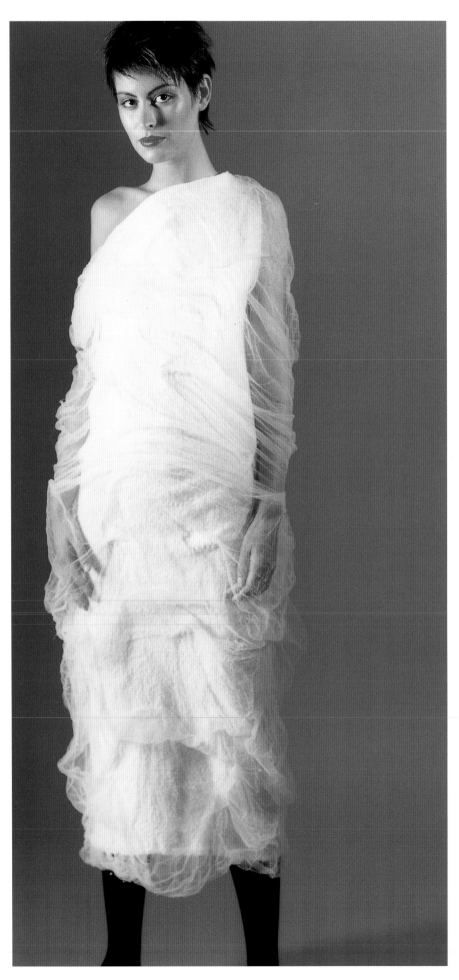

Left Caterina Radvan, 1998. Starting with geometric shapes applied to the body, Radvan has focused on creating seamless knitted garments to develop the unique potential of knitted construction. This seamless dress, made as part of her Masters graduate collection, is knitted in a giant blister stitch on a circular machine in a combination of lambswool and nylon monofilament, then washed to shrink and felt the wool, leaving a ruched layer of nylon attached loosely to the surface.

Opposite left Caterina Radvan, 2000. This seamless dress is knitted in linen, with raw-edged cuffs in rubber yarn. Continuing to develop the seamless theme, Radvan knitted dresses and tops with unconventional asymmetrical and greatly distorted two-dimensional shapes, subverting normal ideas of back, front, sleeves and left-right symmetry. When worn, this produces drape in parts of the garment, and lines of fashioning marks displace normal seams. Radvan is now applying her ideas to unconventional body shapes.

Opposite right Caterina Radvan, 1999. This seamless top is worked on a domestic knitting machine in tubular formation, with integral folds formed by short-row knitting, giving drape to the garment. The lambswool fabric has been felted.

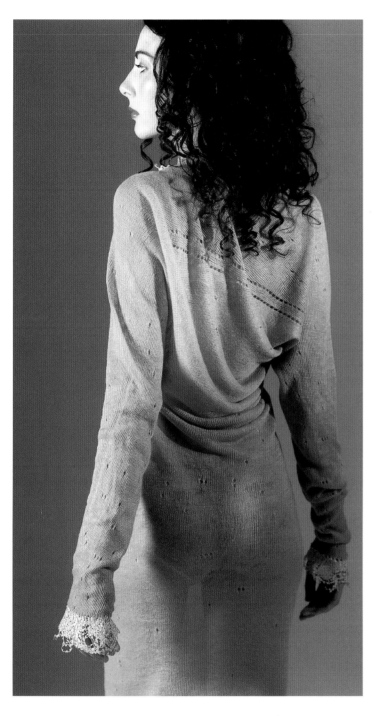
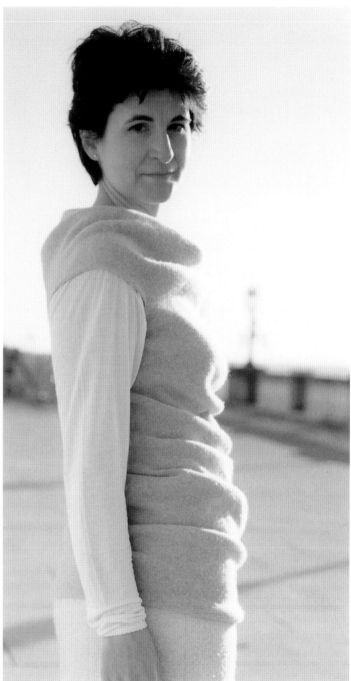

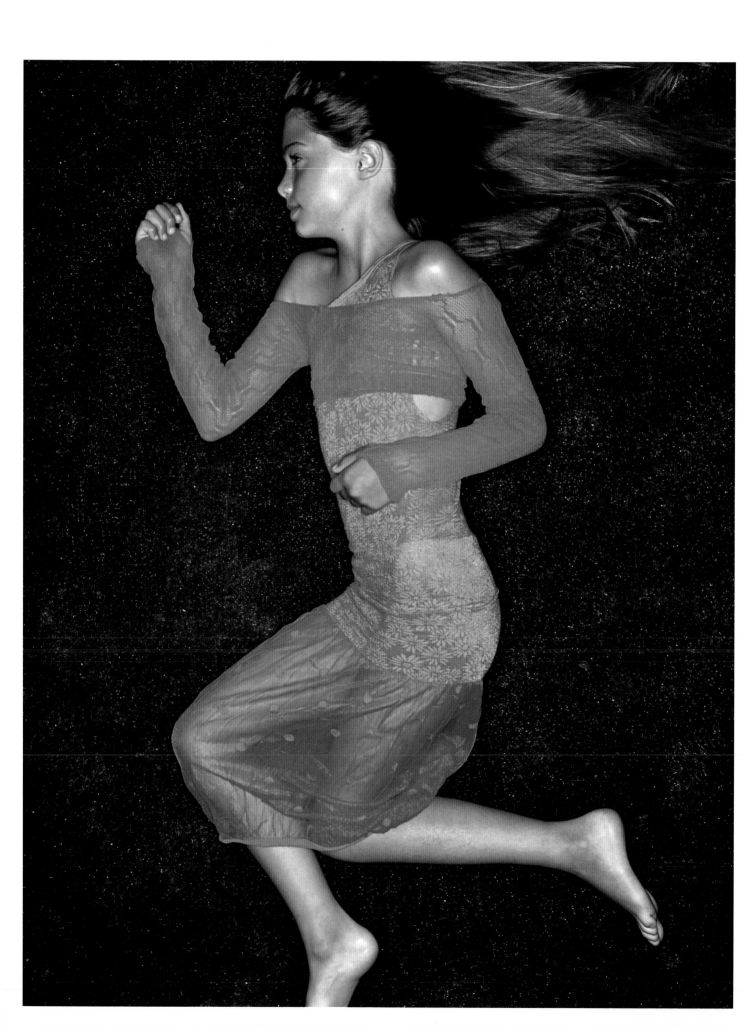

Opposite 'Seamless for Kids', 2001. Machinery manufacturer Matec has developed revolutionary 6- to 10-inch-diameter machines with jacquard capability, which allow for the production of simple 'bodysized' children's garments with minimal seaming and patterned fabrics. The potential for the new technology is shown in this style concept by Emilio Cavallini, using stretch synthetic yarns. Partner company Santoni is at the forefront of 'bodysized' machinery development for adult seamless bodywear, including engineered stitch patterning to create form and structure.

Right Stoll Knitting, seamless dress, 2001. Trend concepts are produced by the design department of this long-established machine builder, which is at the forefront of flat-knitting technology development. These concepts are used to inspire designers and manufacturers, and to promote the newest technologies. This dress combines two-colour knitting and integral knitting in one garment, requiring only neckline and armhole finishing. Note the fully fashioning around the colour divide.

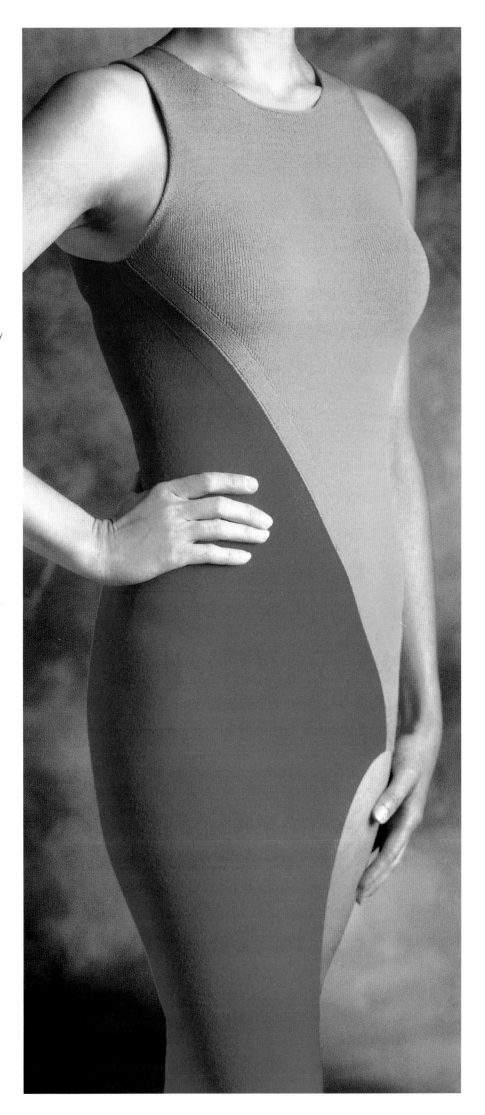

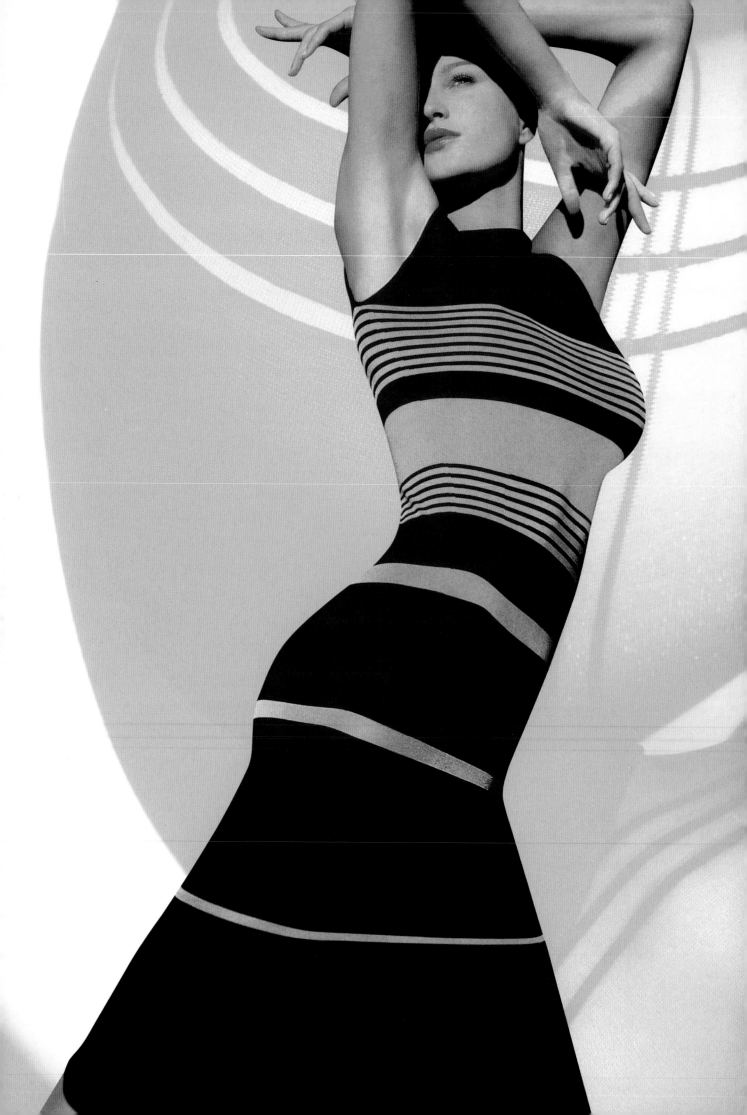

Opposite Wolford seamless dress, spring/summer 2000. Using seamless technology by Santoni, Wolford create bodywear ranges which cross over from intimate wear to outerwear, comprising complex jacquard patterning (such as the tiger-patterned 'Africa' dress) or simple stripes. Wolford have also collaborated with top designers, including Philippe Starck, Hervé Leger and Jean Paul Gaultier, to push the boundaries further.

Background Wolford 'System' tights, autumn/winter 2000/01. Seamlessness became the norm for women's hosiery after the advent of seamfree stockings, then tights, in the 1950s and '60s, although some seaming processes for the body-part and the toes are still generally necessary. Completely seamless tights can now be produced but are not yet widely commercially available. Most design development has taken place in the patterning capabilities applied to hosiery, which are now boundless.

Right Jean Paul Gaultier for Wolford, autumn/winter 2000/01. In this first collaboration, Gaultier designed a range of tights and all-in-one bodies which created the impression of separate pieces of underwear. Further irony was achieved in the seamless tights which were patterned to simulate seamed stockings, complete with suspenders. A second range of designs for summer 2001 featured the Eiffel tower patterned halfway up the leg and across the body.

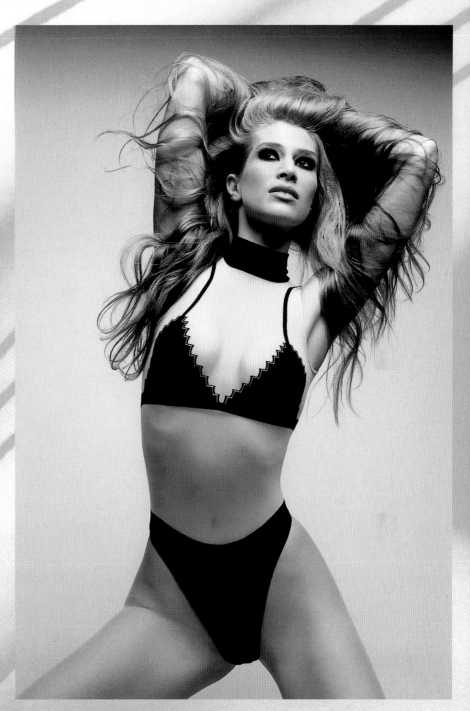

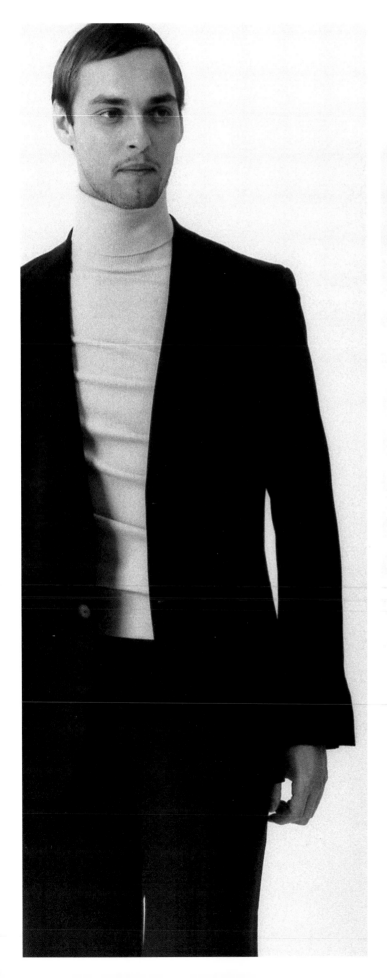

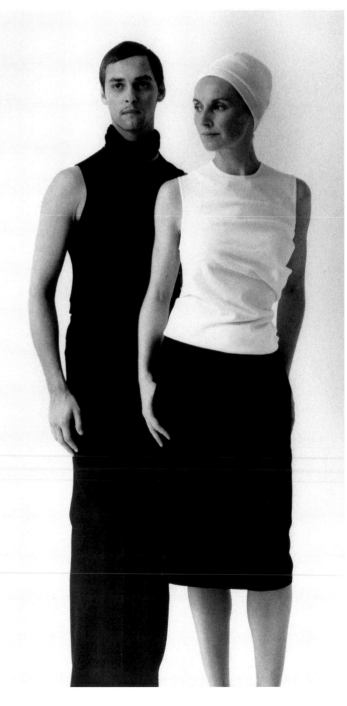

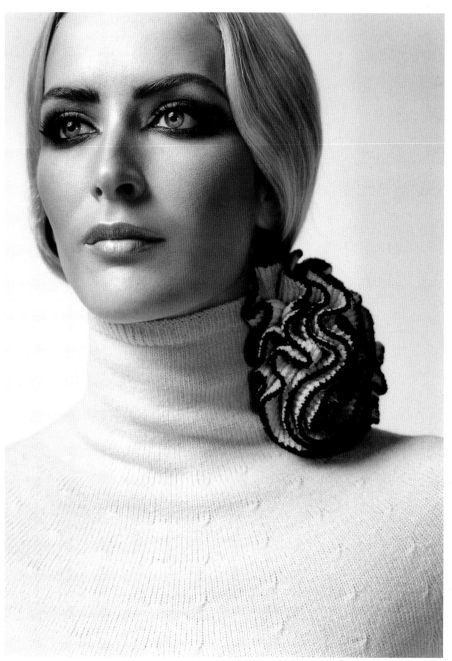

Opposite left and right Testu, spring/summer 2002. Taking a philosophical stance based on a reading of Roland Barthes and the comparability of masculine and feminine clothes, Testu seeks to provide clothing which is gender-neutral but will adapt to either male or female form. The knitwear aspect is based on draping, achieved through a two-dimensional geometry which extends and displaces necklines and armholes as if the body has bent sideways and the clothes carry a memory of the movements. The knitwear is made from viscose with 25% Elité elastane and is side-seamless, forming draped folds on one side of the body. Knitwear items in the collection include sleeveless and long-sleeved sweaters, tops and tubes which can be worn around the neck as collars or around the body.

Below Testu, sleeveless top, illustrating the distorted shape used in the knitwear.

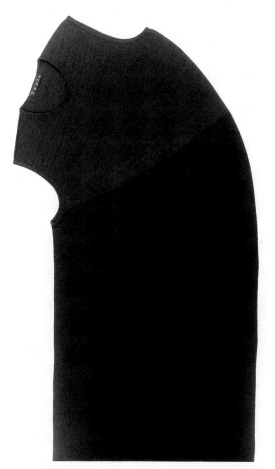

Above Lawrence Steele, autumn/winter 2000/01. The seamless sweater and sweater dress were one of the knitwear looks in this collection, creating a clean and sophisticated, body-hugging silhouette. Steele was one of the first to adopt this technology for designer fashion. The top yoke of the sweater is fashioned by internal wale shaping to give a smooth and three-dimensional shape, ending in an integrally knitted funnel collar. Note the knitted rosette corsage.

Opposite Freddie Robins, installation, Colchester, UK, 2000: 'Headroom', with 'Noway' and 'Headcase' in background. The play on the familiar, both visually and in words, is at the heart of Robins's current work. Her mutant bodies, sweaters and gloves comment on ability and disability. A combination of freak show and genetic engineering, they are at once humorous and disturbing. Utilizing the construction of knitted garments to great effect and taking it to illogical conclusions to create thought-provoking and unwearable pieces, Robins simultaneously puts knitted textiles into a new arena.

Since the Surrealists first adopted fashion as a powerful tool for the communication of their extraordinary concepts, fashion has continued to interpret Surrealism, and now appears within the context of art with increasing frequency. Elsa Schiaparelli believed that 'dress design ... is not a profession but an art', and made the first notable example of knitwear crossing into art with her 1928 trompe l'oeil hand-knitted sweaters. One, adopting the Surrealists' favourite visual trickery, was designed to resemble a tied bow. In the years since Schiaparelli, a number of artists and designers have been engaged in the creation of art objects that involve or interpret clothing, and sculptural or conceptual fashion that can transcend functional clothing to be viewed as art. Issey Miyake has been especially instrumental in bringing experimental textiles and clothing – a significant proportion knitted – into the art gallery and museum, setting standards that few others have met for the presentation of clothing and the body, and moving easily between the worlds of fashion, popular culture and art.

In recent years, the use of clothing – particularly the disembodied form of the dress – as a medium of expression in contemporary art has become a somewhat commonplace but powerful element within artistic vocabulary. Inspired by established artists such as Caroline Broadhead and Annette Messager, practitioners of both art and fashion have increasingly employed the dress, the corset and the shirt to explore the relationship between the body and its adornment and enclosure, the boundary between inner and outer worlds, themes of absence and presence, and temporal and corporeal ephemerality. The neutrality of colour and simplicity of material usually adopted by artists serve to emphasize impermanence and inspire contemplation.

Given impetus originally by the feminist movement, female artists began to address issues of gendered perception associated with textiles and crafts, as noted in Rozsika Parker's book *The Subversive Stitch*. Knitting typifies this perception, with its strong associations of the feminine and the domestic.

German artist Rosemarie Trockel brought knitting into the art gallery with industrially produced knitted 'pictures' and clothing such as balaclavas, leggings, dresses and sweaters, displaying repeating motifs and political logos – the Playboy bunny, the Woolmark, the hammer and sickle, and the swastika. The production of these items, using computer-controlled industrial knitting technology, was in itself a commentary on the familiar associations of knitting as a domestic activity. The shock of exhibiting knitted pictures and knitted clothing in 1986 has been compared in its impact to the Warhol multiples and Pop art of two decades earlier. By the act of being knitted, the logos became stripped of their political status. One art critic of the time was in no

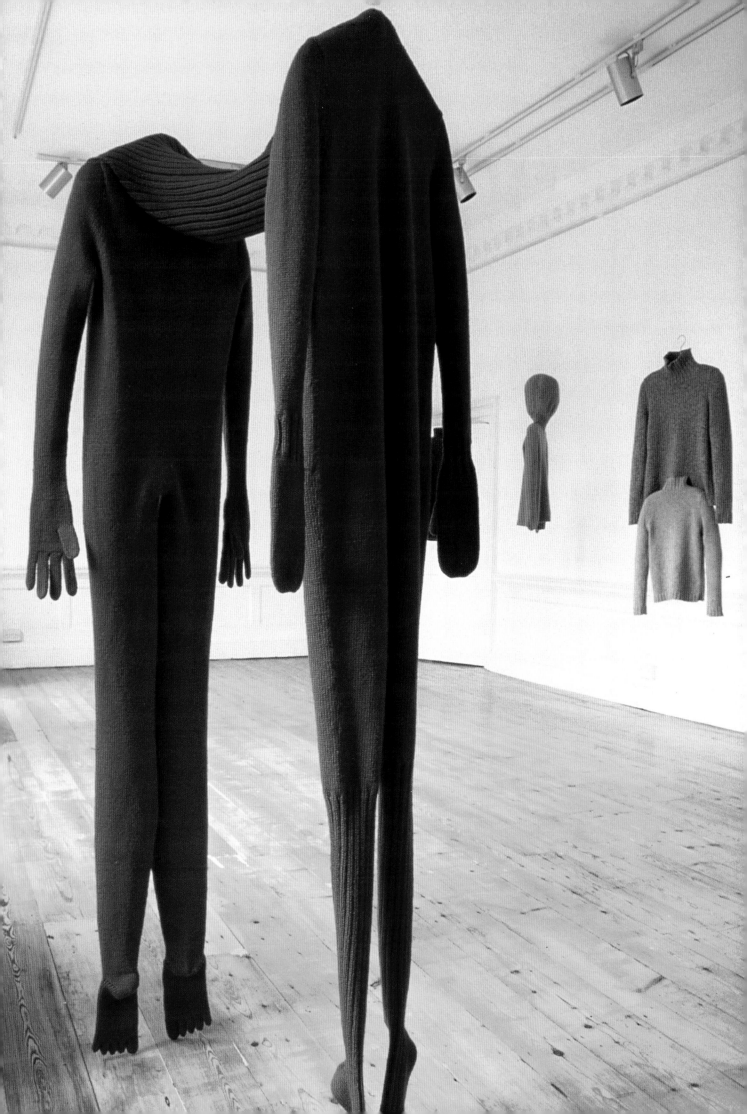

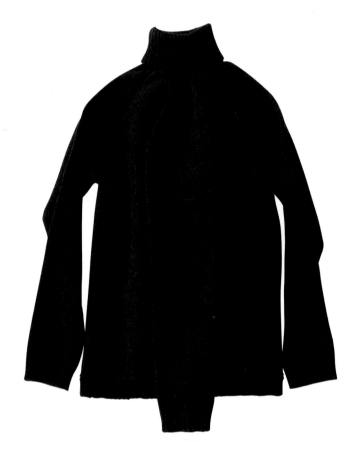

doubt that the act of knitting was inherently feminine. In his piece 'From Icon to Logo' in the *Rosemarie Trockel* catalogue (1988), Peter Weibel wrote: 'As Rosemarie Trockel introduces this artistically inferior material and this aesthetically inferior art form, we become aware of the extent to which the feminine is excluded from culture. For wool as a material, knitting as a method, and knitted motifs as a thema are signifiers of the feminine. If these signifiers are seen as culturally inferior, then the feminine itself must be seen as inferior too.'

In a diverse and evolving body of work, Trockel returns regularly to the medium of knitted textiles, creating new forms which utilize the improving technology – for example, knitted mobiles of circular construction – but also focusing on evocative painted and printed images of knitting.

The crossover between art and fashion, from the direction of the fashion designer, has gained momentum in recent years, with the acceptance of more conceptual design – the work of Rei Kawakubo, Junya Watanabe, Hussein Chalayan and Helen Storey being important examples – although the commercial context of the work varies greatly. Several new artists, including Freddie Robins and Emily Bates, have started out from a textiles and fashion design training. Mutant clothing is a recurring theme. Both Rosemarie Trockel and Freddie Robins arrived at disturbing distortions of the sweater form, but from totally different starting points – Trockel from a highly theorized and varied artistic practice across many media, and Robins from the practice and knowledge of knitting as medium of construction and from the process of knitwear design. Robins creates each of her pieces personally, Trockel hands over the manufacturing process to a third party, yet the meanings are equally powerful.

The basic structure of hand-knitting is immediately recognizable and evocative, keying into personal memories of childhood experiments and mothers and grandmothers knitting at home, creating clothes out of necessity perhaps but also intertwining their knitting with love. Hand-knitting is a metaphor for familiarity, comfort, protection and innocence – or perhaps a tangled web of constraint – all of which are rich sources of implicit meaning for an artwork which uses the knitted structure as a fundamental element. For the general public, knitting still means hand-knitting, with its large, familiar, identifiable loops and uneven texture. The smoothness of machine-knitting is also familiar from domestic knitting machines, but as the scale of industrial knitting diminishes and becomes so fine that we cannot so easily distinguish the knitted loop structure, the associations are broken: jersey knitted fabric, for example, is just fabric and ceases to conjure up the emotional dimension.

If the choice of knitting as a technique gives immediate results, then the choice of materials determines how the structure can be manipulated and formed in three dimensions. Knitting is an ideal sculptural medium. Freddie Robins enjoys the physicality of the knitting process and the mathematical challenge it presents – creating

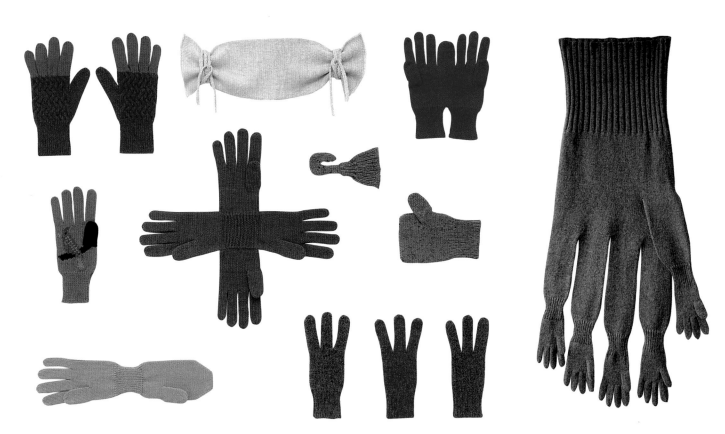

Opposite Freddie Robins, 'Fourway', 1997. One of Robins's earliest mutant sweaters, 'Fourway' has four sleeves evenly spaced around the body. In all Robins's knitworks, the plausibility of the familiar knitwear construction at first takes in the viewer, who then begins to question the image portrayed. In the same series are 'Noway', a sweater with completely enclosed head, and 'Headcase', two sweaters umbilically joined together (see p. 133). Humour and fear of deformity merge in the work.

Above left Freddie Robins, 'Hands of Hoxton' (one of two sets), 1999. Within this piece gloves are used to represent the hand – a universal symbol that transcends age, race, class and culture. The knitted glove is a very ordinary object, here representing the extraordinary lives and stories of the people of Shoreditch in London. For example, the pair of gloves which connect like a book represent children's writer Kate Greenaway, and the four-handed gloves represent Hindu goddess of wealth and good fortune Lakshmi.

Above right Freddie Robins, 'Hand of Good, Hand of God', 1997. An extremely large glove mutates into further gloves at its fingertips, setting up questions of relativity and the place of the individual, whilst amusing with its irony and technical expertise.

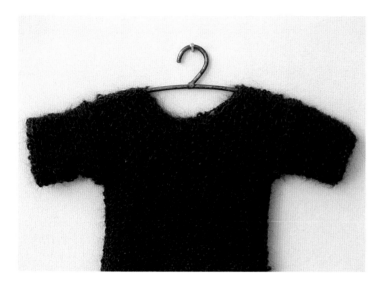

the unfamiliar with a familiar and comfortable medium. Materials which have rigidity such as wire and plastics immediately set up a contradiction: the viewer associates softness and comfort and a certain naïveté with the medium of knitting. Machiko Agano has, however, discovered that it is not necessary to 'use natural material to express natural feelings' in her work with steel wire, whilst Nora Fok exploits the plasticity of knitted nylon when heated to create her intricately formed sculptural body works.

In Japan the tradition of textile art is highly developed, stemming from the skills and processes of weaving and dyeing associated with the making of highly decorated kimonos, and the ancient craft skills of tying, knotting, binding, folding and manipulating that have been applied to sculptural artworks in a range of materials. There is less attention to metaphor and conceptual meaning than is found in European textile art. A simpler, more direct truth to materials can be observed and a sensibility which explores the relationship between the artwork and the surrounding space much as interior and exterior merge in traditional houses of natural materials and no permanent walls. The elements and changing seasons often recur as important influences, and work is created both on macro and micro scales. However, a different sensibility more directly related to fashion and the body can be seen in the work of Suzumi Noda, who, in 'Word Work', has created installations which investigate the materials that wrap and shield the body, and the labels that create the exterior of a product. Clothes and furniture are knitted from strips of printed cloth containing the repeated exhortations of advertising, which become like incantations.

Knitting is associated with useful and practical items and its use outside these norms still has the power to surprise and create visual displacement – a dislocation which can be harnessed for a range of purposes in conveying personal commentaries. The discovery of the versatility, potential and accessibility of knitting will continue to lead to surprising and intriguing results in the hands of a wide range of artists and practitioners.

Right Emily Bates, 'Three Dresses, Blonde, Brunette, Redhead', 1994. 'Growing, styling, dyeing, curling, shorning. Sorting, carding, spinning, knitting.' Bates describes the stages in the making of her impossible dresses. Created from knitted human hair, these dresses simultaneously attract and repulse. The juxtaposition of two evocative elements – material and process – has resulted in a powerful and haunting work (we are reminded of the tale of Rapunzel). The importance of both hair and clothing in expressing our identity has been intertwined; knitted together in a seemingly endless labour of love to create a childlike vision – an idea of a dress.

Opposite Emily Bates, close-up of a knitted human hair dress, handspun and knitted by the artist.

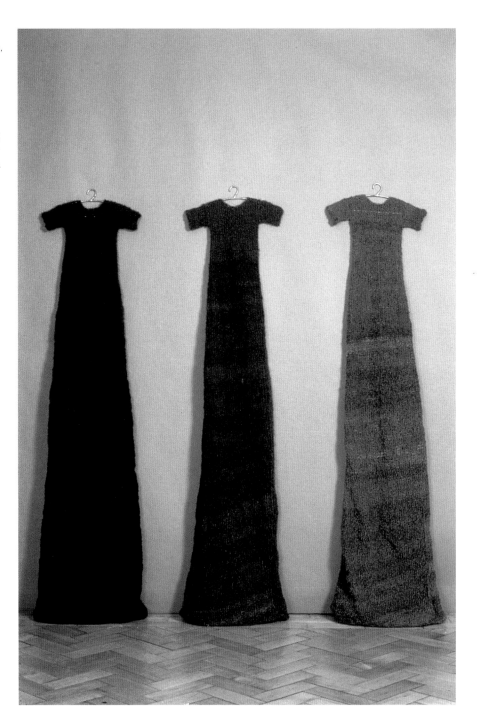

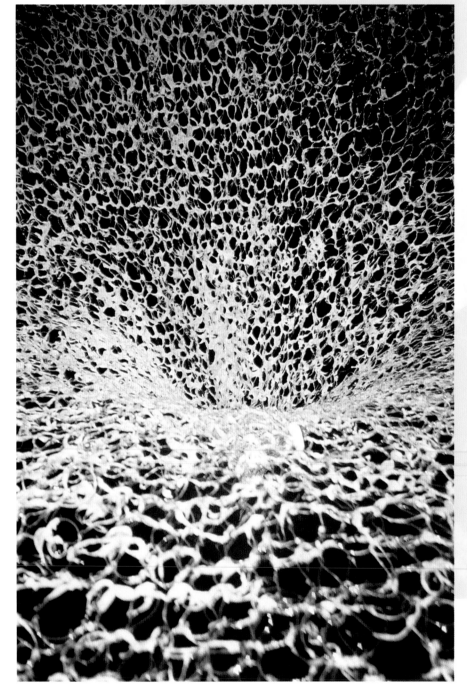

Left Machiko Agano, knitted installation, Brighton, UK, 2001.
A widely exhibited textile artist of international standing, Agano
has recently turned to the technique of hand-knitted construction
using wire combined with yarns such as Lurex and monofilament
nylon. These works are made as site-specific installations and
involve many metres of knitting. Suspension points are formed
through the application of paper pulp, which dries to form a fixed
point. The pieces can be experienced as walk-in environments
and, when illuminated, create a breathtaking visual experience.

Background and opposite Heather Belcher, wall panels, 2000.
Belcher's distinctive artworks play upon the notion of the empty
garment (dress, jacket, cardigan) and the absence of body, within
which a number of resonances can be interpreted – memory,
place, identity... The two pieces illustrated – 'Button Up'
(background) and 'Under My Skin' (opposite) – are constructed
from knitted garments and rolled felt, evoking favourite but
overwashed clothes. Similar works in hand-rolled felt have
been sold and exhibited worldwide.

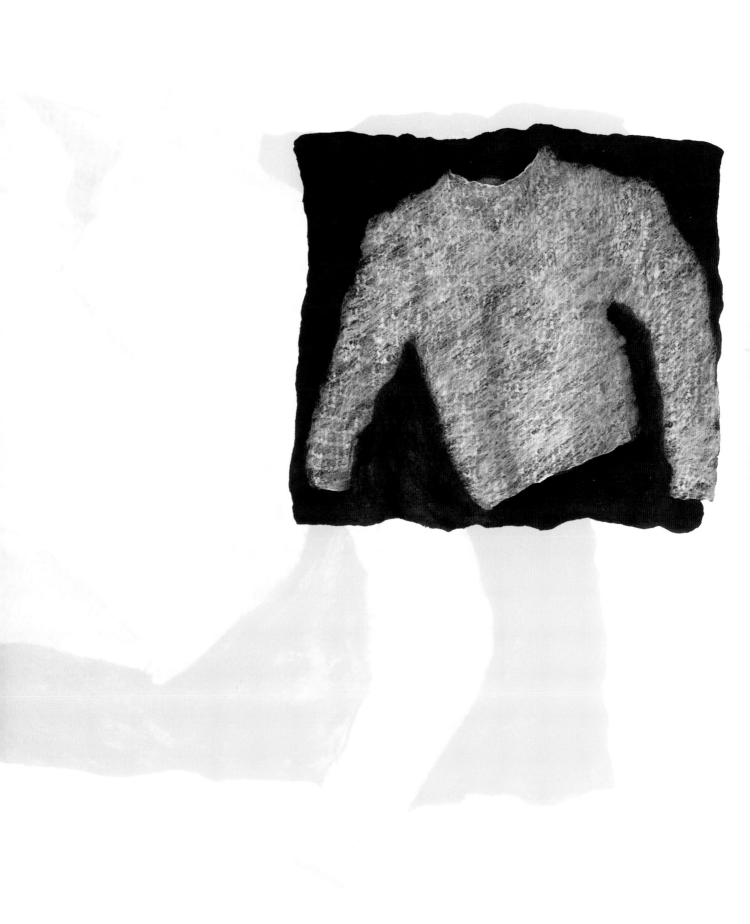

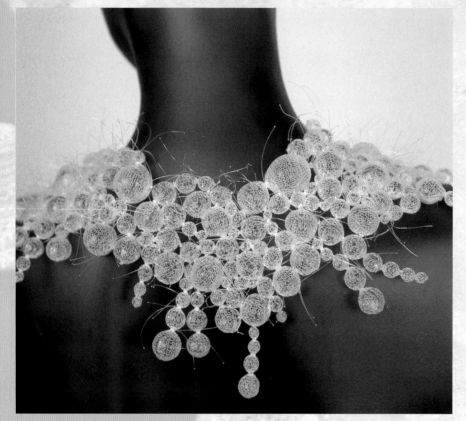

Left and background Nora Fok, 'Bubbles' series, 2001. Inspired by the natural world in both domestic and cosmic spheres, Nora Fok hand-knits, crochets and knots transparent nylon monofilament yarn, which she dyes and heat-forms to create often ethereal body-pieces and idiosyncratic jewelry. Their relationship with the body can be surprising, and many of the sculptural, organic forms are brought to life through movement. The works in the 'Bubbles' series comprise pieces which relate to several parts of the body. Here one work is worn as a neckpiece (left) and another as an amulet for the ankles (background), like stepping into a bubble bath. Each 'bubble' is painstakingly knitted by hand, then heat-moulded around a suitable form, such as a marble, and finally the individual 'bubbles' are tied together.

Opposite Nora Fok, 'Next Generation' neckpiece of knitted, heat-formed and pigmented nylon monofilament, 1996/97. This neckpiece, evoking future beings, is part of a series of body-related works, exhibited under the title 'Galaxies'. Fok's works seem to exist in their own unique universe.

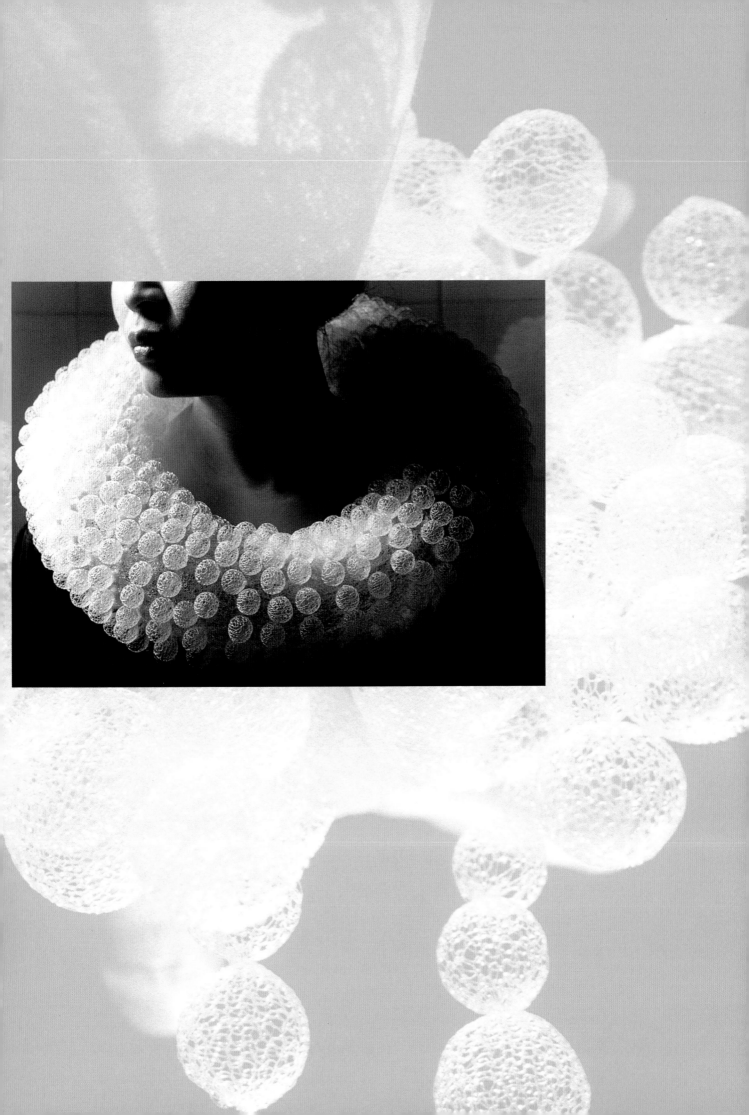

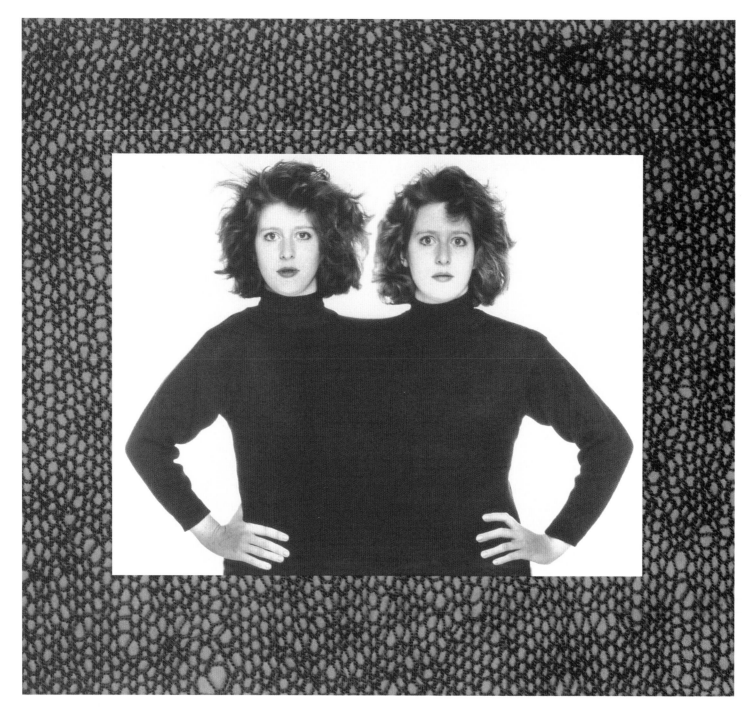

Above Rosemarie Trockel, 'Schizo-Pullover', 1988. One of
Trockel's earlier woolworks, the pullover with two holes for the
head used the sweater form as an absurd but powerful social
commentary. This photomontage shows the sweater worn by
two Esther Schippers.

Background Rosemarie Trockel, 'Untitled (brown)', 1995. A later
series of works focused on the image of knitted fabric in close-up,
either screenprinted on plexiglass (as here) or painted directly
on paper. Slashed knitted 'pictures' reference the work of Lucia
Fontana, and question both the nature of art and the picture itself.
A slashed sweater, 'Lisa', 1993, appears moth-eaten and can be
compared to the deconstructionism in fashion at the time.

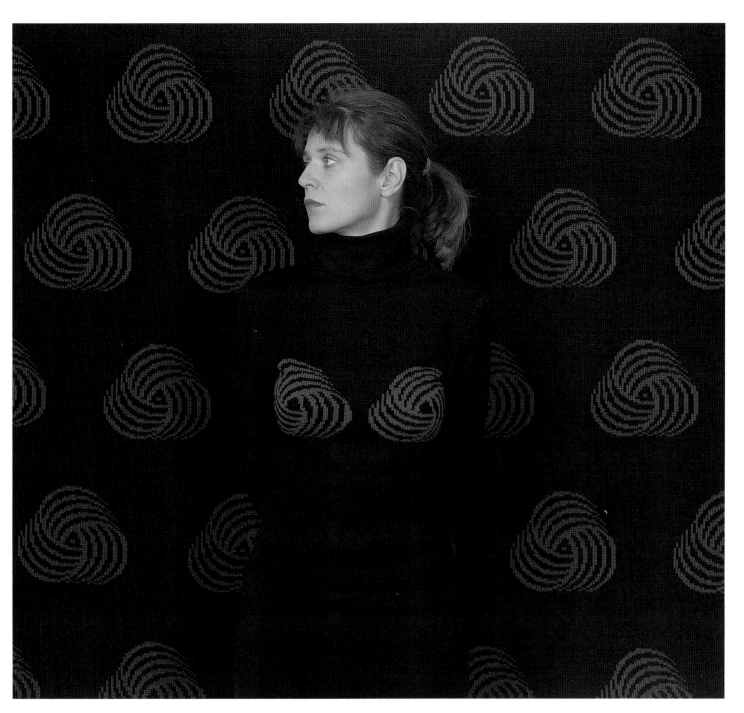

Above Rosemarie Trockel, Monika Sprüth in 'Dress', 1986, in front of 'Untitled', 1986. Trockel's knitted logo 'pictures' set up a contradiction between knitting as an 'embarrassing' (in art terms) handicraft medium and the use of mass-production techniques to create a unique piece of art. Trockel wished to test whether a typically feminine and domestic activity could be classed as art and not as 'women's art', whilst simultaneously challenging the idea of the painted picture.

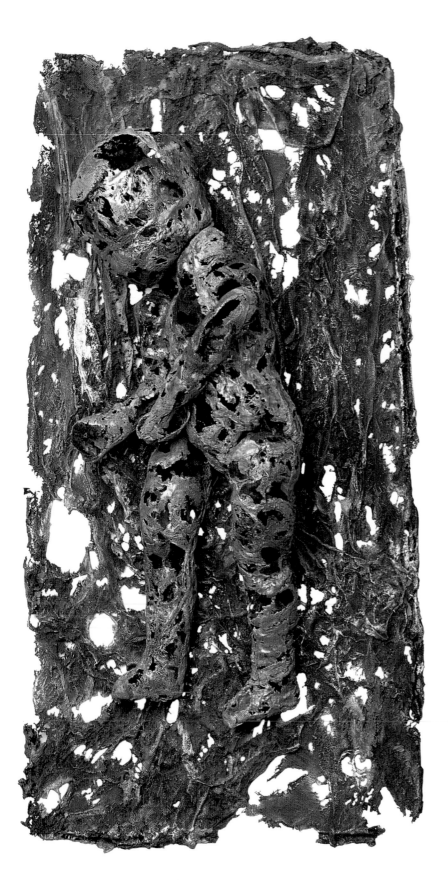

Left Frances Geesin, 'Passage' from 'Revelation' exhibition, 1997. This work is inspired by a found porcelain doll. Combining science and art, Geesin creates three-dimensional forms from manipulated knitted nylon yarn. Her pieces are heat-formed, then metallized in a process of electro-deposition. Representing decay, neglect and patination over time, the beauty of the destroyed surface and surroundings of the doll (one of a series of five) can evoke deep emotions and powerful memories.

Below Frances Geesin, 'Wrapped Stone', 1995. The rigid metallized knitting wraps the space formerly occupied by the stone. Geesin's unique moulding and forming process is like drawing with heat. The multiple hues of the metallic surface have been achieved by a series of patinations with different metals.

Opposite Frances Geesin, 'Zinc Hands', 2000. The theme of the hand – symbolic of making things and interacting with the world – recurs throughout Geesin's work. She likes to create 'pieces people can daydream on'. Her metallizing process has transformative powers, making even mundane objects appear precious.

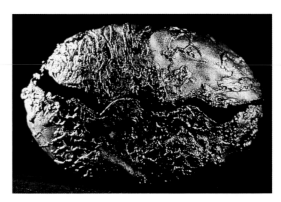

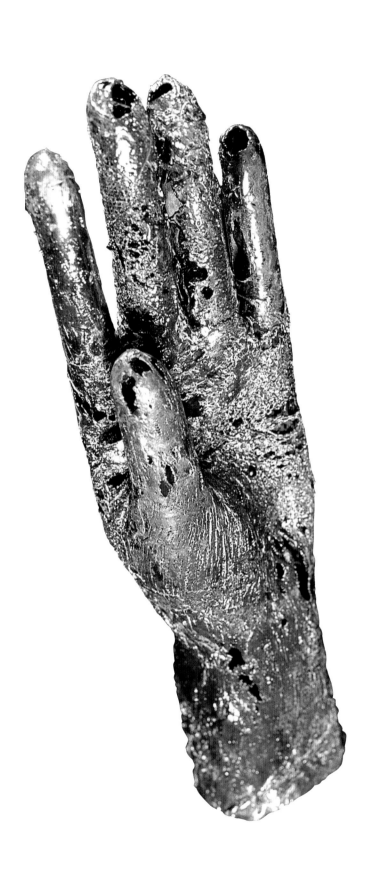
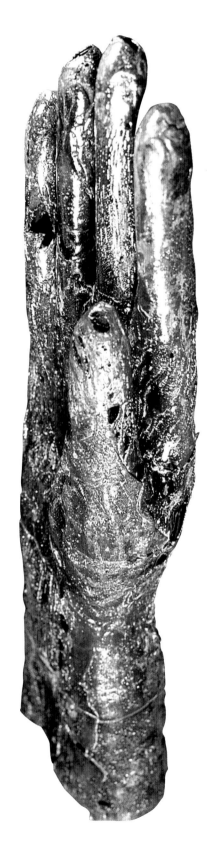

Opposite left, centre and right Mair Joint, 1996. These sculptural pieces, which utilize double-bed knitted fabric in nylon monofilament, viscose and cotton, are given form by metal rods and coloured paper inserted during the knitting. The attitude of the work is exuberant and anthropomorphic. It has been designed in relation to the body with the potential for performance pieces. The medium of knitting is here used for its visual and malleable qualities, rather than in any metaphorical sense.

Background opposite Jan Truman, 'Spiral Gemini Series 1', 2001. Truman has, over recent years, developed her beaded wire knitting technique to create large aerial sculptures for indoor and outdoor use. All are articulated to enable free movement and play with reflection of light. The piece shown is knitted in black and red wire, with rigid steel outer wires and a hand-blown glass droplet.

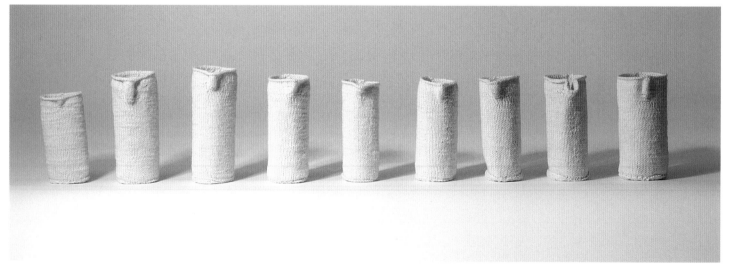

Above Marie Lenclos, 'Knitted Jugs', 2001. Reflecting on the roles of motherhood and women artists, Lenclos explored the use of domestic needlework – sewing, embroidery, knitting – in contemporary art practice, from Louise Bourgeois and Rosemarie Trockel to Tracey Emin. First compelled to knit by imminent motherhood, Lenclos produced her hand-knitted jugs piece as the ironic product of much labour, but without the useful function normally attributed to knitting.

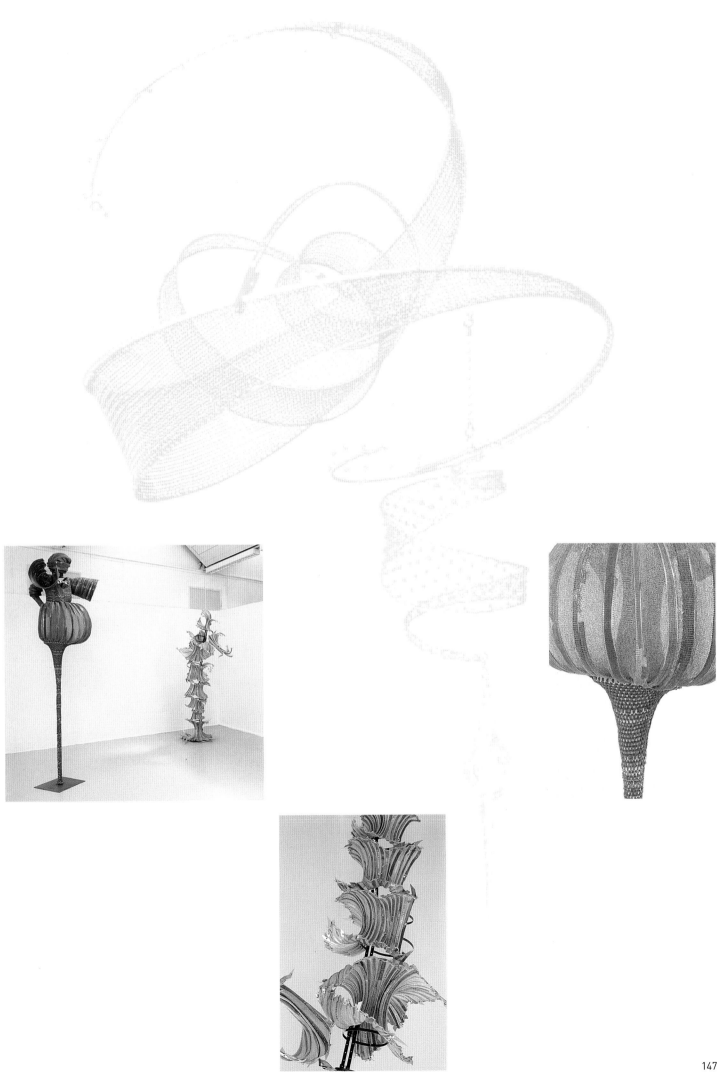

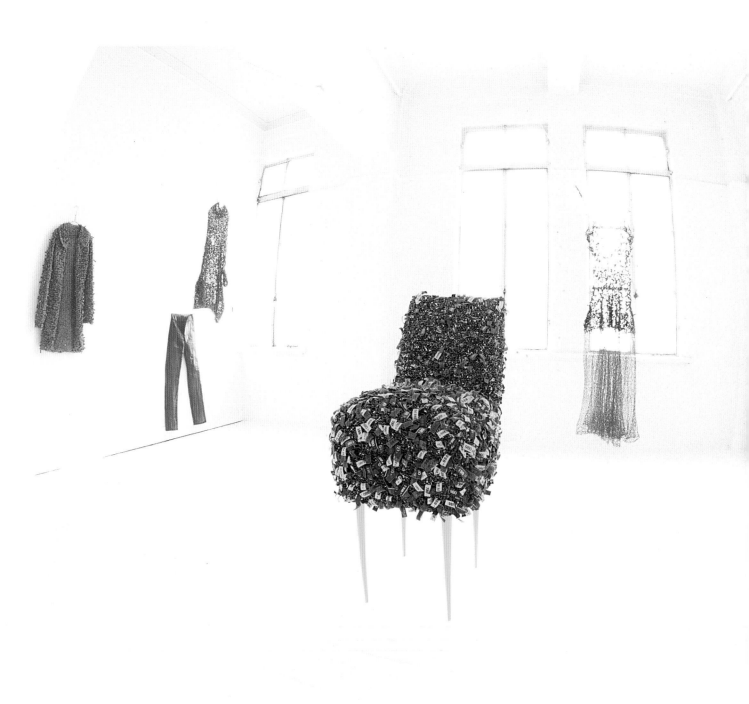

Above Suzumi Noda, 'Word Work', 2000. Working with both clothing and interior design, Noda creates installations in which the viewer often interacts by wearing the clothes and performing in videos. In this series, handbills, clothes labels and packaging were reprinted onto cotton fabric and cut into strips, then hand-knitted into clothes and furniture. Noda seeks to question unthinking responses to the exhortations of advertising, and highlights the consumption of packaging rather than content. 'Cute-Pretty-Diet-Low Calorie; Natural-Secure-Safe-Healthy': according to Noda, the words themselves possess value as commodities. When repeated, they become meaningless mantras. She asks, 'If you wear the clothes knitted with the words, can I free you from the spell?' She also uses names to reflect the origins of her pieces, such as 'Strawberry Milk Coat' and 'Muscle Pants'.

Opposite Suzumi Noda, 'Chair 1980 Yen', 1998. This piece is a commentary on Japanese consumer society on the verge of collapse. Price tags are exposed on the surface of the chair. Hand-knitting is both effective and achievable with minimal tools, whilst highlighting the inherent absurdity of the concept.

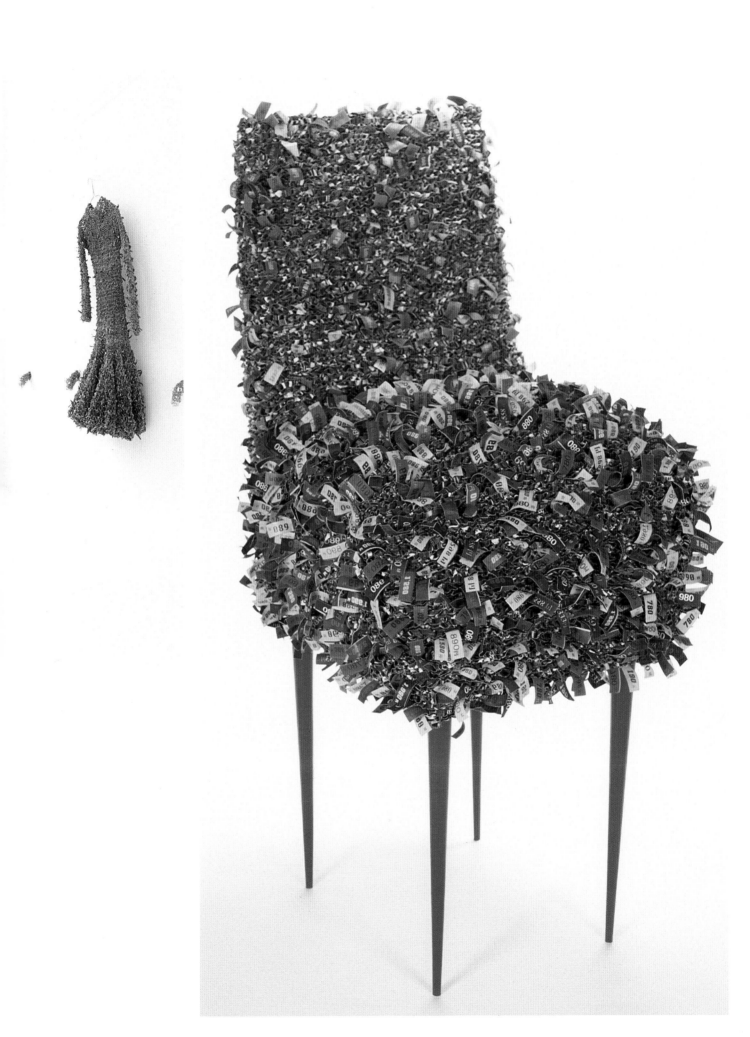

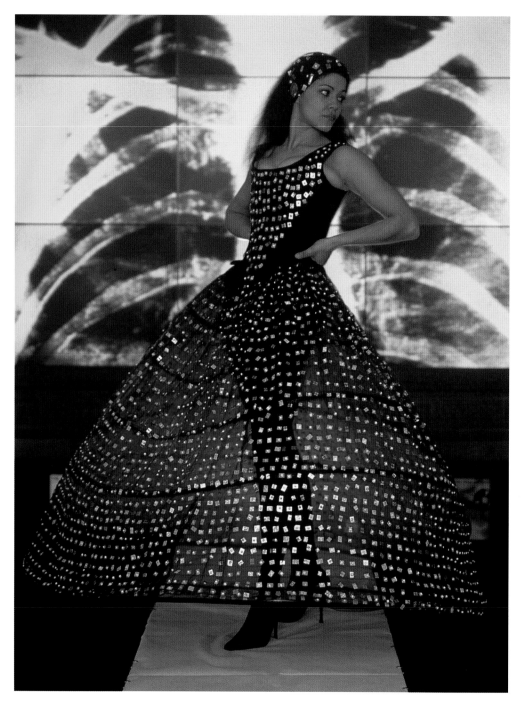

Above Susie Freeman, 'Come Dancing', 1998. The 'Pharmacopoeia' series is a collaboration between knitter Susie Freeman and doctor Liz Lee. Their new 'medico-political art' highlights issues in medicine and comments on medication and treatments, especially from a female perspective. In this ballgown, the first piece in the series, instigated by the Wellcome Trust Sci-Art initiative, the knitted pockets contain 6,550 contraceptive pills, vividly illustrating a lifetime's dependency on drugs.

Background Susie Freeman, 'OTC', 1999. Pocket-knitted veil, containing an assortment of over-the-counter-pills. The attractiveness of the fabric belies its message.

Opposite Susie Freeman, 'A Packet a Week', 1999. This pocket-knitted dress, containing 840 cigarette ends (twenty a week for nine months) worn by a pregnant woman, delivers its medical warning very clearly.

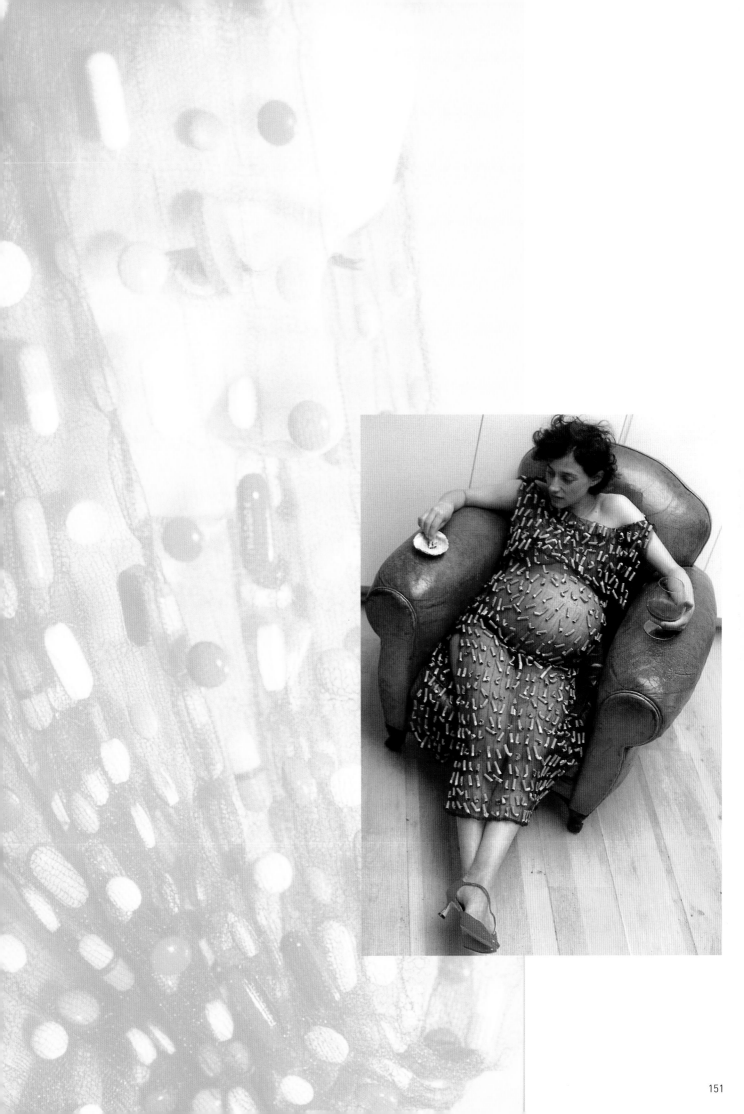

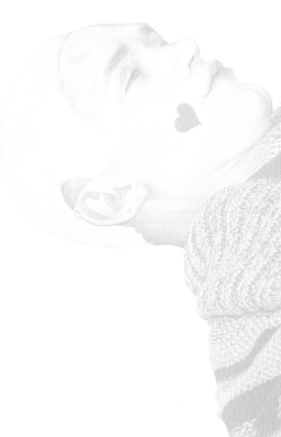

Background Body Map, 1986. Ballet dancer and friend of designers Stevie Stewart and David Holah, Michael Clark performs for the audience on the catwalk of the Body Map winter 1986 fashion show. The 1980s saw great crossovers between the music, popular culture and fashion scenes in London.

Performance fabrics and fibres, designed to enhance functionality in demanding physical circumstances, have become an accepted element of textile and fashion design with the rise of sportswear-inspired clothing. Fine knitted jersey fabrics play a significant part, having been given impetus by the fitness and exercise boom of the 1980s, which created a demand for sleek, body-conscious clothing. The widespread introduction of elastomeric fibres into knitted fabrics created unprecedented stretch and fit in knitwear, and Lycra became a household brand name. Leotards and knitted leggings crossed over from dancewear into fashion during this period, and crossovers were also evident in the opposite direction. Innovative dancer Michael Clark broke away from traditional ballet to form his own company, presenting contemporary ideas and music. In the early 1980s he collaborated with fashion designers and stylists Leigh Bowery and Body Map, who transferred their provocative styling to the stage – outfits which often highlighted the sexuality of the performers in designs with cutouts to reveal the dancer's buttocks or breasts. These designers were also an influential part of the development of club culture, which provided an alternative platform for stylish, body-revealing and glamorous self-promotion through fashion.

Practicality and ease of movement are paramount conditions for dance performance and the use of high-stretch knitted jersey has become a given in the design of costumes. Performers in the musical *Cats*, for instance, started off with handmade knitted outfits but these proved to be impractically heavy and were soon replaced by lightweight printed jersey fabric. Rosemary Moore's groundbreaking Maxxam ruched knitted fabric with Lycra was used in ballet, television and stage productions, and later in swimwear and 'disco' fashions.

The theatricality of catwalk performances, especially in couture and designer collections, has a close affinity with the stage, and it is not surprising that fashion designers have frequently been invited to collaborate in costume design for dance, theatre and film. Chanel was a pioneer with fashionable knitwear designs for the Diaghilev ballet *Le Train Bleu* in 1924. Fashion ideas which are deemed too extreme for public taste can find their expressive niche in a theatrical context. Rei Kawakubo's notorious 'bumps' collection was interpreted in collaboration with the Merce Cunningham dance company in the 1997 production *Scenario*. Jean Paul Gaultier's work with Madonna and the film-maker Pedro Almodóvar is well known; in 1987 he also worked with Régine Chopinot and Courtaulds in the production *Le Défilé*, featuring his signature aran knits. In 1999 Yohji Yamamoto created designs for the twenty-fifth anniversary of Pina Bausch's dance company. Issey Miyake has used dance performers to model his clothes and has created 'Pleats'

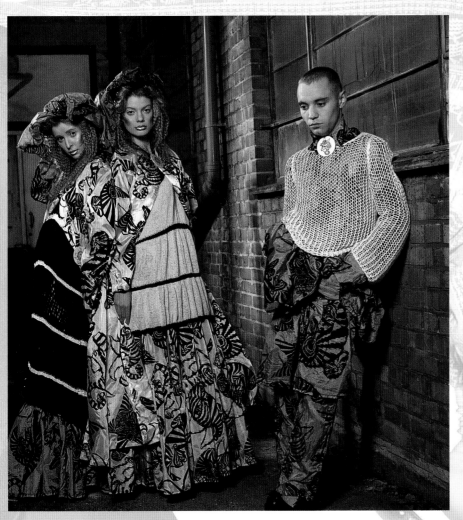

Left Body Map, promotional photograh, 'Comet' collection, spring/summer 1986. Theatre and performance were an integral part of Body Map's presentation. In the early 1980s styling was a growing aspect of fashion in new magazines, such as *i-D* and *The Face*, and photo shoots were staged rather than naturalistic.

Below Michael Clark, 'Mmm...', 1992; stretch jersey fabric bodysuit by Leigh Bowery. During the 1980s the costumes for Clark's ballets were designed by Leigh Bowery and Body Map. Recent new productions have revived the work of the 1980s and have included costumes designed by Stevie Stewart.

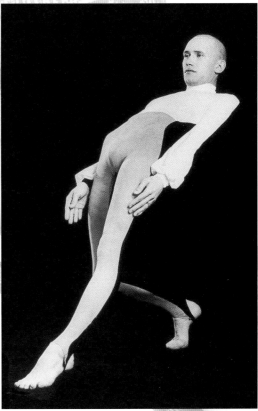

Background and below right 'The Edge of Silence', Birmingham Royal Ballet, mid-1990s; costumes designed by Nadine Bayliss and made by Trevor Collins. Collins specializes in the interpretation and creation of one-off knitted costumes for ballet and theatre. Knitted fabrics are versatile and lend themselves to fantasy and the realization of individual designs, which can be knitted to fit specific body shapes. Here viscose single-bed fabric is inlaid with coloured and textured yarns, lending movement across the dancers' bodies. Techniques include intarsia and tuck stitch, and Lycra yarn is incorporated. Knitted fabric is highly suitable for dance, its fluidity, drape and stretch allowing ease of movement.

Opposite 'Falls Like Rain', London Contemporary Dance Theatre, 1993; costumes designed by Clare Sherliker and made by Trevor Collins. For an acrobatic production requiring the dancers to perform on aerial wires, the costumes had to accommodate a harness. Pleats and patterns were used to disguise the nuts and bolts.

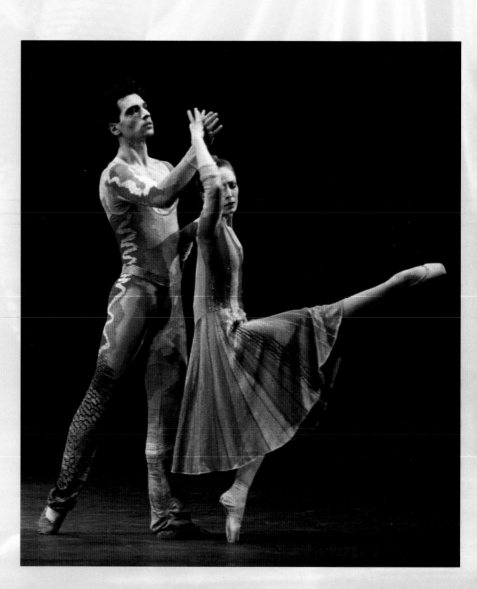

costumes for the Frankfurt Ballet. Sonia Rykiel and Nicole Farhi
have both designed for the stage. Azzedine Alaïa designed costumes
for the actress Arletty and a version of his famous 'bandage' dress for
the dancer Carolyn Carlssen; he has also designed stage costumes
for Tina Turner and Grace Jones.

The malleability of knitting and the immediacy of manual
experimentation lend themselves to the creation of individual pieces
and small production runs. Theatre, television and film costumes are
made by small ateliers working with simple but versatile machinery.
Familiar theatrical artifices such as 'chain mail' and 'fur' – as used
for Jim Henson's 'Muppets' – are often created from knitted fabrics
by makers such as Val Jones, Trevor Collins and Gina Pinnick.

Sweaters feature in a variety of ways in the work of Erwin Wurm,
an Austrian artist who uses installation, video and momentary illusions
in his 'one minute sculptures'. Isolating our everyday experiences, such
as putting on a sweater, he enlarges them to the point of incongruity.
One installation, 'Right Wrong', resulted from a mistake in dressing and
consisted of a series of sweaters on the floor with precise instructions
as to how to put them on, upside down, with legs through sleeves. A
series of Polaroid photos became the record of the work, or disappeared
with the participant. Other similar works give instructions on folding
a jacket or nailing a sweater to the wall. The video '13 Pullovers' shows
a man putting on a sweater, then another on top, then another and then
another ... until his size is grotesque and he is unable to wear any more.

Artist Maria Blaisse also creates performance pieces, as well
as accessories and costumes for designers (including Miyake) and
performance artists. Her new work is based on the unique partial
or short row knitting principle, combined with tubular knitting, allowing
the knitting to change direction or an extra volume of fabric to be
introduced wherever required. Hence a tube of knitting can spiral
continuously or, if opened out, can create frills of varying dimensions.
Enclosure or adornment of the body are both possible, enhanced
by the movement of the body wearing the pieces. For Maria Blaisse,
knitted construction has been a revelation which has helped her
to achieve her vision, and may also be a catalyst for the development
of wearable garments which are comfortable, playful and timeless.

As an artist considers making clothes, so, conversely, the
work of fashion designers – Shelley Fox, for example – is increasingly
being shown in art galleries. Imagination and vision, coupled with
an understanding of knit construction, can undoubtedly result in
new forms. Boundaries are blurring as new hybrids are created.

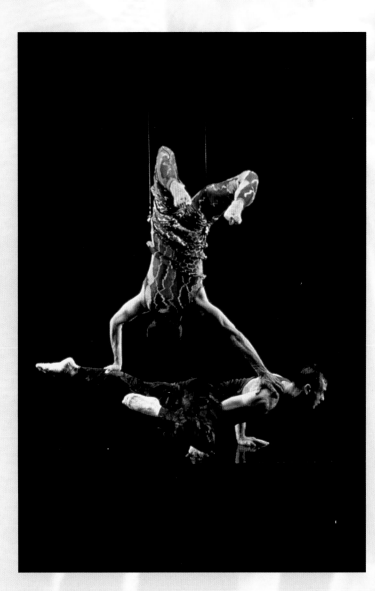

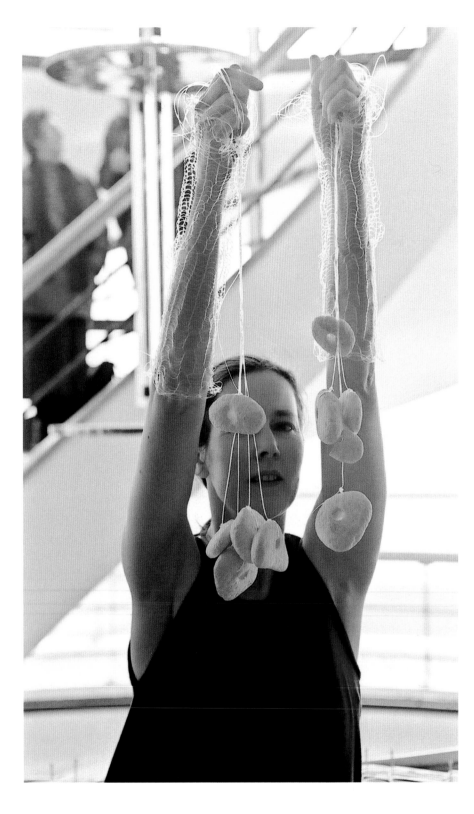

Left, opposite above and below 'Sea Change' performance, 2001. This site-specific piece was developed for the 1930s building, the De La Warr Pavilion, in Sussex, in conjunction with an exhibition, 'Barbara Hepworth and the Sea'. Sculptor Victoria Rance made the enclosure from nylon monofilament, using an enlarged form of circular 'French knitting' (Rance created the large tube of knitting at the start of the performance). The dancer and choreographer, Claire Whistler, wearing knitted armpieces, paid homage to the ocean, then entered the mesh and drew the frame over herself, moving to sounds of songs and the sea. References to the sea and to the feminine – waves, fishing nets, the material of fishing line, tides and cycles – were combined in the textile sculpture and performance.

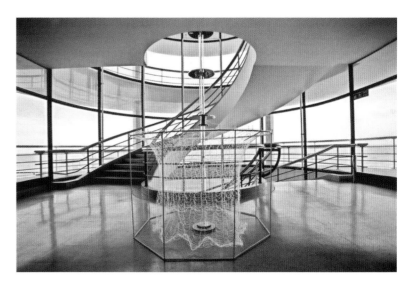

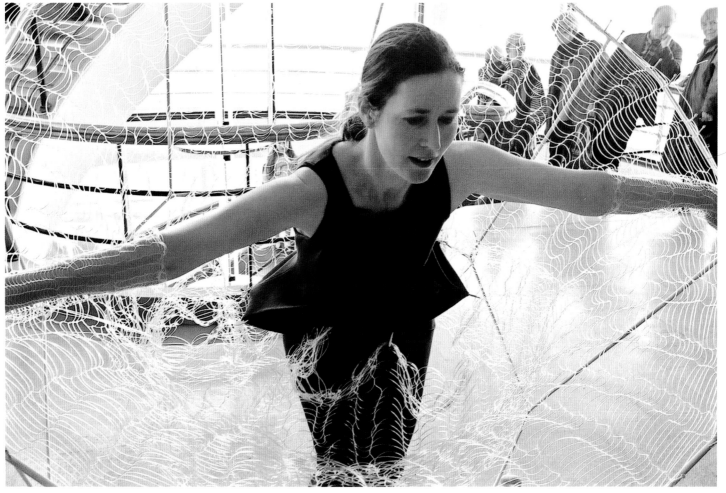

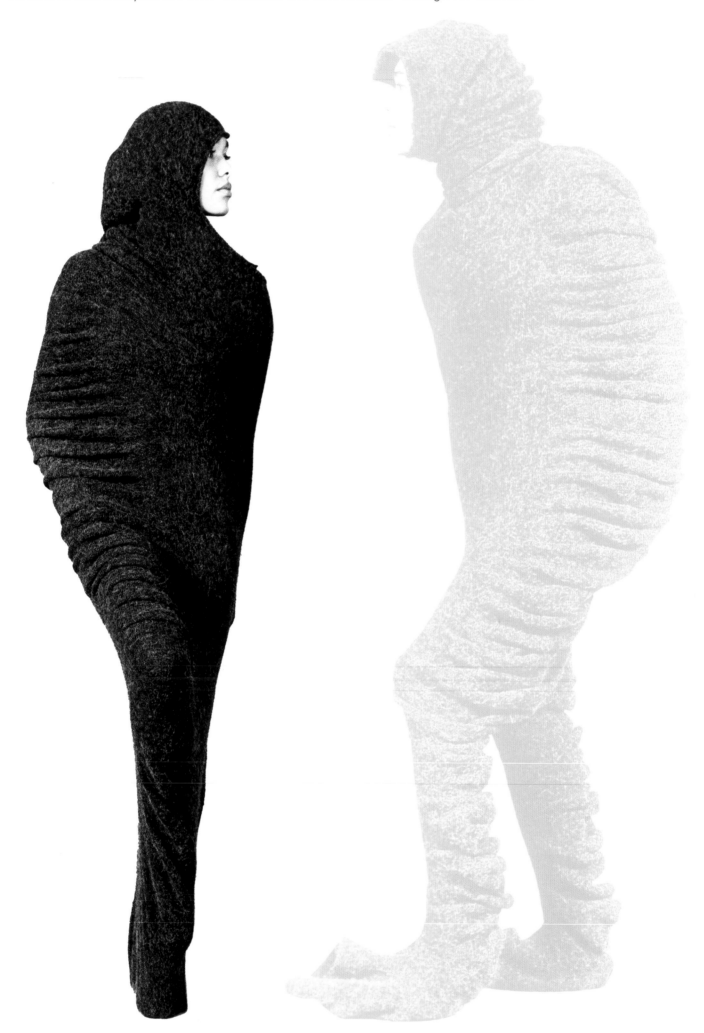

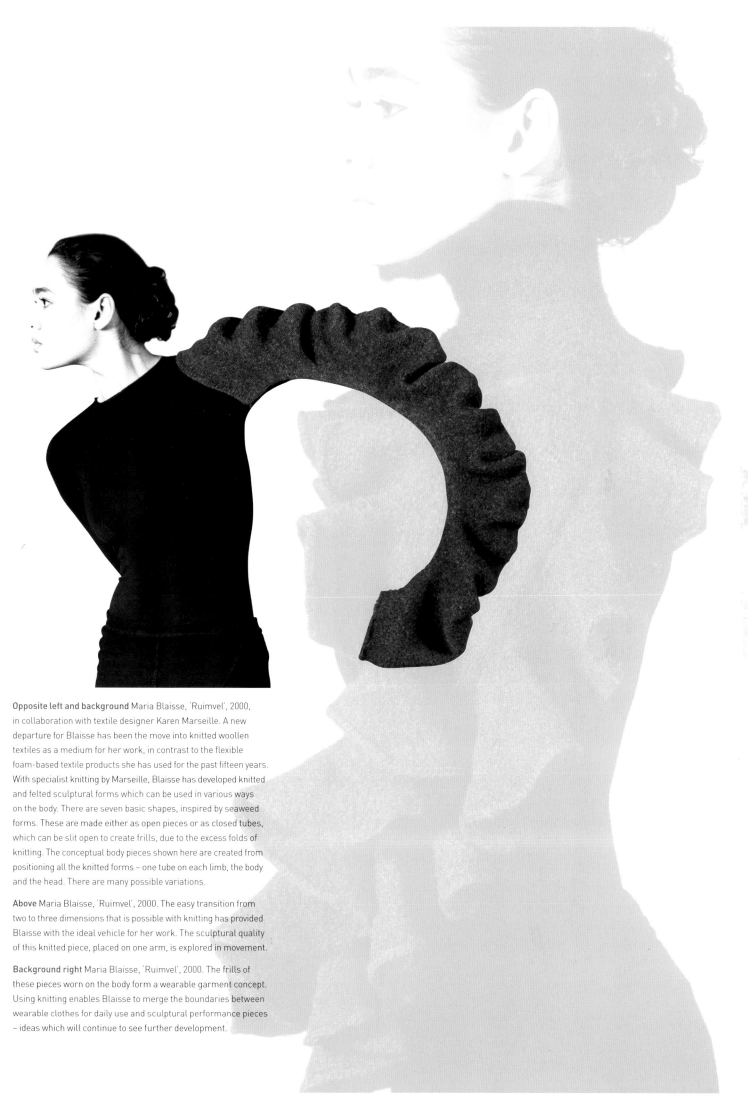

Opposite left and background Maria Blaisse, 'Ruimvel', 2000, in collaboration with textile designer Karen Marseille. A new departure for Blaisse has been the move into knitted woollen textiles as a medium for her work, in contrast to the flexible foam-based textile products she has used for the past fifteen years. With specialist knitting by Marseille, Blaisse has developed knitted and felted sculptural forms which can be used in various ways on the body. There are seven basic shapes, inspired by seaweed forms. These are made either as open pieces or as closed tubes, which can be slit open to create frills, due to the excess folds of knitting. The conceptual body pieces shown here are created from positioning all the knitted forms – one tube on each limb, the body and the head. There are many possible variations.

Above Maria Blaisse, 'Ruimvel', 2000. The easy transition from two to three dimensions that is possible with knitting has provided Blaisse with the ideal vehicle for her work. The sculptural quality of this knitted piece, placed on one arm, is explored in movement.

Background right Maria Blaisse, 'Ruimvel', 2000. The frills of these pieces worn on the body form a wearable garment concept. Using knitting enables Blaisse to merge the boundaries between wearable clothes for daily use and sculptural performance pieces – ideas which will continue to see further development.

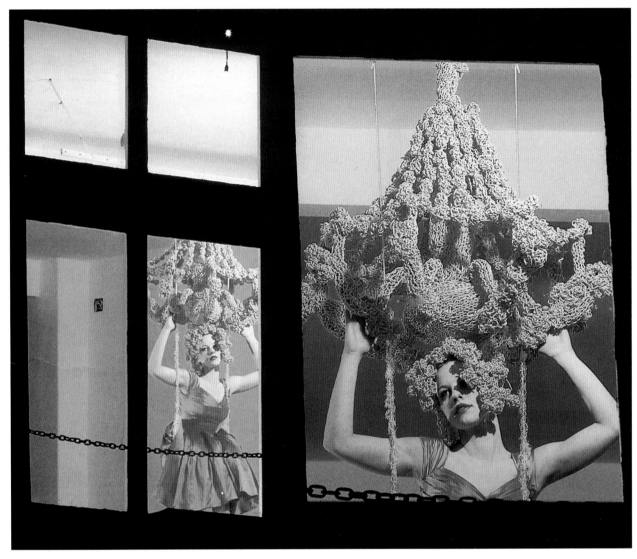

Above Sissi, lampshade installation, 2001. An Italian performance artist, Sissi here becomes an integral part of her knitted sculpture – a chandelier made from flex. In the performance, Sissi draws the piece to her, and herself becomes the last drop of the design – a 'shining pendant of flesh'. The performance took place in the brightly lit window of a gallery in Florence, the artist merging with her creation in a kind of existential ecstasy.

Opposite left Erwin Wurm, 'Right Wrong' from the 'Do It' series, 1998. Instructions to the gallery audience on how to put on a sweater (wrongly) and then pose for a Polaroid picture, to be taken by the gallery keeper. Participants could leave their Polaroid, keep it or send it to Wurm for signature (for a nominal fee). The artwork is the transitory performance of each individual, and the record may or may not be given an art value by the artist's endorsement.

Opposite right Erwin Wurm, '13 Pullovers', 1991. Wurm continually tests the boundaries of sculpture, performance and installation, often through the process of photography or video. By the end of this video performance – seen here at the beginning – the performer's size is grotesque. He becomes an artwork simply through the repeated action of dressing. Other works with pullovers include '59 Positions', in which the audience demonstrates many ways to wear a sweater, and 'The Police Officer's Family Wearing his Jumper' – a photograph of a policeman's wife and daughter in the same sweater.

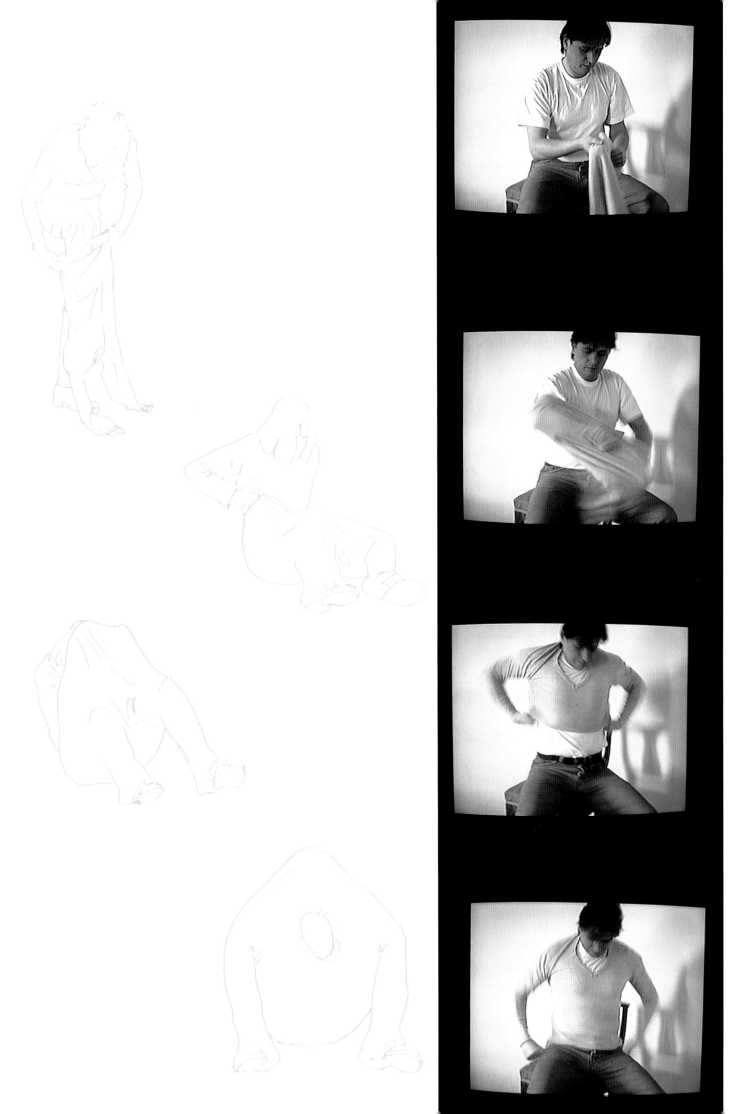

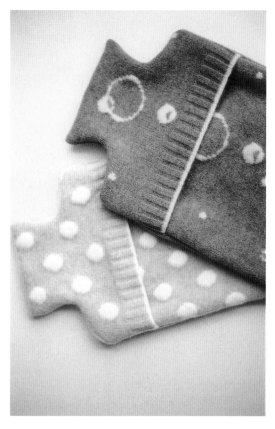

Above Catherine Tough, hot water bottle covers in knitted and felted lambswool, 2000. The old-fashioned hot water bottle has been given a new lease of life in this centrally-heated modern age, as a comforting, back-to-the-nursery accessory for adults and children alike.

Opposite Hikaru Noguchi, in collaboration with Emily Dyson for Couverture, 2001. Throws, cushions and hot water bottle covers in soft wools and optimistic colours help the modern consumer to relax and escape the stressful world outside. The touch of the handcrafted object creates a sense of the personal in an increasingly frenetic and impersonal world.

The soft, cocooning, comfortable characteristics of knitted fabrics have come into their own in the twenty-first-century fashionable interior. As the taste for minimalism and its hard edges and even harder materials has begun to lose absolute sway, colourful materials and fun, offbeat accessories have crept back into the lexicon of interior design style on an international level. From Tokyo and Milan to Paris and London, fashionable interiors – and kitchens, in particular – are home to products with a softer, more childlike and often anthropomorphic feel. Professionals working at home or more flexibly wish to display a more relaxed attitude to the serious and stressful business of everyday life. Advertising campaigns have started to feature cuddly knitted toys (for example Harvey Nichols department store in London and the change of image of a UK digital TV channel). Witness also the revival of the *Clangers* children's series from the 1960s featuring knitted space creatures. When advertising and programming on this scale use this type of quirky imagery it is an indicator of trends coming from the 'cool hunters' who are retained to search out the most unlikely and esoteric ideas by observing young creatives and influential style makers at work and play.

The business of interior design has seen major recent growth and is increasingly aligned with fashion and fashionability. Many international fashion houses have now developed 'lifestyle' interior products for their customers. Old-fashioned knitted bedcovers may survive as heirlooms but in the colour palettes and intensity used by Missoni and other companies in cashmere, 'knitwear' for beds and bedrooms has made a comeback. Cashmere has become a byword for luxury and comfort. Blankets and throws, cushions, pillowcases, bedsocks and wraps all persuade us to stay at home, luxuriate and relax. The bedroom has become the new centre of the home; a sensual haven.

Colette in Paris, situated in the heart of fashionable St Germain, was one of the first 'lifestyle' shops selling fashion and interior products alongside each other in a carefully selected display. The objects one surrounds oneself with in the home – even those hidden from display – have become just as significant as indicators of status and fashion knowledge as designer-label clothes. The influential style magazine *Wallpaper**, founded by Tyler Brûlé (as wallpaper and carpet had long been out of fashion, the title can be seen as ironic), led the way for the integration of fashion and interiors on a popular scale, along with other spin-off magazines aligned to fashion titles such as *Elle Decoration*.

Interior product design, like textiles, jewelry and graphics, is fuelled by a wide range of small businesses creating one-off designs by individual makers. Innovation is the key, and design consultancies have sprung up which create a multi-disciplinary, one-stop

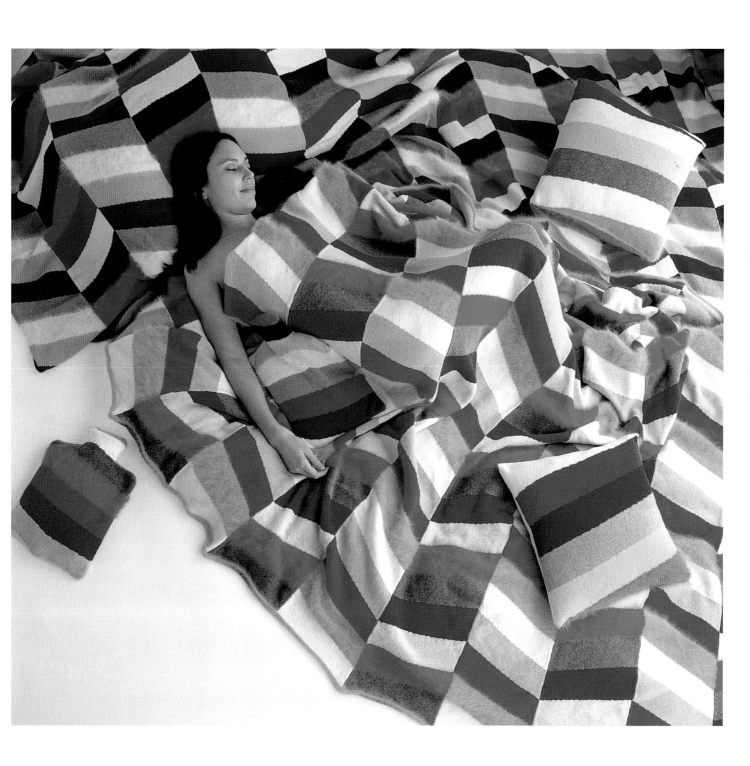

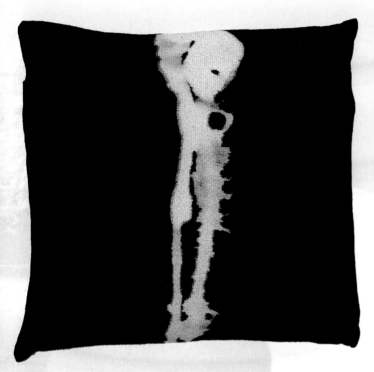

Above Matta, 'Splash' cushion, 2001. Part of a series of designs for interior products which avoid the clichés often applied to design in this area. Matta approach their products with a view to creating individual art-pieces with a raw or random element. Here bleach is splashed over knitted fabric; latex is another alternative.

Background Catherine Tough, sculptured-surface woollen cushions, with raised upholstered cubes or blocks, 2001. The distinctive effect is based on pocket knitting, the pockets being stuffed during the knitting process.

shop for architects and clients who want to generate a creative buzz. Under the umbrella of Droog Design, many young Dutch designers have quickly built a reputation for innovative and witty product design and fashion. Notable in this context are Gijs Bakker's 'Knitted Maria' coffee pot with ceramic crochet cover, Marcel Wanders's knotted carbon and aramid fibre sling chair and Aukje Peters's stockinette-covered, wire-frame laundry basket.

Humour and playfulness are strongly evident in Hikaru Noguchi's exuberant upholstered chairs, cushions and throws. She was one of the first textile-trained designers to apply handmade knitted fabrics to upholstery, working to specific commissions.

Distortions of scale and textural form are fundamental to Catherine Tough's collections of cushions and accessories, hence the giant-stitched knitted cushions made from coarsely twisted wool with their strikingly three-dimensional surfaces.

The openwork structure of knitted fabric, together with the flexibility available in design and construction, is beginning to be exploited in interior furnishings. Karina Thomas and June Swindell's company salt offers a bespoke service in knitted and woven window blinds and screens for modern interiors. Deceptive in their simplicity but mathematically precise in their execution, the screens can provide a textured calm, or a humorous quality when bright colour and hairy yarns are used, or they can give a three-dimensional effect when combined with metal rods.

As other areas of design have been subjected to a softening design influence, so too have light fittings and lamps become a favourite field for reinvention and experimentation with materials. Silicone and unfired ceramics are malleable substances which, with the right formulation, can be manipulated into knitted fabrics and then formed into three-dimensional shapes which diffuse light. The juxtaposition of a soft, domesticated, home-made fabric with the intensity of light and heat creates a strong impact. Stretch fabrics are commonplace in fashion but when used as the basis for lighting are taken out of context and have a striking effect. The lights designed by Christian Dufay utilize stretch jersey fabric to clothe a simple frame, creating characterful objects that reflect a new sense of modernity whilst echoing the optimistic design of the 1950s. As in other fields, the pace of change in interior design is quickening. Interior design style has become a matter of fashion.

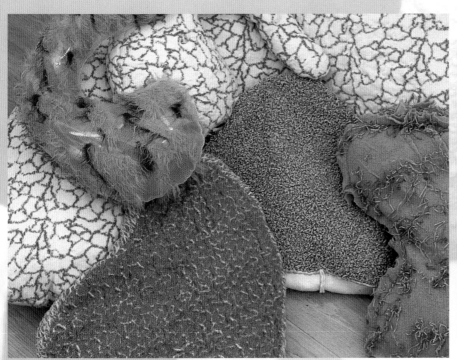

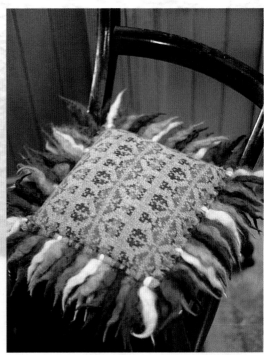

Above left Cristina Brown, textured floor cushions, 1999. Strong tactile qualities and witty organic shapes (banana- or comma-shaped cushions) mark out these prototype designs. The fabrics are knitted from modern synthetic fancy yarns mixed with lambswools that have been felted to give density and enhanced textures. The hairy cushion (top left) is a covered inflatable.

Above right Tait & Style, fringed cushion, 2001. Accessories for fashion and the home give an opportunity for quirky humour and bold statements, creating little conversation pieces. Tait & Style use bold textures mixed with traditional elements from the founder Ingrid Tait's Scottish roots.

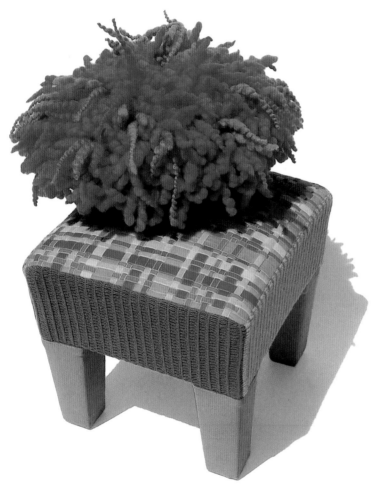

Left Hikaru Noguchi, shaggy cushion and woven ribbon and knitted footstool, 1995. Noguchi started her textile design career in the early 1990s and came to prominence for her original and inventive chairs, sometimes made in collaboration with interior designers. Knitted handmade fabric had not previously been forefronted for upholstery, therefore the furniture has a unique character.

Opposite above Hikaru Noguchi, nursing chair made in wool, cotton and silk, with rippled seat and rolled knitted strips as decoration, 1995. Juxtaposition of colour and texture with quirky detailing is a recognizable Noguchi signature. In addition to various knitted constructions – including jacquards, bobbles and loops – Noguchi also often incorporates silk and velvet ribbons and tassels, giving a sumptuous quality to the pieces.

Opposite below Hikaru Noguchi, deep button chair in wool with jacquard stripe patterns, 1995. Having started making chairs to commission (some for stately homes), Noguchi now produces clothing and accessories, too. Her interiors work has been widely exhibited around the world and her fashion is sold internationally.

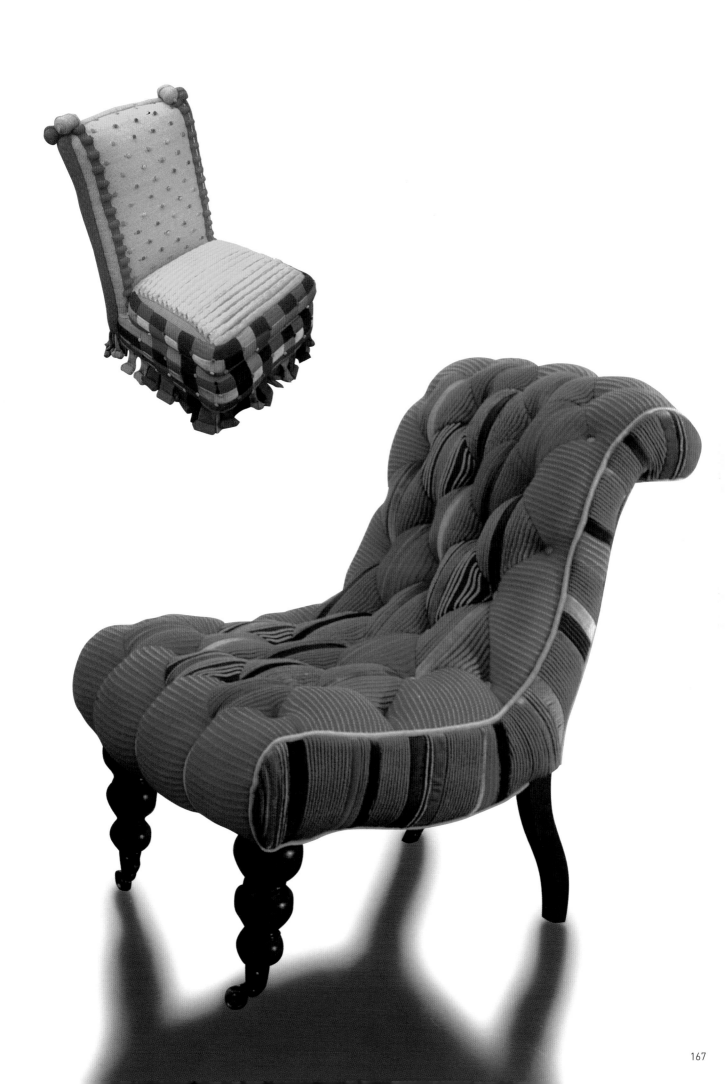

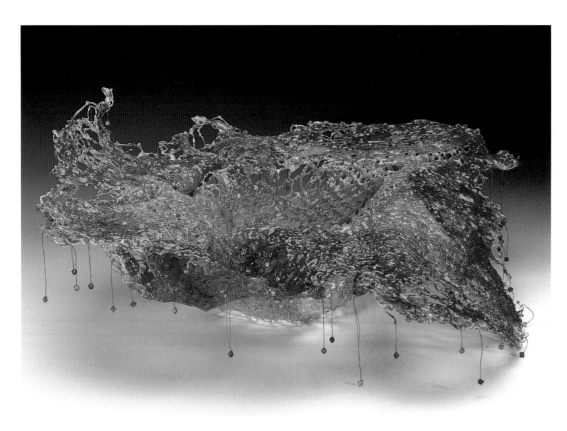

Above Marcia Windebank, knitted bowl, 2000. Windebank
celebrates the visual and chaotic qualities of random lace and
openwork knitting by embedding knitted fabric into resin to form
three-dimensional decorative bowls and two-dimensional panels
(see p. 7). Each bowl is a unique combination of cotton and viscose
yarn, treated with paper pulp, resin and beading.

Right Nichola Gowing, glass plate, 1997. Gowing's experimental approach in mixed media resulted in the embedding of metallic knitting between layers of glass. With its attractive filigree effect, this completely contradicts the usual function of knitting. The transposition from functional use to aesthetic image creates great decorative possibilities.

Below Judit Kárpáti-Rácz, wire bowl, 2001. One of a range of objects and accessories produced by Kárpáti-Rácz using an ancient knotting technique executed with a needle but bearing a strong similarity to modern knitting. The steel wire material takes on a rigid shape after being formed around a block, and is perfectly functional.

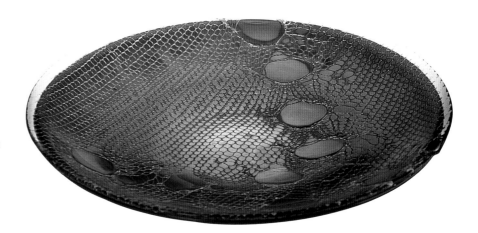

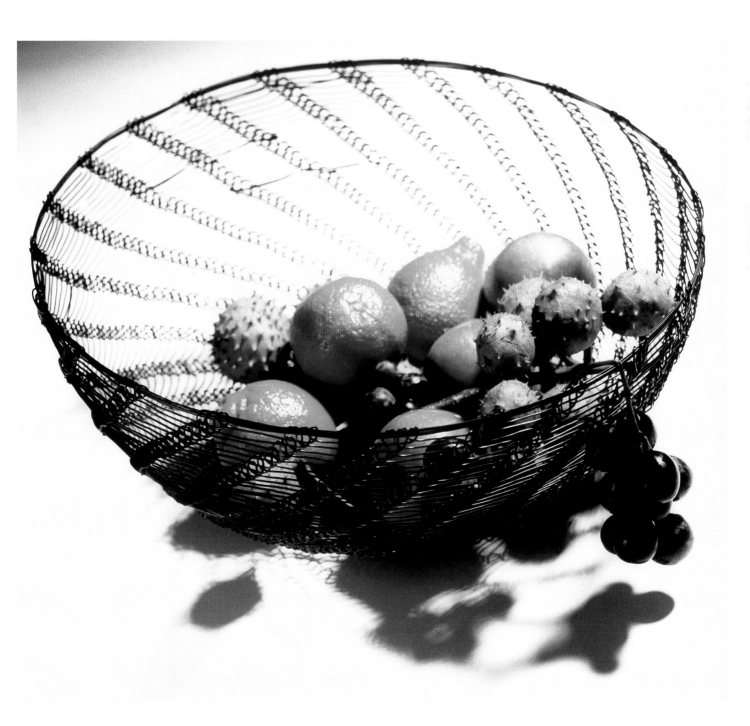

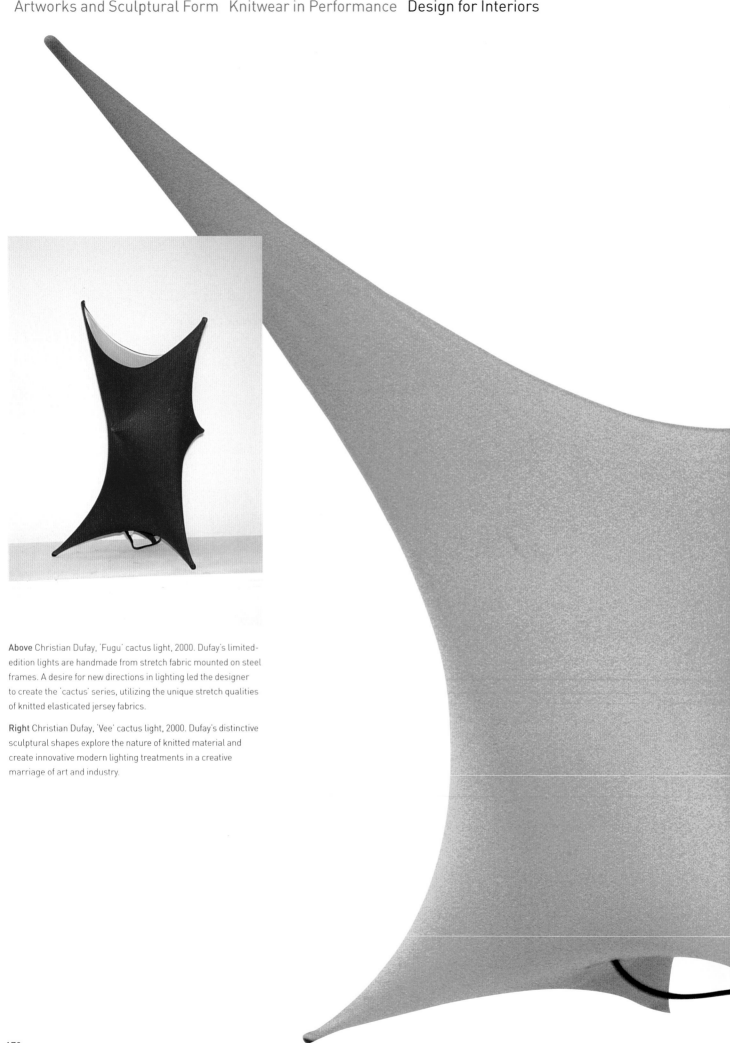

Above Christian Dufay, 'Fugu' cactus light, 2000. Dufay's limited-edition lights are handmade from stretch fabric mounted on steel frames. A desire for new directions in lighting led the designer to create the 'cactus' series, utilizing the unique stretch qualities of knitted elasticated jersey fabrics.

Right Christian Dufay, 'Vee' cactus light, 2000. Dufay's distinctive sculptural shapes explore the nature of knitted material and create innovative modern lighting treatments in a creative marriage of art and industry.

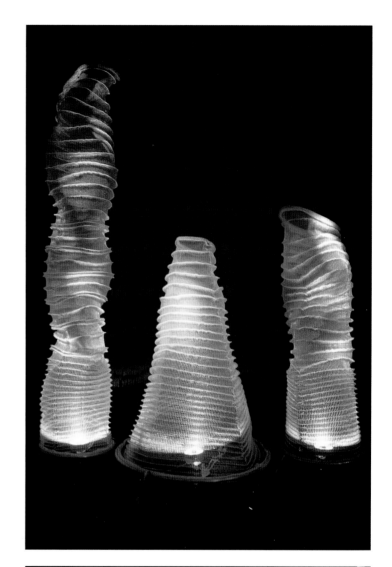

Above right Niki Jones, 'Stalaglights', 1998. These prototype knitted light-cones have been formed seamlessly on the knitting machine by integrating shape and structure. The materials are nylon monofilament and organsin, which has been dip-dyed to impart subtle colour. Experimentation with crossovers between fashion and interiors, and the feel for organic shapes, is continuing to gather momentum.

Right Lisa Gatherar, 'Bag' light, 2001. Exploration of materials, coupled with the simplicity of hand-knitting, led to this intriguing lighting concept. Knitted from silicone 'rope' – an industrial product that can withstand heat – the knitting filters the light inside, creating a subtle glow and a visual paradox.

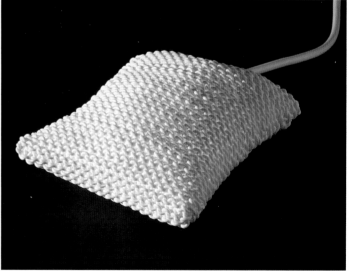

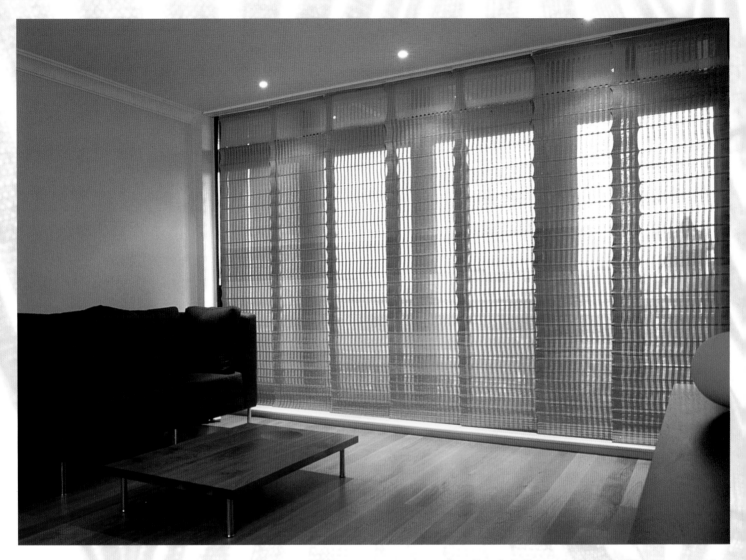

Above Karina Thomas of salt, 'Totem', 2000. This panel-glide blind is made of knitted cotton with a spaced rib structure. salt partners Karina Thomas and June Swindell studied knitted textiles and woven textiles respectively, and create bespoke fabric panels for windows and screens.

Background Karina Thomas of salt, 'Creased Totem', 2000. These cotton rib panels have bent metal rods inserted to create dimension. salt's textile solutions to light-filtering and control are both sculptural and innovative.

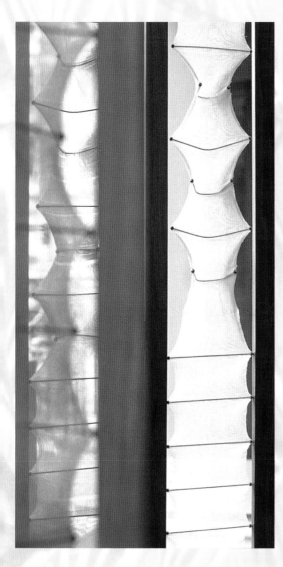

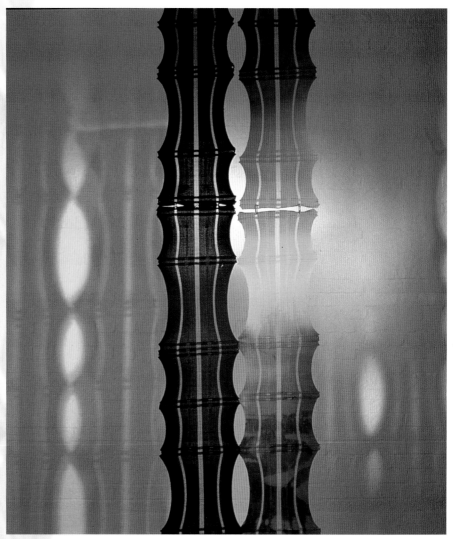

Above left Karina Thomas of salt, detail of knitted screen, 2000. salt's window treatments and screens have a minimal architectural aesthetic: a fusion of design, technology and technique, in tune with contemporary interior spaces. The panels shown here feature metal rods within a wooden frame screen.

Above right Karina Thomas of salt, 'Totem', 2000. These knitted panels can be combined to any width. 'Totem' modular knitted blinds are now available through a commercial collaboration. salt's recent work has included diversification into graded colours and surface textures.

Classes of knitted fabric and machinery

Knitting is formed from the intermeshing of individually made loops to create a fabric. This fabric is made either in tubular or flat form. Uniquely, it can be shaped whilst in construction. Industrial knitting technology can be divided into two main areas – weft knitting, which encompasses circular knitting, and warp knitting. Each has a different principle of construction. The majority of knitted fabrics for clothing are weft-knitted and this is therefore the main focus of this section.

Weft knitting: comprised of loops formed in horizontal 'rows', technically referred to as 'courses', each loop linking to a loop or stitch below and to each side. The vertical lines of stitches are called 'wales'. The knitted loop is symmetrical, side to side and top to bottom. Basic fabric structures – such as plain knitting (stocking stitch) and ribs – are created from one thread. Weft knitting by machine was derived from hand-knitting and the structures are identical. The final courses of loops must be secured by binding off so that the loops do not disconnect from the stitches below, hence unravelling the fabric. A wale of loops which has unravelled is known as a 'ladder' – a term familiar from hosiery.

In hand-knitting, the two fundamental stitches are described as knit and purl, depending on the direction of the loop formation, front to back or back to front. In machine-knitting, the direction of loop formation is fixed, unless the stitch is mechanically transferred from front to back needle bed or vice versa. Weft knitting can be constructed as flat fabric with selvedges, created by knitting to and fro across a fixed number of stitches, or as circular fabric, formed in a continuous spiral. The basic properties of weft-knitted fabrics are extensibility and recovery, which can be accentuated by yarn choice and stitch structure, speed and versatility of production, and the ability to create shaped garment pieces or integral garments knitted and shaped at the same time.

There are three fundamental knitting actions undertaken by all weft-knitting machine needles: a) to knit, i.e. form a new loop and drop the previous loop to form a stitch; b) miss, i.e. hold the previous loop for that course of knitting, making a float appear on the back of the fabric (loops may be held for several courses, creating puckering effects and surface pattern: this action also forms the basis

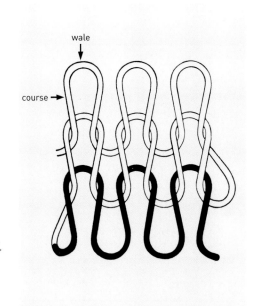

Above Weft knitting

Above Warp knitting

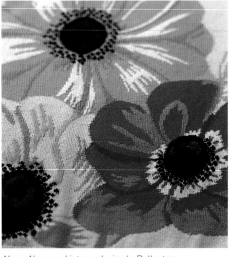

Above Aberangel intarsa design by Ballantyne

of float jacquard colour knitting sequences); c) tuck, i.e. take a new loop up but also hold the previous one, thereby holding two loops on the same needle until a subsequent knitting course (this action produces gathering and spreading of the fabric, but, depending on the gauge, loops may not be able to be built up for many courses).

Flat-bed machines can be fine gauge to heavy gauge (E14 to E3) and knit a wide range of garments, but mainly outerwear.

a) V-bed machines: two parallel needle beds with needles facing in opposite directions, inclined at an angle in inverted V-formation, for rib fabrics and variations. The majority of these machines are now electronically controlled (e.g. Stoll, Shima Seiki and Protti) but some are hand-operated (e.g. Dubied hand flat machines). There are also some domestic hand-operated or motorized versions (e.g. Passap and Pfaff). Many electronic V-bed machines can now knit geometric intarsia patterns (a specialist intarsia V-bed machine has been developed by Zamark).

b) Single-bed: machines with one horizontal needle bed, particularly hand intarsia machines (now almost obsolete) and domestic knitting machines (an additional needle bed can be attached for rib fabrics).

c) Cottons Patent machines: single-bed machines with bearded needles arranged vertically, specially adapted for automatic fully fashioned garment shaping.

d) purl machines, also known as links-links: specialist machines with two needle beds in a horizontal plane which share one set of double-ended latch needles, enabling plain and purl stitches to be created in the same wale and on the same face of the fabric. The needles slide between the two needle beds according to the programme. These machines were created to simulate hand-knitting effects and are slow in operation. They are gradually being replaced by the electronic V-bed machine.

Circular machines produce jersey fabric, normally in fine gauges from E18 to E30.

a) Single jersey: one set of needles arranged vertically around a cylinder (e.g. Bentley), capable of knitting plain fabric and variations such as stripes and tuck-stitch effects. The emphasis is on speed of production, using multiple yarn feeders to create efficiency. The resulting tubular fabric is slit vertically into flat fabric, finished, then used for cut-and-sew knitwear.

b) Double jersey: two sets of needles at 90 degrees, one set aligned vertically – the cylinder needles – and the other radiating horizontally – the dial needles – for double-bed fabric production, particularly jacquard and interlock fabrics, or for specialist production (e.g. Moratronic and Wildt Mellor Bromley). Fabrics are stable and can be used for cut-and-sew outerwear or underwear.

c) Specialist circular machines (e.g. Santoni and Sangiacomo) are used to knit other fabrics, such as fleeces and plush or pile fabrics, or are used in smaller diameter to knit bodysized, seamless garments for swimwear, lingerie and underwear. Small-diameter, specialist, fine-gauge machines are also used for knitting stockings and tights.

Warp knitting: the principal direction of warp knitting is vertical. The fabric comprises wales of loops, each formed from a separate warp thread knitted vertically and interlinked to adjacent or other wale loops by the horizontal movement of the yarn feeders after each knitted course. The feeders underlap or overlap each needle to form the new stitch. If each thread continued to knit only in its own wale, the fabric would be split into separate chain lengths. Each needle has one or more yarn feeders, therefore different colours or textures can be knitted along the length of the fabric, parallel to the selvedge. Reels of warp threads are wound prior to knitting and form a warp beam, similar to woven fabric production. A wide range of fabrics, including mock crochet, and complex lace and embroidery effects can be produced, depending on the knitting sequence and number of warp beams and corresponding feeder guide bars employed. Warp-knitted fabrics are more stable than weft-knitted, and will not ladder or unravel. Fabrics produced by warp knitting are used for household textiles, such as sheets and net curtains; mesh fabrics, including string vests; and clothing, including scarves with integral fringes.

Two principal classes of warp machine are tricot and raschel, although there is now less distinction between the two and many fabrics can be produced on both.

Tricot: previously used bearded needles only, but now a compound needle is more common. Fabric is drawn away horizontally under very little tension, allowing high-speed production and soft-handle fabric to be produced that is suitable,

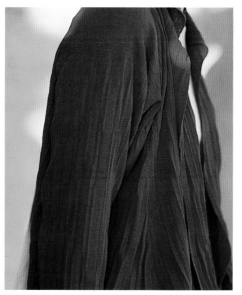

Above Uneven pleated fabric by Jürgen Lehl

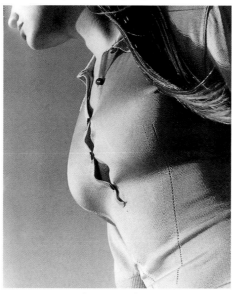

Above Internal dart (wale shaping) by Azzedine Alaïa

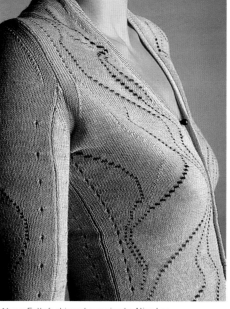

Above Fully fashioned seaming by Alice Lee

for example, for lingerie. The simpler warp structure fabrics are generally produced on tricot machines, requiring only two beams and guide bars.

Raschel: the knitting action, based on the latch needle, is different from that of the tricot machine. The raschel (e.g. Karl Mayer, leading manufacturer of warp machines) allows more versatility and commonly uses twelve beams and guide bars, though there can be up to 36. Fabrics are drawn away vertically under greater tension, allowing complex fabric structures, such as openwork laces, to be produced. The crochet machine is a specialist type of raschel machine. This works on a principle of warp chains linked by a separate weft inlay yarn. It is often used to produce decorative braids.

Developments are taking place in the warp-knitting industry, in particular adaptation to tubular knitting, and investigation of shaping possibilities.

Some types of knitted fabric
This section lists some of the fabrics commonly used in fashion (the majority weft-knitted) and featured in the book, but it is not a comprehensive list of knitted fabric structures (see Further Reading). It is included to facilitate fabric recognition within fashion garments and other end products.

Plain fabric, also known as stocking stitch, single jersey, stockinette: the basic weft-knitted structure is simple to knit by hand or on a single-bed machine, and has good elasticity. The fabric has a natural tendency to curl, the sides towards the back, the top and bottom towards the front. The two sides of the fabric appear different: the technical face appears as knit loops, the technical back as purl loops, though many designers use the back as the right side (see Yohji Yamamoto, p. 101).

Intarsia: plain fabric traditionally knitted manually on a single-bed knitting machine. Blocks of colour are laid over the horizontal needle bed according to a geometric, graphic or pictorial design, built up course by course. The technique is very labour-intensive as each colour is laid across the needles by hand. Each area of colour is worked only within its own boundary and does not cross any other colour area. Adjacent colours are linked together where they join by crossing threads or by knitting a stitch in both colours. The back and the front are almost identical. There is unlimited scope for patterning and intricate imagery using the manual technique, but finishing can be laborious.

Modern V-bed machines now have the facility to create true intarsia patterns using multiple yarn feeders and precision control to position the feeders to knit exactly where required, rather than across the entire needle bed. Geometric patterns such as the classic argyll diamond (called a Ballantyne in Italy) are simplest to knit. Mock intarsia is knitted with floats across the back of the motifs. Intricate patterns are still made by hand in a number of factories to meet a specialist demand.

Purl fabric, also known as links-links fabric: this structure is either hand-knitted or made on special purl machines. It has both knit loops and purl loops on each side of the fabric, both occurring in the same wale. The basic purl fabric (garter stitch in hand-knitting) shows as purl loop courses alternating with knit loop courses, which are slightly hidden. The fabric is the same on both sides, and stable, being particularly extensible in a vertical direction. Many variations of purl fabrics exist, including designs of textural purl stitches on a plain ground, which appear in reverse on the back of the fabric. Tensions within the knitted loops can give unexpected three-dimensional effects in some designs (see Nuala MacCulloch, p. 87).

Rib fabric: comprises knit and purl stitches in the same course, arranged in alternating wales. The basic rib structure – an elastic, stable fabric that appears the same on both sides – is 1 x 1 rib (also known as English rib), consisting of one knit wale and one purl wale alternately. The fabric can be hand-knitted or made on a double-bed (V-bed) knitting machine or double jersey circular machine, with alternating needles selected to knit on each needle bed. Many variations are possible, the most common being 2 x 2 or 2 x 1 ribs. These have great elasticity and are used to give stability to knitwear in the form of welts at the lower edges of classic sweaters or cardigans, or to form entire garments which cling to the body. Many other wide rib variations can be devised, such as 5 x 5 or 3 x 6, with varying elasticity.

Tuck rib fabric, also known as half or full cardigan or fisherman's rib: one of the basic knit structures, this is a simple variation on 1 x 1 or 2 x 2 rib, in which either one needle bed (half cardigan) or both needle beds alternately (full cardigan) form tuck stitches. Half cardigan looks different on each side; full cardigan looks the same. The ribs are broadened and the fabric is wider than conventional rib. Cardigan stitch is often used for heavy knitwear.

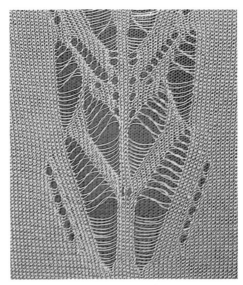

Above Stitch transfer lace by Marina Spadafora

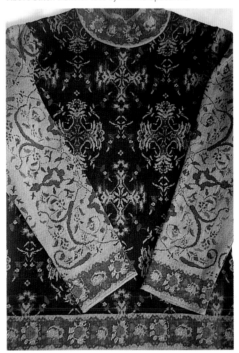

Above Four-colour jacquard by Kenzo

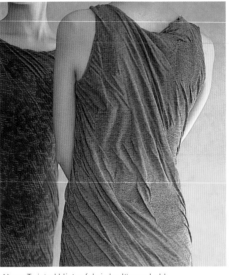

Above Twisted blister fabric by Jürgen Lehl

Pleated fabric: particular arrangements of needles can create clear pleated effects, particularly effective in fine natural wool or cotton yarns knitted in 1 x 1 rib structure, with single needles left out of knitting action on alternate needle beds at regular intervals. The removal of a needle creates a 'bend' in the fabric along the wale which has been removed.

Edge shaping and wale shaping: narrowing or widening of the fabric can be achieved at the edges or – on modern industrial machines (or by hand) – within the width of the knitted fabric piece. On the machine, to narrow the width of fabric, loops are transferred from one wale to an adjacent wale (creating one double loop and an empty needle) over a predetermined sequence, reducing the total number of wales in the fabric width. At the edge this creates shape but within the fabric it creates an internal dart and interesting visual effects where stitches have been moved and others fill their place. The effects are accentuated in rib-structured fabrics. Loops can be transferred for decorative effect without reducing the overall fabric width, giving rise to contour lines of wales which follow the fabric movement. If loops are transferred outwards onto an empty needle at the edge, this will have the effect of widening the fabric as the empty needle is knitted. Where edges are shaped by a movement of a constant group of two or three wales to widen or narrow the fabric, this is known as 'fully fashioning'.

Cable stitch fabric and 'aran' fabrics: traditionally made by hand-knitting, these three-dimensional effects can be produced on V-bed machines, with the cabled face loop wales being formed on one needle bed and the backing loops on the other. The cable cord is formed of two or three wales which twist around each other, achieved by physically changing the place of the two sets of stitches. On modern machines this is facilitated by additional transfer points to hold the loops (see Jean Paul Gaultier, pp. 17, 42). Similar procedures produce honeycomb and other textural stitch effects.

Stitch transfer lace: commonly created on single-bed machines or by hand-knitting on a base of plain fabric. The action of transferring a loop to an adjacent needle leaves an empty needle, which when filled in on the next knitting course creates an eyelet hole which is secure (i.e. it will not ladder). Geometric or more random design effects can be achieved (see John Rocha, p. 47). Shetland lace shawls are fine examples of the hand-knitted version.

Colour effects: the simplest introduction of colour, in any technique, is through striping. Regular stripes in up to four colours pose no problems, whereas irregular stripes or single row stripes create more difficulties in aligning yarn feeders, and are usually avoided in commercial work. Colour can also be introduced by mixing different yarns together to create random marl effects. More systematic colour mixing is produced in machine-knitting by the use of a plating technique in which two different coloured yarns are held consistently in the same relative position to the front or back of the knitted loop. A bi-colour effect is produced dependent on structure: in a plain fabric, the back will appear mainly one colour, the front mainly the other; in rib fabric, when stretched, all the knit loops appear one colour and the purl loops another.

Jacquard fabric: colour patterning in geometric, floral or any other design can be created in jacquard fabrics, using two, three or four colours per course and individual needle selection. It is produced either as single jersey float jacquard, or double-bed or circular rib jacquard. Float jacquard is based on the principle of knit and miss: each colour is knitted according to a needle selection, and the remaining needles miss during that pass of the knitting carriage. During the next pass the second colour is knitted according to its needle selection, and so on. Two-colour jacquard takes two passes of the carriage to build up one knitted course, three-colour takes three passes, etc. The colour pattern is made up of face loops; the reverse of the fabric shows float threads. This limits the extensibility of the fabric.

Rib jacquard is composed of coloured face loops creating the design on one needle bed (or cylinder in circular machines), with the other needle bed forming a knitted backing. In three-colour jacquard with 'striper' backing, the knitting sequence creates six backing rows for two pattern design courses, which can be cumbersome. 'Birdseye' backing is more balanced, knitting alternate needles on each backing row to produce three backing rows for two design courses.

With clever design, jacquard can introduce many colours over the pattern design area (which, with advanced technology, can now extend to the width of the machine) whilst maintaining no more than three or four colours in each design row.

Blister or cloqué fabric: variations on jacquard fabric can result in relief stitch fabrics,

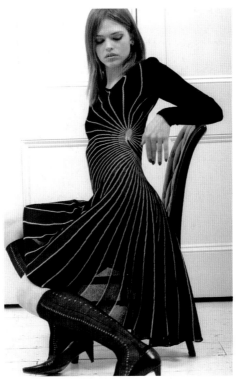

Above Short-row knitting by Alice Lee

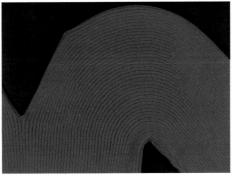

Above Curved rib in short row knitting by Hiroaki Oya

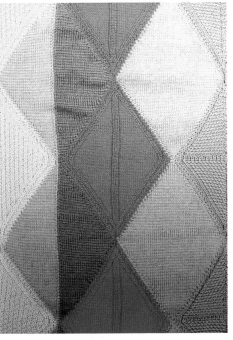

Above Multiple patterning by Comme des Garçons

either in self-colour or in two-colour. A ground yarn knits across both needle beds, then the blister yarn knits a selected pattern on one needle bed only, creating a separation between front and back. This results in more fabric build-up on the surface, giving a raised effect. Further dramatic effects can be created by working a quilt technique, in which groups of adjacent needles are knitted on the face needle bed only, and the fabric is joined only intermittently to the backing fabric (see Susie Freeman pocket fabric, pp. 150-1).

Three-dimensional effects using elastomeric fibres: the use of a stretch fibre under tension can create strongly sculpted surfaces when the fibre relaxes. Such effects are often achieved with jacquard techniques, one of the yarns being elastomeric (see Kate Carrick, p. 82).

Short row knitting, also known as flèchage, partial knitting, course shaping or wedge forming: this machine-knitting technique is usually worked on single jersey fabrics. It is highly versatile and can be applied to create three-dimensional structures, to introduce colour effects, or a combination of the two. It is also the principle under which sock heels and pouches are formed. It may be carried out at one side of a knitted fabric, across the entire width, or in a central section (as for a heel pouch). The number of loops knitted in each course is reduced or extended by regular steps, according to the angle required. When repeated, a spiral fabric formation occurs, from successive 'wedges' forming an angle with previously held courses (see Alice Lee, p. 97). No loops are lost during the process, which can be used to create additional fabric (frills) or to remove excess fabric (darts and spirals). Rib and other double-bed fabrics can be produced in a similar manner, but with greater attention to pressing or weighting the loops. The effect can also be produced in hand-knitting: one example is the entrelac technique, which gives a basketweave look.

Multiple patterning: with computer control and advanced pattern preparation systems, the scope for mixing techniques within one fabric has been exploited in high-level design (production of multiple techniques is slow and hence expensive). Shima Seiki machines first demonstrated this potential. They form the basis of the Australian company Coogi's products (see p. 21). Other multiple techniques, such as intarsia with stitch pattern effects, can be seen in Comme des Garçons menswear, produced on Stoll machinery.

In the post-war years, knitting machine industries built up around the world, in particular in Germany, Italy and Japan, with Germany becoming dominant in warp-knitting. The transition from mechanically controlled machines to electronic control was the defining development of the modern industry. By the 1970s, most circular double jersey machines incorporated electronic patterning systems, linked with a computer-aided-design (CAD) unit. Electronic control, later applied to flat knitting machines, with individual needle selection, gave immense scope for patterning and opened up design potential beyond the mimicking of hand-knitting, through increasingly sophisticated CAD pattern preparation systems linked directly to machine production.

With electronic machine control, pattern preparation data from design systems can be transferred into machine language and knitting sequence data can be transmitted directly to the knitting machine. Global communication links mean, in addition, that information can be transmitted across the world so that design can function remotely from the site of production.

Flat knitting machines now predominate worldwide, due to their versatility. The two major players have emerged as Stoll of Germany and Shima Seiki of Japan. Both have recently developed machinery for integral garment knitting, based on similar principles. Shima Seiki's FIRST machine, for example, has four complete needle beds – two additional ones positioned just above the normal beds in exact alignment, to facilitate transferring of loops – and uses a newly developed slide compound needle. Such innovations represent the state-of-the-art of flat-bed knitting at present. Knitting sequences – key to design originality – are also increasingly being patented to protect competitive advantage.

Design developments can clearly be linked to technological developments: technology can lead design, or design and fashion can lead technology. For example, the early twentieth-century hosiery industry was predicated on fully fashioned – i.e. flat, shaped – stockings with a sewn seam at the back. With the advent in the 1950s of the bare-legged fashion, a new seamless production method was adopted – knitted circular tubes of nylon, heat-set to the leg shape. The fully fashioned hosiery industry had totally declined

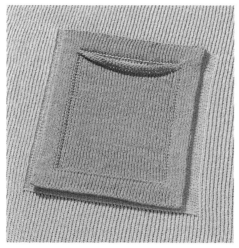

Above Integrally knitted pocket by Stoll

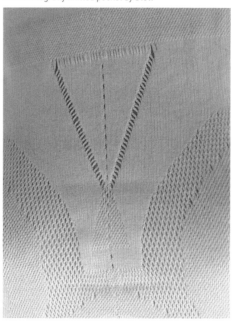

Above Warp knitting, A-POC design, by Issey Miyake

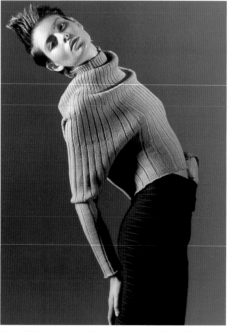

Above Stitch shaping with gradated rib by Atsuro Tayama

when the mini-skirt came in, but was replaced by the development of tights, which stimulated machine innovations in seamless construction.

Knitwear is constructed in one of three ways: 1) from knitted-to-shape (fully fashioned) flat pieces, requiring seaming and some trims; 2) from cut-and-sew fabric, requiring overlocking, trims and seaming; 3) by integral knitting with integrated trims, requiring little or no seaming.

Integral garments are based on tubular knitting. A basic sweater knitted on either Stoll or Shima Seiki patented systems is made of three tubes – two for the sleeves and one for the body. Each is positioned in the correct relationship on the needle beds, and the three are knitted simultaneously from three feeder carriages, with gradual widening of the sleeves until they meet the body tube. Narrowing occurs to create a raglan or circular yoke, finishing usually with a funnel collar which is automatically cast off on the machine (another recent innovation). The fabric may be plain or ribbed and can include intarsia patterns, stitch effects and complex details, such as pockets. Intricate styling details for collars and necklines within traditional production can also be achieved. Unique to knitwear production is a subtle variation of integral knitting, which comprises stitch-shaped items. These use variations in stitch structure and size to develop shape and form. The focus for integral garment research has now moved from lingerie and swimwear to outerwear.

New research in warp knitting has centred on creating seamless items from warp-knitted circular construction. Mesh fabrics and nets have been adapted to circular form to create fishnet tights and net bags. Tubular warp knitting is based, in a similar way to flat V-bed weft knitting, on two sets of needles, aligned vertically and knitting in tubular formation. Each tube requires four guide bars and sets of feeders, one for the back bed, one for the front bed, and one each to form the join between front and back at each side, enabling the tube to be formed. In order to create a sweater, two tubes are required for sleeves and a third for the body, using separate but simultaneous knitting actions, in a similar manner to weft knitting. Mesh patterning can be programmed into the fabric, as in Issey Miyake's A-POC tubular clothing. This is a unique process and has also been patented.

The potential, in design terms, resulting from new knitting technology is enormous.

This section gives a brief introductory look at the fundamental material of knitwear – yarns and fibres. Fibres fall into two distinct categories – natural and manmade/synthetic – and two distinct forms – staple fibres (short lengths) and filament fibres (continuous length).

Natural fibres have remained consistently popular for high-quality classic knitwear and are classified in three main types: 1) animal staple fibres, including wool and hairs such as mohair, angora, alpaca, cashmere, and so on, either alone or blended with other fibres; 2) plant staple fibres, such as cotton (a seed fibre), which can be fine to coarse, or flax (stem fibre), a strong fibre from which linen is made; and 3) the only natural continuous filament fibre, silk, which is either cultivated or wild, and can be spun to a matt or lustrous finish.

Cotton and wool are most commonly used for knitwear. Yarns such as fine combed cotton or worsted spun wools have proved highly suitable for underwear and fine gauge knitwear, which ideally requires smooth, strong but fairly elastic yarns. Thicker, coarser woollen yarns are knitted on coarser gauge machines or by hand for outerwear of all types, from heavy, slightly oily, aran-style sweaters to tweed-effect coats knitted from multicoloured 'fancy' yarns, for example those pioneered by Bernat Klein in the 1950s. Hair fibres are classed as luxury fibres due to their high cost of production, and are often blended with wool. Hand-knitting in mohair became popular in the 1960s and again in the '80s, when prices fell and it was widely available. Silk is less commonly used for knitwear, except in fine gauge fabric. Jersey fabrics are made in a wide range of yarns, from basic cotton to silk and viscose blends for wonderful fluid drape characteristics.

The transition from natural fibres to synthetic fibres has taken place over the relatively short period since the end of the nineteenth century, when the first synthetic fibre – rayon – was invented. Nylon (polyamide) was the next to emerge in 1938. The purpose of the first generation of synthetics was very much to simulate the qualities of natural fibres – rayon was known as artificial silk, and acrylic yarns were designed to mimic wool. The continued development of rayon has produced a range of fibres, structures and finishes, dependent on the chemical processes used in their manufacture.

Rayon is a cellulose fibre, produced from wood pulp, and is therefore made from renewable resources, unlike oil-based polymer fibres. The cellulose is made into a liquid and extruded through holes (spinarets) into continuous filaments. Depending on the chemicals and the production process, the result is viscose rayon, acetate rayon, cupramonium rayon (used in a popular woven fabric, 'cupro') or solvent spun rayon, which is the latest development. Viscose rayon (commonly just called viscose) accounts for the vast majority of production. Its drape and lustre have made it a popular choice for knitwear.

Since the 1980s, great technological developments have taken place in the design of manmade yarns, pioneered above all in Japan, and a second generation of synthetics has evolved, focused on very fine polyester, polyamide and viscose, made into yarns which have highly attractive handle and finishes. Many of the newest synthetics are designed to have high performance qualities, giving rise to 'high-tech' fibres with very specific characteristics, such as high tensile strength, bulk without weight and moisture absorption. They may insulate from or conduct electricity; be biodegradable, resistant to odour or ultraviolet rays; they may change in response to heat. These fibres have applications in clothing for extreme conditions; automotive, aerospace and geotextiles industries; and, increasingly, in architecture and medicine.

Both the historical importance (the Silk Road) and the desirable properties of silk – such as lustre, drape, ability to take dye, softness of touch and attractive handle, together with its unique rustling and 'scrooping' sounds – have driven the development of synthetic fibres. One of the fundamental aspects of manmade fibres is the ability to create specific textures during the manufacture. Firstly, the cross-section of the individual filament fibres can be controlled by the shape of the spinarets (silk has a triangular cross-section filament, hence this was the first to be reproduced). Early synthetic fibres had circular cross-sections and were therefore smooth, but texturizing processes to provide bulk and surface interest were applied, such as crimping (as in Crimplene by Courtaulds) or knit-de-knit (knitting, heat-setting and unravelling).

The development of extremely fine microfibres has created more opportunities.

Synthetics can be given textures – a soft, silk-like touch, for example, or a 'peach-skin' feel – to provide the comfort increasingly demanded by the market.

A new variation of cellulose fibre – lyocell, made by Courtaulds in 1988 under the name Tencel – is a yarn in which all the solvent used can be reprocessed: it is therefore more environmentally friendly. Tencel has a circular cross-section and cotton-like properties, and is particularly suitable for texturing treatments. Many companies, such as Kanebo and Toray in Japan, have produced 'high-touch' fabrics from combinations of fibre structures and yarn finishing treatments which create totally new aspects, not achievable with natural fibres – a new category, given the name *shin-gosen*, to denote a new aesthetic quality.

Fine microfibre and stretch yarns are finding increasing applications in the new seamless lingerie and bodywear markets. Brand names, such as DuPont's Lycra elastane and Tactel polyamide, Nylstar's Meryl polyamide and Elité elastane, promote qualities of comfort, fit and softness. The use of elastomeric stretch yarns in knitwear and bodywear has continued to grow since their development in the 1950s. DuPont were the first to invent an elastomeric fibre made from polyurethane (also known as spandex). Branded Lycra, it was at first used as a replacement for rubber in corsets, in knitted collars and cuffs, and later in stockings, but was slow to be taken up in knitwear. The fibre has a molecular structure similar to coiled springs, giving it the ability to expand greatly in length and then return to its relaxed state. It is usually combined in a small proportion with other yarns, or is covered with another yarn, such as cotton, and used as a yarn itself.

All fibres have their own intrinsic properties and, increasingly, sophisticated fibre blends are being spun together in order to best achieve desired effects. It is increasingly hard to distinguish individual components, and accurate textiles labelling is crucial. Many companies produce yarns from similar raw materials and of similar types, and the consumer may not differentiate between a generic name and a particular brand name. Indeed, some brand names, such as Lycra, have almost become generic.

Yarns are formed in two main ways: from relatively short lengths (staples) of fibres spun together, or from continuous lengths (filaments) of fibres. All manmade yarns are of the filament type, extruded from chemical bases, but these can be processed in many ways, including chopping into staple lengths. Staple yarns usually appear more hairy and coarse than filament yarns. Most yarns contain many fine filaments, except in the case of monofilament yarns, which consist of one filament only. Continuous filament yarns tend to be smooth and lustrous, unless a texturizing process is applied to introduce crimps, snarls and crinkles into the filaments.

The basic twisted fibres form a single strand or 'ply' of yarns, but this is rarely used alone. Strands of yarns are folded together to make two-fold, three-fold and so on yarns (called two-ply, three-ply, etc. in hand-knitting), which are much more balanced. Yarn or thread thickness (count) is designated either by weight per unit length (direct system) or length per unit weight (indirect). Many different systems have evolved over time but these are now more streamlined. Examples are the tex system, which measures grams per kilometre (direct – the coarser the yarn, the higher the count) or the metric count, which is the number of metres per kilogram weight (indirect – the coarser the yarn, the lower the count).

Combined with fibre content and thickness (count) of yarn, a further variable is yarn structure created during the spinning. Common structures are slub yarns which are of uneven thickness, bouclé yarns which have a loop structure, and knop yarns which incorporate tight coils of thread at intervals. Further highly specialized 'fancy' or 'novelty' yarns have interesting effects: chenille, for example, has a furry pile which results from cutting a special woven fabric along its warp threads.

Metallic yarns, for example the brand Lurex, are an example of a different yarn technology. They are produced from metal sheet, often aluminium, which is laminated by applying plastic film on both sides and bonding the layers together. This is then cut into strips and wound as a yarn. The flat surface gives great light reflection. A recent development – split film technology – can create yarns from strips of polyethylene or polypropylene film: under certain conditions, such as extreme tension, the film is induced to 'fibrillate', that is, break into fibres naturally.

Colour in design can be of major importance, as in the space-dyed effect which became popular in the 1970s . To achieve these results, yarn is

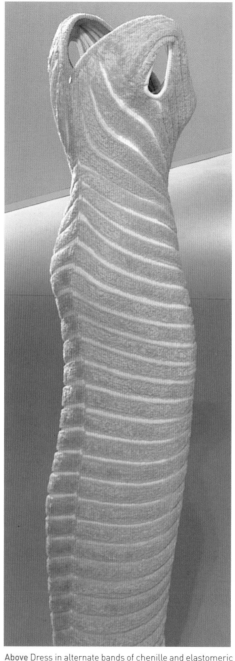

Above Dress in alternate bands of chenille and elastomeric yarn by Azzedine Alaïa

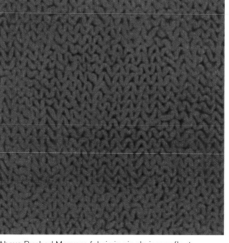

Above Ruched Maxxam fabric in single jersey float jacquard with Lycra by Rosemary Moore

wound into hanks and sections are immersed in different coloured dye-baths according to a predetermined sequence, until the hanks are all dyed. This is a laborious process but creates unique effects in two or more colours. When knitted simply in a straight piece without shaping, a distinctive pattern, reminiscent of ikat in weaving, appears – broad, broken, diagonal lines or 'flame' effects moving over the piece. When shaping occurs or when a new batch of yarn is introduced, the sequence is broken and changes constantly. This effect has become a signature of Missoni knitwear, either on its own or mixed with plain stripes (see pp. 2-3, 23, 30).

All the variables – yarn, machine gauge and stitch structure – must work in harmony before any real design development can begin. Machine gauges commonly used range from 3 (coarse) to 30 (fine jersey), and yarn thickness has to be compatible for successful fabrics.

Although extensibility is a benefit in knitting, it can make fabric prone to distortion when knitted too loosely – an effect capitalized upon in punk and grunge knitwear. Unwanted effects are sometimes turned to advantage in designer-level knitwear: for example, highly spun and twisted yarns can create spirality in single jersey structures, and this produces an angular twist of the seams – an effect regularly utilized in Yohji Yamamoto knitwear (see p. 98). Spirality can be avoided by using the yarns in a balanced structure, such as a rib fabric or double jersey. Jürgen Lehl, however, deliberately uses high twist yarns to create particularly 'lively' fabrics, which may have unpredictable results (see p. 45).

Successful combination of yarn and structure is paramount to the success of a knitted garment. For example, early rayon yarns proved to be very heavy, and tended to sag and grow in length. Stitch structure and stitch density (tightness or looseness of construction) play a major role, and several prototypes may be prepared to test out whole garment effects, making design development a costly process.

Machiko Agano b. Japan, 1953. Following a series of pieces constructed from twigs, handmade paper and twine, Agano recently turned her attention to articulating interior space through mesh constructions made from hand-knitted steel wire combined with yarns such as silk, nylon and Lurex. Her site-specific installations, often experimenting with new materials, have been exhibited worldwide.

Azzedine Alaïa b. Tunisia, 1940. Christened the 'king of cling', Alaïa uses Lycra-rich knitted fabrics to make the sexiest of garments, including his infamous stretch dresses. Alaïa was the first to use elastomeric fabrics in such an extreme way, exploiting their ability to mould the body like an invisible corset and create a smooth silhouette. Considered to be the last great couturier to work directly on the body, he drapes, cuts and sculpts fabric precisely to the figure, emphasizing it with contouring seams. The knitted fabrics he has favoured include fluid silk and wool jerseys, and medium- to heavy-weight viscose and wool blends.

Alice Lee founded by Alice Smith and Lee Farmer, London, UK, 1996. Smith trained in knitwear and Farmer has a background in fashion illustration. Taking a radically new approach to the construction of the knitted dress, and working three-dimensionally around the body, they have established a signature look. This derives from a sophisticated application of the short row knitting technique to create intricate sunburst effects centering around one point, such as the waist. Each dress is made in one piece. Every season further variations of fabric and complexities of structure are created.

Artwork design company founded by Jane and Patrick Gottelier, London, UK, 1977. Jane trained in fashion and Patrick in painting. Together they launched one of the first of the British 'designer knitwear' labels, with hand-knitted sweaters featuring graphic motifs, stitch textures and thematic collections of beaded, studded, fringed and embroidered knitwear, as well as hand-printed intarsia hand-knits, co-ordinated with non-knitted separates. Artwork first introduced their denim knitwear in 1984, since when it has featured consistently in the range.

Ballantyne knitwear manufacturer founded Innerleithen, Scotland, 1920s. The business was expanded in the 1930s to produce fully fashioned knitwear in cashmere. It exports the majority of its production around the world. The company is one of the last to produce manually made intarsia knitwear, and manufactures for designers including Clements Ribeiro, Ann-Louise Roswald and Chanel (qq.v.).

Emily Bates b. Basingstoke, UK, 1970. Bates plays on the layers of meaning associated with fetish objects. She uses human hair and fine threads as her materials, thereby making the familiar uncomfortable. She has exhibited widely: her 1997 exhibition 'Denier' focused on appropriations of the stocking and its use as a simulacrum of the body – a foot, an arm, a hand – and its sexual taboos.

Heather Belcher b. Nottingham, UK, 1960. The trapped image of a dress, cardigan or jacket within Belcher's felted wall-pieces plays with contradictions between image and reality. The pieces seem to have a life of their own, caught in time and space.

Laura Biagiotti b. Rome, Italy, 1943. Having manufactured for other designers since 1965, Biagiotti launched her own label in 1972. An early exponent of feminine Italian style, she is known for her comfortable easy dressing in, for example, cashmere knitwear, including trousers and dresses.

Sarah Bigley graduated from the University of Brighton (BA Fashion Textiles) in 1996.

Dorothée Bis design house founded by Jacqueline and Elie Jacobson, Paris, France, 1962. Designer Jacqueline became known for her cropped skinny sweaters and co-ordinates, and her fast-changing, fashion-led sportswear collection for working women with a wide variety of total knitwear looks. This incorporated at various times layered volumes, graphic chunky knits and a slim, lean silhouette. In the mid-1970s the ultimate layered look could include a cardigan-coat over a tunic over a skirt over loose trousers.

Maria Blaisse b. Amsterdam, Netherlands, 1944. Material, form and movement are the building blocks of Blaisse's work. Since 1982 she has created sculptural, flexible forms for fashion and dance, researching new fabrics and often starting from an industrial source. Originally inspired by the inner tubes of tyres, she uses rubber and synthetic foams, exploiting their thermoplastic qualities by vacuum-moulding and laminating. Since 1999 she has developed her 'Flexible Design' project through the ideal medium of knitted wool fabrics in collaboration with knitter Karen Marseille.

Body Map design house founded by David Holah and Stevie Stewart, London, UK, 1982. Body Map's hugely influential designs (no longer in production) epitomized a young and fun fashion zeitgeist, centred on London and merging the 'New Romantic' ethos with punk elements and a new, daring, body-conscious silhouette. Knitwear featured in several ways – as hand-knitted cardigans, dresses and tweed suits; as machine-knitted graphic or shapely designs; and as printed tights and stretch jersey bodywear. Frills, eclectic use of colour and accessories completed the often bizarre but directional picture.

Maya Bramwell graduated from the Royal College of Art, London (MA Fashion) in 1999, and is now a designer for Tse.

Leonie Branston graduated from the University of Brighton (BA Fashion Textiles) in 1994.

Cristina Brown graduated from Central St Martins, London (BA Textiles) in 1999.

Kate Carrick graduated from the University of Brighton (BA Fashion Textiles) in 1995.

Ernestina Cerini b. Italy. Cerini began her career as a freelance designer in the Reggio Emilia area – the centre of knitwear production in Italy. She first showed her own label in 1988 and quickly built a reputation for highly complex and unusual textural pieces, often using braiding techniques to create meandering 'laces' and openwork fabrics. Her line (no longer in production) included knitted coats, jackets and dresses, and particularly favoured a trapeze shape, which sometimes appeared to unravel into chaotic braids.

Hussein Chalayan b. Nicosia, Cyprus, 1970. Chalayan has gained a respected place in fashion based on his highly intellectual approach to experimental design and the breathtaking moments of fashion theatre in his catwalk shows. His clothes are created with meticulous attention to cut, detail and proportion, incorporating both fine jersey fabrics and, more recently, heavier-gauge knitwear, usually with a 'twist', such as extra long sleeves, transparent areas or integrated pockets. He designed collections for Tse (q.v.) New York in 1999 and 2000.

Chanel design house founded by Gabrielle ('Coco') Chanel, Paris, France, 1915. In addition to her famous tweed suits and accessories, legendary designer Coco Chanel pioneered casual knitted dressing in jersey fabric appropriated from underwear. She also created the leisure sweater ensemble, borrowing the style of men's sports sweaters, as worn by her on vacation in Deauville. The house of Chanel still produces classic knitwear, some of which is manufactured in Scotland. In 1996 Karl Lagerfeld (q.v.) commissioned Julien Macdonald (q.v.), who created elaborate couture knitted dresses.

Clements Ribeiro design house founded by Suzanne Clements and Inacio Ribeiro, London, UK, 1993. Having met at Central St Martins College of Art and Design in London, the husband-and-wife team have developed a fashion-forward, feminine style, based on eclectic fabric and pattern mixes with an individual application of colour. Their range of recoloured and restyled classic cashmere knitwear, created in collaboration with Barrie of Scotland, was highly influential and much copied. Knitwear has featured as a constantly updated part of the collection, with geometric patterns, Lurex yarns, army styling and a very successful 'rugby shirt' for women. Clements Ribeiro now also design the Cacharel collection.

Trevor Collins b. Wycombe, UK, 1953. Collins makes one-off costumes for ballet, opera, theatre and television, often combining machine- and hand-knitting, crochet and weaving. Working to commissions, he has worked with choreographers such as Siobhan Davies, and has created unique fabric lengths for special uses.

Comme des Garçons design house founded by Rei Kawakubo, Tokyo, Japan, 1973. Kawakubo has consistently challenged accepted notions of fashion and the fashionable body. Slicing through classic silhouettes; juxtaposing and layering seemingly incongruous combinations of fabrics; boiling textiles to create incomplete- or unfinished-looking garments, replete with frills, pleats and ruched details – these are all innovations which have been influential. Knitwear is always a strong component of the Homme Plus collection and, off the catwalk, the Robe de Chambre and Tricot lines (the latter designed by Junya Watanabe, q.v.). Techniques have included combining intarsia

with overprinting, and piecing together garments from knits of different structures, qualities and weights, whether heavy hand-knit, medium sweatshirt fabric or fine jersey.

Gina Conquest graduated from Nottingham Trent University (BA Textiles) in 1999.

Coogi knitwear company founded by Jacky Taranto, Abbotsford, Australia, 1970s. Coogi is known for its unique, distinctive, multicoloured and multipatterned knitwear, which uses advanced technology from Stoll Knitting (q.v.), with whom it is a knitwear development partner. Taranto views the product as 'wearable art' and samples of the fabric are in the Cooper Hewitt Textile Museum in New York.

Sarah Dallas b. Bristol, UK, 1951. Dallas designed her fashion knitwear collection from 1976 to 1988 – simple, fashionable shapes with bold, graphic details. She was given the British Design Council Award in 1987 for 'New Classics'. Dallas now lectures at the Royal College of Art, London.

Dior design house founded by Christian Dior, Paris, France, 1946. Following Dior's death in 1957, the house has maintained its position in high fashion by engaging a series of artistic directors, namely Yves Saint Laurent, Marc Bohan, Gianfranco Ferre and, from 1997, John Galliano (q.v.), who is chief designer for both haute couture and ready-to-wear. Galliano has increased the use of knitwear in the Dior collections, which recently included oversized mohair textured knits. His outrageously theatrical creative statements are part of the successful repositioning of the image of the house.

Dolce & Gabbana design house founded by Domenico Dolce and Stefano Gabbana, Italy, 1982. Knitwear was an early part of the now wide-ranging collections for men and women. It has varied from oversized chunky cable knits and patchwork for men and fine crochet evening cardigans for women to sexy transparent tops and '50s-style graphic cardigans for men.

Susan Duckworth b. UK, 1950. Duckworth is a painter who turned to hand-knitting whilst waiting for a job in costume design. The combination resulted in finely detailed and beautifully coloured knitwear with floral or geometric patterning. She was one of the new wave of British designer knitters of the 1970s, when colour and yarns transformed the dowdy image of knitting.

Christian Dufay b. Geneva, Switzerland, 1961. Dufay trained as an architect in America and worked in New York before setting up his design studio, Abode, in Los Angeles in 1994. Now located in Europe, Studio Christian Dufay produces innovative designs which focus on the potential of materials and their expressive applications, with a growing range of lighting designs.

Rebecca Earley b. UK, 1970. Earley developed her heat photogram printing technique in 1994, whilst at college, and has gone on to show her fashion and accessories collections in catwalk shows, exhibitions and galleries in the UK and Europe, under the label B. Earley. Her product is environmentally sound, as she uses recycled polyester as her base material, and the printing process creates no wastage.

Fake London design house founded by Desirée Mejer, London, UK, 1995. Mejer's irreverent take on all things British caught the eye of London's fashion, art and media 'in-crowd', and business success followed. The contradiction of luxury cashmere recycled and cut up in patchwork designs with roughly overlocked edges was a breath of fresh air in knitwear design, since much copied.

Nicole Farhi b. Nice, France, 1946. After designing for the French Connection chain, Farhi set up her own label in 1983, using her personal style philosophy of casual understated dressing to inform her ranges of highly wearable clothes for women and – from 1989 – men. Comfort and ease are expressed throughout in unstructured designs, and particularly in the knitwear ranges of sweaters in natural mixture yarns, long relaxed cardigans and simple dresses.

Fendi design house founded by Adele Casagrande, Italy, 1918. This family business, now run by the five Fendi daughters, is renowned for its furs, leatherwork and accessories. Since 1965, Karl Lagerfeld (q.v.) has designed the 'haute fourrure' and clothing collections. The accessories have come to the forefront, perfectly in tune with high fashion trends, and achieving cult status.

Marion Foale b. UK. One half of Foale and Tuffin, whose boutique came to prominence in the Carnaby Street of the swinging '60s, Foale has now built an international fashion knitwear business based on fine hand-knitwear. She works three-dimensionally to integrate shape and minimize seams, with details such as pockets and collars knitted integrally. She has consulted for Marks & Spencer to bring items of her knitwear to a wider market.

Nora Fok b. Hong Kong, 1953. Fok has perfected the manipulation of knitted and knotted monofilament nylon, and her larger work describes and circumscribes the body, often centering on the neck. Themes may be cosmic or microscopic, or may arise from more parochial observations of nature. She exhibits internationally.

Shelley Fox b. Scunthorpe, UK, 1967. Fox's textiles and fashion training, together with her experimental approach, has led to quietly innovative work. Early pieces were developed from felted knitted wool, embossed with subtle patterning. However, when a piece of fabric felted wrongly into creases and ripples, this sparked off further development into one-off effects. Often inspired by scientific and medical research, Fox has also developed unorthodox 'circle cutting' techniques and has created intricately constructed skirts, which can be worn in several ways. Classic knitwear in the form of twinsets features regularly but (mis)treated to processes of scorching, bleaching or spraying with paint or candle wax.

Susie Freeman b. London, UK, 1956. Susie Freeman discovered the technique of 'pocket knitting' whilst studying at London's Royal College of Art. Transforming the method with the use of transparent nylon yarn, Freeman created intricate magpie-nest-like textiles, accessories and clothing, which entrapped a treasure trove of found objects, including shells, scraps of fabric, beads, sequins and minute buttons, into the knitted structure as it was made. Recently Freeman has been working in collaboration with Dr Liz Lee, their 'medico-political' work forefronting social commentary and informed by the crossover between scientific disciplines and textile design.

Alan Gallacher b. Scotland. Whilst also lecturing at Glasgow School of Art, Gallacher has, since 1994, created a range of distinctive knitted felted wool scarves and wraps which, through carefully controlled construction and dyeing, scintillate with colours and are reminiscent of African beading and hair braids.

John Galliano b. Gibraltar, 1960. After an early career filled with critical acclaim for his romantic, theatrical and historically inspired collections, but beset by financial difficulties, Galliano became the first British designer to be appointed to a French couture house. After only a year at Givenchy he moved to Dior to design haute couture and ready-to-wear, whilst also maintaining his own label. Galliano introduced hand-knits into his early British collections and continues to design evening dresses using fine knitted fabrics.

Lisa Gatherar graduated from the University of Brighton (BA Three-Dimensional Design) in 2001.

Jean Paul Gaultier b. Arceuil, France, 1952. Gaultier has consistently featured knitwear in his collections, whether playfully reinventing ethnic and cultural traditions or reworking classic elements with his own inimitable styling. He often juxtaposes fabrics, and uses refined industrial knitted textiles as well as hand-knitting. A key look is the mixing and layering of many elements – of which knitwear is usually one. The result is always a riot of colour, texture and innovative silhouettes. The couture line, started in 1997, features more intricate techniques and more inventive use of cross-cultural and cross-gender references. The aran sweater, Peruvian knitted hat, fair isle slipover and Norwegian snowflake sweater have all made an appearance, albeit radically transformed.

Frances Geesin b. London, UK, 1941. Combining science and art, Dr Geesin creates 3-D forms from knitted nylon yarn and other fabrics, then metallizes them in an electro-deposition process she herself has developed. Opulent juxtapositions of surface and structure are formed: a soft, malleable piece of fabric becomes rigid and precious. Geesin also uses modern synthetic materials, in particular a special form of nylon, known as Grilon, which is knitted then moulded-to-form with heat – sometimes to the point of destruction – enabling the creation of intricate surfaces on which layers of different metal oxides are built up, giving shimmering, multi-hued effects. Geesin has collaborated with fashion, millinery and jewelry designers. She also works in interactive fabrics and consults for Philips Research.

Genny design and manufacturing company founded by Arnoldo and Donatella Girombelli, Ancona, Italy,

1961. One of the most prominent fashion companies in Italy, designing, manufacturing and distributing ranges including the labels Genny, Complice and Byblos. A strong design element is maintained by engaging leading designers, who have included Gianni Versace in 1974 and more recently Dolce & Gabbana for Complice, and Varty and Cleaver for Byblos.

Jo Gordon b. UK. Gordon started her career with dramatic millinery and developed knitted hats, gloves and scarves as a sideline. These have now become her major business, resulting from anticipation of the right time to relaunch traditional woolly accessories, such as long striped scarves, with carefully considered colours, proportions and witty detailing.

Nichola Gowing graduated from the Royal College of Art, London (MA Constructed Textiles) in 1999.

Shirin Guild b. Tehran, Iran, 1946. Guild has designed new knitwear classics that give unique proportions (especially the width of the body, which can be up to 90 or 100 cm) to traditional sweater and cardigan shapes. When seen in two dimensions, her garments are based on rectangles, but they hang from the shoulders and drape over the body – an undulating shape first inspired by the traditional clothing of Turkish women. This volume of fabric and generous sizing means that the clothes are flattering and easy-to-wear by women of many proportions. The collection is knitwear-led but complemented by woven jackets, skirts and especially trousers, which also play with proportion and drape. High quality yarns such as sea island cotton and cashmere lend added value to Guild's sophisticated but understated simplicity.

Isabelle Harman graduated from Central St Martins, London (BA Textiles) in 1998.

Iben Høj b. Copenhagen, Denmark, 1970. Knitwear and textile designer for Bruuns Bazaar, Høj also supplies knitwear ideas to many companies, including Marc Jacobs, Calvin Klein, Donna Karan, Kenzo (q.v.), Ralph Lauren and Hervé Leger.

Tracy Hunt b. Rochford, UK, 1971. Hunt knits simple fabrics in mixtures of synthetic yarns, including polypropylene, which is then heat-set and laminated to create semi-rigid but flexible fabrics. These lend themselves to many new end uses for interior products, including lighting. Other fabrics

Hunt has designed contain insertions within the knitted construction which dictate folds and pleated effects. She is currently developing products for commercial production.

Mie Iwatsubo b. Japan, 1977. Iwatsubo has developed intricately textured accessories through combining Japanese shibori (shaped resist dyeing) technique with knitted and felted fabrics, inspired by patterns in nature. Fabrics are knitted in pleats or ripples in a combination of different yarns, such as wool with cotton; the pleats are then stitched together, and the fabric is dyed and felted simultaneously, creating unpredictable effects. In 1999/2000 Iwatsubo created accessories for designer Jürgen Lehl (q.v.).

Betty Jackson b. Bacup, UK, 1949. Jackson's relaxed style of dressing incorporates a high proportion of knitwear: decorative sweaters featured in the 1980s, giving way to more sophisticated, longer line cardigans, dresses and skirts, layered with linen pieces. Recently the line has begun to target a younger clientèle, with the silhouette closer to the body, and raw-edged effects.

Jan & Carlos design house founded Italy, mid-1980s. The knitwear collection is now produced by Linea Più, specializing in engineered garments using advanced knitting technology.

Lisa Jansen graduated from the University of Brighton (BA Fashion Textiles) in 1997.

Mair Joint graduated from Goldsmiths' College, London (BA Textiles) in 1996 and is now working in a dance and performance context.

Adam Jones b. UK, 1966. Jones has worked in Paris since 1989, first as knitwear designer for Kenzo (q.v.) womenswear. He moved to Dior (q.v.) in 1995 and in 2001 launched his solo label. His individual look uses a seductive mix of knitted and woven fabrics spliced together in unconventional juxtapositions.

Niki Jones graduated from the Royal College of Art, London (MA Textiles) in 1998.

Joseph (Ettedgui) b. Casablanca, Morocco, 1936. Always on the look-out for ideas and talents, Joseph has been responsible for introducing many new names to London fashion, including Kenzo and Azzedine Alaïa (qq.v.). He started his retail career in the early 1970s, selling Kenzo sweaters

in his hairdressing shop. By 1984 he had developed the Joseph Tricot line – a mix of classic knitted separates and graphic hand-knitted sweaters designed by Martin Kidman. Joseph's influential 'lifestyle' concept mixed fashion with art and café society, and created a blueprint for retailing in the 1980s and '90s.

Kei Kagami b. Japan. Combining an education in architecture and fashion, Kagami has, since 1996, created a sculptural collection which pushes at boundaries between fashion, performance and art. His innovative use of materials has resulted in a 'glass' skirt and clothes made entirely from transparent zips. He has collaborated with many makers, including experimental knitwear designer Fatima Saifee (q.v.).

Sasha Kagan b. UK. Based in Wales, Kagan is a self-taught designer and producer of colourful handmade knitwear in natural fibres. She came to prominence in 1977 as part of the British designer knitwear boom. Known for humorous graphic motifs and floral designs, she sells internationally, particularly in America.

Judit Kárpáti-Rácz b. Budapest, Hungary. Kárpáti-Rácz's work has developed from a traditional technique of Hungarian knotting, originally used to create decorative necklaces in horsehair. Kárpáti-Rácz uses modern nylon yarns or steel and copper wires. She has invented shapes which have evolved in empathy with the technique, which is highly labour-intensive, to create attractive bags, necklaces, hats and body-pieces.

Tamara Kemoklidse graduated from Central St Martins, London (BA Textiles) in 2001.

Kenzo b. Hyogo, Japan, 1939. Kenzo designed hugely influential collections from the early 1970s (he retired in 1999). His relaxed style in the early years gave women more freedom of movement and initiated the knitted layering and multiple patterning that is synonymous with the Kenzo label today. Knitwear has played a prominent role throughout, especially in the intricate, multicoloured jacquard patterning, often over-embroidered. The breathtaking visual feast of colour and the mix of floral and geometric designs are inspired by a mix of cultures both eastern and western.

Lainey Keogh b. Old Town, Ireland, 1957. Keogh is inspired by yarns and texture, creating tactile,

handcrafted, couture knitwear, crochet and hand-woven pieces. Although she started designing in 1984 and has a celebrity client list, Keogh did not make her London catwalk debut until 1997, when her voluptuous and sensual knitwear, treating each woman as a goddess, had a stunning impact. After three seasons Keogh decided to retire from the fashion limelight to continue her couture business from her own spiritual standpoint.

Krizia design house founded by Mariuccia Mandelli, Italy, 1954. Krizia's prolific output covers a wide range of both evening and daywear. Mandelli's personal preference for wearing sweaters led to the formation of the Kriziamaglia line in 1967, which specialized in casual holidaywear and witty animal graphic intarsia sweaters and dresses. These became a trademark of the company and a zoo of animals has been produced season by season – wolves, bears, elephants, tigers, and so on. Other images have been inspired by Magritte (winter 1989) and Dick Tracy (winter 1991), all painstakingly intarsia-knitted. The extremely varied knitwear collection has included beaded sweaters and sweaters with slotted ribbon for evening, heavily textured daywear sweaters and coats, and brief summer dresses.

Christian Lacroix b. Arles, France, 1951. The sumptuous extremes often found in couture are expressed in the house of Lacroix, established in 1987. Lacroix's collections work through rich juxtapositions of colour and texture, some achieved through intricate jacquard knitwear – multicoloured sweaters to accessorize, or knitted suits and coats in multiple patterns.

Karl Lagerfeld b. Hamburg, Germany, 1938. Involved over a long period with many design houses, including Fendi (q.v.), Krizia (q.v.) and Chloe, Lagerfeld has been artistic director at Chanel (q.v.) since 1983, establishing his KL labels at the same time. He seeks out fresh talent through a student competition run at London's Royal College of Art.

Jürgen Lehl b. Poland, 1944. Lehl, a German national, has been based in Japan since 1971. His textile-led womenswear is rooted in the Japanese aesthetic of paring ideas down to their essence and in traditional craft skills of weaving and dyeing. However, he embraces modern technology for his sophisticated knitted fabrics, many of which are produced in layers of colour and texture, including embroidery, often sourced in Asia. Approximately half of the collection is knitwear, spanning a range from textural jersey and fine knitted fabrics to heavier weights with a handmade feel and experimental approach, such as winter 2000's 3-D knitwear twisting around the body, which was developed by Lehl's knitwear designer Ricarda Heubel.

Marie Lenclos graduated from the Royal College of Art, London (MA Communication Art and Design) in 2001.

Winni Lok b. UK, 1972. Lok studied fine art and fashion, and started her own label in 2000. Although designs under her own name are likely to be deconstructed and raw-edged, she collaborated with Hussein Chalayan (q.v.) in the design of his knitwear for three seasons, from winter 1997/98.

Nuala MacCulloch graduated from Birmingham Institute of Art and Design (MA Textiles) in 1998.

Julien Macdonald b. Merthyr Tydfil, Wales, 1974. Macdonald has produced his signature lacy knits for several designers, including Koji Tatsuno (q.v.), Alexander McQueen (q.v.) and Antonio Berardi. In 1996 he became knitwear designer for Karl Lagerfeld and Chanel (qq.v.), and went on to stage his own spectacular shows. He transforms machine-knitted fabrics into extraordinary cobweb dresses, and makes minuscule but sensational dresses by hand, encrusting and weighing them down with crystals and other objects. The two extremes of intricate but wearable manufactured designs and highly theatrical, hand-made couture have continued in his own-label collections. He was appointed designer for Givenchy in 2001.

Emma Maloney graduated from the University of Brighton (BA Fashion Textiles) in 1997.

Martin Margiela b. Genk, Belgium, 1957. Margiela's vision for his collections can appear uncompromising, but it is underpinned by a systematic logic of transformation and taxonomy. The collections are now numbered according to strict principles and the basic womenswear collection '6' is pared down to bare essentials. Knitwear is consistently featured in the ranges, based on classical items such as plain sweaters and cardigans, but they undergo transformations of finish or construction detail which render them unique. Margiela also designs for Hermès.

Matec machinery manufacturer founded Italy. Part of the Santoni Group (q.v.), Matec have developed a revolutionary 10-inch-diameter machine with jacquard capability, which allows for the production of simple bodysized childrenswear with patterning and minimal seaming.

Matta design company founded by Bill Campbell, UK, 1998. Campbell has created a range of interior textile products such as cushions, throws and wall-pieces, using a wide variety of materials and processes. The company also collaborates with artists and makers for one-off pieces.

Alexander McQueen b. London, UK, 1970. Knitwear pieces have recently become a feature of McQueen's catwalk shows, for example the oversized knits of winter 1999 and the deconstructed dark knits of winter 2001. For these showpieces, McQueen commissions knitwear designers such as Sidney Bryan and Alex Gore-Browne, whose graduate collection of felted appliqué knits was developed for winter 2000.

Simone Memel b. Netherlands, 1967. Having had a combined education in fine arts and shoemaking, Memel creates shoes as art objects, using materials to define the shoe and express ironic commentary on issues of gender and perception. Her work has been exhibited widely in Europe.

Missoni design house founded by Ottavio and Rosita Missoni, Italy, 1953. The Missonis have, with an artist's eye for colour and pattern, worked their myriad textures and designs into the most instantly recognizable knitwear in the world. With Rosita's family business's old warp-knitting machinery, previously used to manufacture shawls, they reinterpreted the textiles for fashion and created their signature zigzag and stripe effects. Space-dyed yarns enhance the fabrics' unique qualities and produce the characteristic 'flame' effect and movement of colour over the garment. Striking multi-coloured jacquard designs in stylized floral and mosaic patchwork patterns contribute to the total look. After almost fifty years, the creative baton has now been handed to the Missoni children, Angela (womenswear) and Luca (menswear).

Issey Miyake b. Hiroshima, Japan, 1938. Miyake's output of innovative ideas for clothing and fabric development has been prodigious throughout his long career. Knitwear has played a significant role and is often used for its fluidity and suppleness in enveloping the body with volume. Appreciating other qualities of knitted fabrics, such as stretch-to-fit, Miyake has also evolved a parallel strand of design, using stretch knit to outline the body in powerful and dynamic sculptural forms. Miyake's main collection is now designed by Naoki Takizawa, whilst he concentrates on A-POC.

Georgina Naish graduated from the University of Brighton (BA Three-Dimensional Design) in 1998.

Suzumi Noda b. Osaka, Japan, 1951. With training in both interior design and textiles, Noda creates participative art installations questioning outward appearance in the form of clothing and elements of packaging. 'Word work' (2000) consists of clothes and furniture hand-knitted from cut-up handbills Noda reprinted from advertising and packaging. She currently leads a fashion course in Osaka.

Hikaru Noguchi b. Tokyo, Japan. Noguchi moved to England in 1989 to study textiles, having previously studied graphic design. She produces a wide range of handcrafted knitwear, accessories and furniture, all with a quirky, individual look based on a mix of traditional fabrics and motifs, such as the Nordic star and fair isle patterns. She also applies fun elements, such as fringing, updated with contemporary colours and styling.

Monika Olszynska graduated from the University of Brighton (BA Fashion Textiles) in 2000.

Karl Pinfold graduated from the University of Brighton (BA Fashion Textiles) in 2000, and went on to study Mixed Media Textiles at the Royal College of Art, London.

Gina Pinnick b. Birmingham, UK, 1956. Pinnick creates one-off knitted costumes for a wide range of theatre, opera, film and television, working mainly by manual machine production methods. The work usually involves a great deal of interpretation and origination of technical and design ideas in order to meet a commission brief.

Stephanie Piogé b. Aix-en-Provence, France, 1975. Combining fashion, photography and conceptual art, Piogé has realized a range of conceptual clothing which looks at issues of femininity and restriction. Piogé works freelance with trend-forecasting agencies, such as Peclers and Li Edelkoort, making predictions for colours and materials.

Prada design house founded by Mario Prada, Italy, 1913. In 1978 Miuccia Prada took over the directorship of her grandfather's leather goods firm and has transformed it into a fashion leader in accessories and clothing. Recent collections have reintroduced the ladylike chic of the 1950s. 'Classic-with-a-twist' knitwear co-ordinates with each collection.

Pringle knitwear manufacturer founded by Robert Pringle, Scotland, 1815. Pringle began with hosiery and underwear, but a century ago turned to knitwear as outerwear. They took a lead in fashion by appointing a designer in 1933 (Otto Weiz from Austria), who is credited with the origination of the twinset for both men and women, and argyll golfing sweaters. The company is now owned by the Hong Kong-based Fang brothers, and new energy has been injected to appeal to a younger market, with classics being updated from the company's extensive archive of past designs.

Caterina Radvan b. Brighton, UK, 1961. Research into seamless knitwear is at the core of Radvan's work, which now forms the basis of a doctoral study in design for disabled women. A geometric approach is often applied to the construction of unconventionally shaped clothes, which build upon knitted fabric's potential for 3-D shape.

Victoria Rance b. Streatley, UK, 1959. Rance trained as a sculptor and has exhibited widely in the UK. She makes site-specific works which define ordered and patterned spaces, often relating to the body. Her sculptures, many of conical form, use interlacings or spokes within a structural framework which can sometimes be entered.

Patricia Roberts b. UK. Roberts started her knitwear business in 1972, designing and selling her intricately detailed, graphic, often humorous hand-knits. She was at the forefront of the British designer knitwear movement of the time, and four years later opened the first of three shops in London, which also sold her brand of Woollybear yarns. Her designs are known for their technical complexity, with a mix of stitch structures, colour intarsia patterns and 3-D details, such as bows and the famous 'bunch of grapes'. Together with stylist Caroline Baker, she brought fashion styling

to knitting patterns, and also pioneered the publishing of fashion knitting pattern books. She continues to design and sell worldwide.

Freddie Robins b. UK, 1965. Robins trained as a textile designer, working with Tait & Style (q.v.) until 1997, but now produces more conceptual and personal pieces using knitting. At present she makes all her artworks herself on a domestic knitting machine but is seeking to create work on a larger scale, using the latest technology. Robins takes familiar forms of knitwear, such as sweaters and gloves, and subverts them to make impossible clothes for imagined bodies – elongated, headless, connected bodysuits, a four-sleeved sweater, gloves with dismembered fingers, sweaters connected at the abdomen like mother and child. Sometimes witty, sometimes disturbing, the work can be read as a commentary on ability, disability and notions of normality.

John Rocha b. Hong Kong, 1953. Rocha based his business, founded in 1979, in Dublin, Ireland, in preference to a fashion capital. This has an influence on his approach to design – a blending of tradition with modernity. However, his knitwear has little to do with traditional handcraft. Gossamer-fine knitted lace and transparent filigree crochet dresses were shown for summer 1995 and 1997, and the autumn/winter 2001 collection included rag knitting in torn muslin.

Ann-Louise Roswald b. Gothenburg, Sweden. Roswald established her label in 1997, designing printed cashmere knitwear, which gave top-to-toe possibilities of pattern through sweaters and cardigans, skirts, and her specially made knitted fabric clogs. The garments are knitted to shape and half made up so they can be opened flat and printed by hand, garment by garment, in bold, graphic, stylized floral designs with unusual colour combinations.

Sonia Rykiel b. Paris, France, 1930. The first Sonia Rykiel shop opened in 1968 and immediately gained a reputation for its chic and wearable knitwear. The sweater is Rykiel's emblem – even used as the shape of her perfume bottle. Distinctive aspects are the ever-renewed striped knitwear, much of it black with sherbet or bright colours, rhinestones and applied lettering. Her catwalk shows exemplify Parisian sophistication, and always include an

army of models dressed in all colour variations. Although Rykiel is still in overall control, daughter Natalie is now Creative Director.

Fatima Saifee graduated from Chelsea College of Art and Design (BA Textiles) in 2000, and went on to study knitwear at the Royal College of Art, London.

salt interior design company founded by Karina Thomas and June Swindell, UK, 1996. salt is a unique service, making to commission specially designed fabrics for innovative light-filtering and window treatments in specific interiors.

Santoni hosiery machinery manufacturer founded Brescia, Italy, 1919. In 1988 Santoni became part of the Lonati Group (foremost producer of machinery for socks and stockings). Santoni have developed sophisticated technology applied to circular systems for knitted fabric, and now occupy a leading position in machinery for seamless complete garments with end uses in underwear, beachwear, sportswear and medical wear. Further developments into outerwear are also taking place.

Shima Seiki knitting machinery manufacturer founded by Masahiro Shima, Wakayama, Japan, 1962. With a company philosophy of 'ever onward', Shima Seiki has become a leading exponent of integrated systems of computer-controlled flat knitting machines. The business was founded on the success of the first fully automated glove knitting machine and continues to innovate advanced knitting technology.

Julie Skarland b. Trondheim, Norway, 1960. Skarland studied architecture and then moved to Paris to study fashion, showing her first collection in 1991. Although inspired by romantic legends and fairy tales of trolls and princesses in snowy landscapes (Skarland's studio is called the Princess Factory), her work has a modern feel. The clothes are concerned with opposition of fabrics and a modern use of artisanal techniques of painting, embroidery, printing and knitting. Hand-knitted fabrics are pieced together with woven fabrics in simple geometric forms.

John Smedley knitwear manufacturer founded by John Smedley and Peter Nightingale, UK, 1784. The second John Smedley took over in 1825, setting up a company to spin, knit and manufacture knitwear under one roof. The company's first products were fine gauge, fully-fashioned underwear, gradually moving to outerwear in the 1930s. Most knitwear is made in high quality merino wool or sea island cotton, and the company has prided itself on its 'unshrinkable' garments. John Smedley have consistently manufactured for designer labels, including Yves Saint Laurent, Paul Smith, Vivienne Westwood (q.v.) and Antonio Berardi. In 2000 they opened their first shop in London.

Marina Spadafora design house founded Italy, 1925. Marina Spadafora is one of three sisters now running the family firm, whose collections consist primarily of knitwear. Previously a costume designer, Marina delights in experimenting with a wide range of fabrics, materials and finishes, and often uses skilled hand-workers in Tuscany to create unique, demi-couture pieces. Stitch structures for evening, day and sportswear range from lace and mock fur to brushed jacquards and braided knit fabric.

Lawrence Steele b. Hampton, VA, USA, 1963. Based in Milan, Steele worked with Prada (q.v.) and Moschino, then launched his own line in 1994. He has built his distinctive 'vocabulary of clothes' into a signature look of sophisticated but sensual chic, with great attention to detail and a certain edge. His innovative knitwear utilizes 3-D features, such as gauges graduated from fine to heavy to create integral shaping; he was also one of the early adopters of seamless knitting technology. His experiments with knit fabric have included gold printed fur fabric and double-layered knitwear.

Stoll knitting machinery manufacturer founded by Heinrich Stoll and Christian Schmidt, Riedlingen, Germany, 1873. The company is now run by the fourth generation of the Stoll family and has developed into Europe's largest manufacturer of electronically controlled flat knitting machines. They offer a pattern service and trend collection, and have exhibited at the influential Pitti Filati yarn fair in Florence since 1995, reinforcing the link between design and technology.

Anna Sui b. Dearborn Heights, MA, USA, 1955. Sui formed her New York-based company in 1983. She is known for her hippy chic and grunge styles of the early 1990s, in which an eclectic mix of styles of clothing referenced the casual rag-bag dress of 1960s youth. Several elements of the collections were knitted, such as Peruvian-style garments and sweaters which appeared to be unravelling.

Tait & Style accessories company founded by Ingrid Tait, London, UK, 1989. Tait & Style specialize in imaginative and witty accessories using a range of textile techniques, including needle-punch felts, embroidery, and coarse and fine weaving and knitting. Scarves, gloves, socks, hats and quirky pieces, such as knitted necklaces, are regularly produced and sold in fashion outlets internationally. For several years design ideas were contributed by Freddie Robins (q.v.).

Koji Tatsuno b. Tokyo, Japan, 1964. Tatsuno came to London around 1982 and started working with old kimono fabrics, combining them into opulent shirts and waistcoats. Although he had no formal training in fashion, he used his clear vision and strong artisan skills of manipulation to build up a bespoke tailoring business (backed by Yohji Yamamoto, q.v.) which branched into highly creative one-off pieces. By 1993 he was fêted as a 'poète de vêtements'. He used unconventional materials, including safety pins, to build couture pieces, and developed chaotic web-like knitwear with Julien Macdonald (q.v.). In 1999 he launched a new label, Trace, using knitwear in several ways: recycled cardigans, oversize knitting and intriguing circular garments which fold around the body.

Atsuro Tayama b. Tokyo, Japan, 1955. After fashion college in Tokyo, Tayama worked as assistant to Yohji Yamamoto (q.v.), then became his European design director in Paris. He went on to design for Cacharel before showing his own collection in Paris in 1992. He is known for his asymmetric, wrapped and pleated silhouettes, occasionally in knitted fabric. Some of his sweaters have intriguing folded construction, others wrap the body in swathes of knit bandage. Even the simplest have built-in features, such as double layers and mittens. The autumn/winter 2000 collection included cut-up aran knit skirts, and pocket belts created from a cut-off cardigan worn round the hips.

Testu founded by Jean-Luc Testu, France, 2001. Having previously worked with Azzedine Alaïa (q.v.), Testu spent ten years designing menswear (for Thierry Mugler from 1996). He then launched his solo label, using modern yarns and knitting technology combined with architectural wovens to create clothes that are comfortable in movement.

Catherine Tough b. Cambridge, UK, 1975. Whilst maintaining a sense of playfulness, Tough explores

the broader application of knitted textiles within interiors. The work ranges from accessories, such as hot water bottle covers and bedsocks, to one-off upholstered pieces. Texture, comfort and desirability are the key factors.

Rosemarie Trockel b. Schwerte, Germany, 1952. Regarded as one of the most important contemporary German artists, Trockel brings a wide-ranging background to her work, having studied anthropology, theology, mathematics, sociology and painting. Her complex body of work includes sculptures, mixed media installations and painting. The original knitworks (balaclavas, repeating motif pictures, dresses) were created between 1985 and 1989, with further work (mobiles and screenprints of knitted fabric, and 'moth' pictures of slashed knitting) between 1992 and 1996. In 1992 she made a video, 'Wool', of a female wearing a sweater which eventually unravelled to nothing.

Jan Truman b. Birmingham, UK. Since 1986 Truman has worked in enamelled copper wire, glass and gemstones. The interplay of movement and light is explored through dancing spiral structures for interior and exterior use. The laborious but highly effective technique centres on machine- or hand-knitted wire, threaded with beads incorporated into the knitting process. Truman also creates a range of jewelry with characterful shapes, and has exhibited widely.

Tse design house founded by Augustine Tse, Hong Kong, 1989. Originally a Hong Kong-based manufacturing company, Tse now produces a range of lines, with a specialist focus on cashmere and other knitwear. Tse New York is the fashion-forward range, which recently collaborated with high profile fashion designers such as Narciso Rodriguez and Hussein Chalayan (q.v.) to create concepts for leading-edge collections. Fine gauge intarsia production is a speciality of the company.

Twincinc by Cinc, design company founded by Christophe Cottin and Christophe Contentin, Paris, France, 2000. The company creates modern twinsets for men, which offer an alternative to the traditional shirt and jacket. The two pieces of fine gauge knitwear are completely co-ordinated and include new details and finishes little used in knitwear, such as integral collars and ties, scarf collars and removable collars. Fabrics are all knitted jersey and range from fake fur to merino wools. Contentin previously worked for Dior (q.v.) and Lanvin.

Dries Van Noten b. Antwerp, Belgium, 1958. Known for his eclectic and confident treatment of colour, print and embroidery, Van Noten inspires a loyal following. Within the womenswear collections, knitwear is ever-present, not leading the way but accessorizing – a pretty ruched top, a patterned metallic yarn gilet. There is a tremendous attention to detail, for example the asymmetric fine cashmere tops from summer 2001, which drape at one side. Menswear always includes a range of knitwear – for winter 2001 chunky, slightly feminized, hairy yarns, and for summer 2002, a radical departure in space-dyed and bleached loose cardigans and sweaters, evocative of the hippy trail of the 1960s.

Joaquim Verdu b. Barcelona, Spain. Since 1991, Verdu has concentrated on fashion made from knitted fabrics, with woven fabrics playing a complementary role. Key factors are well-defined volumes, fluid lines and immaculate detailing. Colour is mostly plain, with variations in texture predominant. Verdu is unusual in keeping personal control of the entire design process.

Lynsey Walters graduated from the Royal College of Art, London (MA Constructed Textiles) in 2000.

Junya Watanabe b. Japan, 1961. A prodigious talent nurtured by Rei Kawakubo and working under the Comme des Garçons (q.v.) label, Watanabe has an uncompromisingly radical approach to clothes. He designs for the 'Tricot' range of Comme des Garçons in addition to his own line, which ironically does not involve much knitwear.

Sharon Wauchob b. Ireland. Wauchob approaches fashion from both a textile and silhouette viewpoint, creating extreme contrasts and juxtapositions. She worked with Koji Tatsuno (q.v.) and subsequently designed for Louis Vuitton. From 1998 she started her own label, s. wauchob, shown in Paris. Although untrained in knitwear, she conceives unusual knitted pieces, including the classic reinvention of detached trims in plain V-neck sweaters shown on the Vuitton catwalk.

Rebecca Webber graduated from Winchester School of Art (BA Textiles) in 2001.

Vivienne Westwood b. Glossop, UK, 1941. Following her punk era, Westwood turned to costume history, reworking the historical clothing of the English, Scottish and French aristocracy. In the late 1980s she appropriated classic weekend and sporting knitwear, such as the twinset and the argyll sweater and socks. She also reintroduced the corset and bustle. Westwood's knitted outfits (often complete with exuberant accessories) have incorporated many techniques, including complex lace stitching, applied embroidery and crochet, and have been made of many materials, including heavy cotton and chenille hand-knits as well as fine knitted jersey. Recent collections have included oversized hand-knitted cable sweaters, as well as innovative trompe l'oeil beaded 'sweaters' and 'cardigans', cleverly created in the image of cable knits.

Bernhard Willhelm b. Ulm, Germany, 1972. A 1998 graduate of the famed Royal Academy of Fine Arts in Antwerp, Willhelm has already forged his own path with two recent collections, both strongly themed but in completely contrasting styles. The first, spring/summer 2001, was faux-naïve, with a mix of 1950s advertising for home and kitchen with childlike pictorial designs for men and women in jacquard patterns and embroidery. These had a strong handcrafted feel and referenced the pictorial knit designs of the 1970s. The next collection was a mix of Arabic, Turkish and Afghan influences, but featuring eclectic knitwear, including co-ordinated stockings and socks, with a home-knitted retro feel.

Delphine Wilson Wilson sculpts hand-knitting to echo and contour lines of the body's musculature and bone structure. The fabric grows, divides and rejoins itself in ever-new configurations, intertwining patterns and forms to accentuate and expose areas of the body, or wrap it like a neverending moebius strip. Often using the natural weight and drape of viscose yarns, Wilson continually reinvents the notion of the sweater and the cardigan.

Marcia Windebank graduated from Central St Martins, London (BA Textiles) in 1999.

Wolford hosiery company founded by Reinhold Wolff and Walter Palmers, Bregenz, Germany, 1950. Manufacturers of luxury products for leg- and bodywear, with a strong focus on design and fashion co-ordination. Working with Santoni

(q.v.), the company is at the forefront of seamless technology for bodywear, which has extended to placement of motifs such as Fornasetti images. Wolford have collaborated with high-profile designers Philippe Starck and Jean Paul Gaultier (q.v.) to develop innovative products.

Erwin Wurm b. Austria, 1954. Wurm tests the boundaries of what can be termed 'sculpture' by using photography and video to cross between performance, art and document. His series of 'one minute sculptures' takes place in the street, choreographed into witty and absurd situations of objects and people (balancing on two oranges, for example). The pullover (sweater) is used repeatedly in Wurm's work – pulled over a pedestal, a trash-can, a head, two people... It becomes a catalyst for intervention, performance and ironic commentary.

Xuly Bet design label founded by Lamine Kouyate, Paris, France, 1989. Mali-born Kouyate's recycled 'shabby chic' clothes made from 'pre-worn' flea market finds caused a sensation in the winter 1992/93 season in Paris. His shows and studio were, in the tradition of contemporaries such as Margiela (q.v.), in abandoned Parisian buildings. Cut-up knitwear was overlocked together with external seams, and threads were left trailing – now a familiar deconstructionist sign.

Yohji Yamamoto b. Yokohama, Japan, 1943. Yamamoto approaches knitwear boldly and with few preconceptions. His Y's label includes a wide range of knitwear that plays with proportion and, particularly, construction, using layering and reversibility. A notable feature is the use of unusual garment shapes: they may have an asymmetrical silhouette or curved arms. Many designs feature a twisted, distorted look, with seams in the 'wrong' place – often simply the result of the natural characteristics of a high-twist, single-spun yarn knitted in single jersey. Yamamoto has also favoured the use of large-scale knits for outerwear in both men's and women's collections. Surprising configurations often mark these out: off the body it can be unclear how a piece is to be worn, or how extra fabric is to be used. The collection utilizes the natural structure of knitted fabrics, such as curling edges, combined with the designer's agile imagination, which can visualize inside, outside and their possible interconnections, in an almost topological manner.

beam part of a weaving loom or warp knitting machine around which the warp threads are wound, set horizontally in position

bearded needle the original type of knitting element used on the earliest knitting machines and still used today on some straight bar and warp knitting machines. This knitting element, made from one piece of sprung steel with its tip bent back, requires the use of a presser bar to form knitted loops.

circular knitting a type of weft knitting by hand or circular machine in which the direction of knitting is constant, creating a seamless tube of continuous spiral formation

compound needle knitting element, used in specialist machines, similar to a latch needle but with a sliding latch movement which opens and closes the hook of the needle

course sequence of loops formed in horizontal direction across a knitted fabric during the knitting process. In hand-knitting this is known as a 'row' of knitting.

cut-and-sew knitwear fully cut from jersey fabrics or from garment blanks, which may have some trims included. Garment-length knitting sequences are produced on both circular and flat-bed machines, separated by 'draw threads' in continuous production. A typical sweater may have back and front cut from one piece and sleeves from another, creating wastage.

double bed knitting machine with two needle beds

double jacquard jacquard fabric based on rib structure created on a double-bed flat knitting machine or circular rib machine, in which one needle bed knits the colour pattern on the face of the fabric and the other knits the yarn which would otherwise float on the back of the fabric

float jacquard created on a single needle bed machine, with floats of yarn at the back of the fabric where needles of each colour are missed in the pattern selection

fully fashioned the shaping of individual garment pieces during knitting so that each edge is a selvedge. Shapings are often decorative, especially at the armholes, forming characteristic marks near the edge of the fabric, and leaving a clean edge for seaming. Used in high quality knitwear. The fully fashioned markings where stitches have been transferred are regarded as a mark of quality. As there is no wastage, luxury knitwear in yarns such as cashmere are produced in this manner. The recent trend for trimless knitwear has removed some of the adding of welts, collars and edgings after knitting, thus reducing labour costs.

garment blank unshaped piece of knitted fabric from which garment shapes are cut, created from a garment knitting sequence usually incorporating a welt at the lower edge and other design features.

gauge system of measuring the linear spacing of needles in a knitting machine needle bed, either in needles per inch or per 1.5 inches. The larger the number, the finer the gauge and the finer the resulting fabric. Known as the English system (used worldwide) and denoted by the letter E.

guide bar component of a warp knitting machine which contains multiple yarn feeders threaded with the warp threads from a beam. Feeds yarn to all the needles across the width of the machine simultaneously, one feeder per needle.

intarsia single-bed weft fabric with coloured pattern formed of solid areas of colour through which no other colour passes

integral knitting garments – complete with finishing details – based on tubular knitting, requiring a minimal amount of cutting or seaming, and produced entirely on either a circular or specialized flat V-bed machine

jacquard term originating from woven fabrics, also applied to knitted weft fabric in which two or more coloured yarns each knit a selection of needles to create a pre-determined colour pattern; variations use contrast in texture rather than colour

jersey general term for fine weft-knitted fabric (usually above gauge 16) made on circular machines as bulk fabric: either single jersey (one set of needles) or double jersey (two sets of needles)

latch needle knitting element consisting of a hooked needle with a moveable latch which opens and closes the hook during the knitting cycle to form knitted loops

making up general term for the processes involved in creating a garment from pieces of knitted fabric. Making-up techniques include:
   cup seaming cup seamer grips fabric vertically between two feeder wheels and produces a two-thread lock stitch, using feeding and guiding mechanisms specifically designed for knitted fabric with selvedges
   link overlocker combines both random linking and overlocking functions. Being a dial machine with points, which also cuts and overlocks the edges, it is suitable for a wide range of knitted fabrics and is excellent for pattern matching.
   mock/random linking uses point-to-point machinery but without accurate correspondence of points to stitches, thus requiring less skill
   overlocking most often used for cut-and-sewn knitwear to cover cut edges and seam simultaneously. There is considerable flexibility in the resulting seam, which is essential for knitwear.
   point-to-point linking uses a machine with a dial of points that corresponds to the stitch gauge of the fabric and sews with matching yarn in single chain stitch. Used mainly for very high quality attaching of neckline trims, resulting in an elastic seam. The knitted fabric is introduced vertically to the points to avoid stretching.

microfibre very fine manmade fibre, with a thickness of less than 0.1 tex – about 60 times finer than human hair. Made by splitting filaments into finer components.

monofilament a yarn which is formed of only one continuous length of fibre, and not twisted or spun. A common example is nylon monofilament, as used for fishing line.

needle bed set of knitting elements of a knitting machine arranged either in linear or circular formation

polymer general class of compounds with molecules arranged in long chain formation, suitable for textile fibres

selvedge closed edge of a knitted or woven fabric resulting from the yarns changing direction at each edge of the cloth width

shibori Japanese shape or stitch resist dyeing technique in which fabric is drawn up and stitched tightly in areas, before dyeing. When dyed, the stitches are removed to create a pattern where the dye has not penetrated through the layers.

single bed knitting machine with one needle bed

space-dyeing method of dyeing yarns in several colours or shades, in which the colour changes along the length in a repeating sequence, giving a variegated appearance to the final fabric

tuck stitch incomplete knitting action resulting in a loop or loops held in the hook of a latch needle for several rows or courses of knitting, used for decorative or textural effect. Tends to spread the width of the resulting fabric.

wale line of stitches flowing vertically through a fabric, parallel to the selvedges, formed by one needle or stitch

warp term applied to vertical threads running the length of the fabric on a weaving loom or in woven cloth

warp knitting process of machine-knitting in which multiple threads running the length of a fabric are formed simultaneously into vertical chains of stitches interlinked to each other to create a fabric

weft term applied to horizontal threads running across the width of a woven fabric, or the thread used during weaving

weft knitting process of hand- or machine-knitting in which the fabric is built up in horizontal rows of loops knitted sequentially by a single thread or a small number of threads passing across the width

worsted method of spinning wool in which the staple fibres are combed parallel to each other, resulting in a smooth yarn

Textiles and Textile Technology

Anstey, Helen, and Terry Weston, *The Anstey Weston Guide to Textile Terms*, London, 1997

Brackenbury, Terry, *Knitted Clothing Technology*, Oxford, 1992

Braddock, Sarah E., and Marie O'Mahony, *Techno Textiles*, London, 1998

Colchester, Chloë, *The New Textiles, Trends and Traditions*, London, 1991

Corbman, Bernard P., *Textiles: Fiber to Fabric*, New York, 1983

Feder, Ruven, and Jean-Michel Glasman, *Socks Story*, Paris, 1992

Hatch, Kathryn L., *Textile Science*, Minneapolis, MN, 1993

Hongu Tatsuya, and Glyn O. Phillips, *New Fibres*, Cambridge, 1997

Lewis, Susanna E., and Julia Weissman, *A Machine Knitter's Guide to Creating Fabrics*, Asheville, NC, 1986

Macintyre, Jane, and Paul N. Daniels (eds), *Textile Terms and Definitions*, The Textile Institute, Manchester, 1995

Millington, John, and Stanley Chapman, *Four Centuries of Machine Knitting*, Bradford, 1989

Paling, D. F., *Warp Knitting Technology*, Manchester, CT, 1965

Philips Electronics, *New Nomads: An Exploration of Wearable Electronics*, Rotterdam, 2000

Spencer, David J., *Knitting Technology*, Cambridge, 2001

Tao, Xiaoming (ed), *Smart Fibres, Fabrics and Clothing*, Cambridge, 2001

Taylor, Marjorie A., *Technology of Textile Properties: An Introduction*, London, 1990

Thomas, Mary, *Mary Thomas's Knitting Book*, London, 1985

Walker, Barbara G., *A Treasury of Knitting Patterns*, New York, 1968

— *A Second Treasury of Knitting Patterns*, New York, 1970

— *Charted Knitting Designs*, New York, 1972

Fashion Designers and Directories

Alaïa, Azzedine, *Alaïa*, Göttingen, 1998

Azzedine Alaïa Livre de Collections, Eté 1992, Paris, 1992

Baudot, François, *Alaïa*, London, 1996

— *Christian Lacroix*, London, 1996

— *Elsa Schiaparelli*, London, 1997

— *Yohji Yamamoto*, London, 1997

Bénaïm, Laurence, *Issey Miyake*, London, 1997

Buxbaum, Gerda (ed), *Icons of Fashion: the 20th Century*, Munich, 1999

Callan, Georgina O'Hara, *Dictionary of Fashion and Fashion Designers*, London, 1998

Chenoune, Farid, *Jean Paul Gaultier*, London, 1996

de la Haye, Amy, and Shelley Tobin, *Chanel: The Couturiere at Work*, London, 1994

Derycke, Luc, and Sandra van de Veire (eds), *Belgian Fashion Design*, Amsterdam, 1999

The Fashion Book, London, 1998

Frankel, Susannah, *Visionaries: Interviews with Fashion Designers*, London, 2001

Holborn, Mark, *Issey Miyake*, Cologne, 1995

Issey Miyake Bodyworks, Tokyo, 1983

Issey Miyake and Miyake Design Studio, 1970–1985, Tokyo, 1985

Issey Miyake by Irving Penn, Miyake Design Studio, Tokyo, 1989, 1990, 1992, 1995, 1997

Irving Penn Regards the Work of Issey Miyake, London, 1999

Koike, Kazuko, *Issey Miyake East Meets West*, Tokyo, Japan, 1978

Koren, Leonard, *New Fashion Japan*, Tokyo, Japan, 1984

Krell, Gene, *Vivienne Westwood*, London, 1997

Martin, Richard (ed), *Contemporary Fashion*, London, 1995

Mauriès, Patrick, *Christian Lacroix: The Diary of a Collection*, London, 1996

Mazza, Samuele, and Mariuccia Casadio, *Missoni*, London, 1998

McDowell, Colin, *Jean Paul Gaultier*, London, 2001

Menkes, Suzy, *The Knitwear Revolution*, London, 1983

Mulvagh, Jane, *Vivienne Westwood: An Unfashionable Life*, London, 1998

Notebook on Cities and Clothes: film about Yohji Yamamoto, directed by Wim Wenders, 1989

Sainderichin, Ginette, *Kenzo*, London, 1999

— *Kenzo*, Paris, 1989

Sheard, Stephen, *Rowan's Designer Collection: Summer and Winter Knitting*, London, 1987

Street Magazine, Maison Martin Margiela Special, Volumes 1 & 2, Paris, 1999

Sudjic, Dejan, *Rei Kawakubo and Comme des Garçons*, New York, 1990

Takada, Kenzo, *Kenzo*, Tokyo, Japan, 1985

Tucker, Andrew, *The London Fashion Book*, London, 1998

— *Dries Van Noten*, London, 1999

Vercelloni, Isa Tutino (ed), *Missonologia: Il Mondo dei Missoni/The World of Missoni*, Milan, 1994

White, Palmer, *Elsa Schiaparelli, Empress of Fashion*, London, 1986

Windels, V., *Young Belgian Fashion Design*, Amsterdam, 2001

Worsley, Harriet, *Decades of Fashion* (The Hulton Getty Picture Collection), Cologne, 2000

Fashion Theory: Culture and History

Ash, Juliet, and Elizabeth Wilson (eds), *Chic Thrills: A Fashion Reader*, London, 1992

Barthes, Roland, *The Fashion System*, London, 1985

Bolton, Andrew, *The Supermodern Wardrobe*, London, 2002

Breward, Christopher, *The Culture of Fashion: A New History of Fashionable Dress*, Manchester, 1995

Craik, Jennifer, *The Face of Fashion: Cultural Studies in Fashion*, London, 1993

Entwistle, Joanne, *The Fashioned Body: Fashion, Dress and Modern Social Theory*, Cambridge, 2000

Italian Fashion, Vol. 1: The Origins of High Fashion and Knitwear, Milan, 1987

Macdonald, Anne L., *No Idle Hands: The Social History of American Knitting*, New York, 1988

Martin, Richard, *Fashion and Surrealism*, New York, 1987

McDermott, Catherine, *Street Style: British Design in the 80s*, London, 1987

McRobbie, Angela, *British Fashion Design: Rag Trade or Image Industry?*, London, 1998

Müller, Florence, *Art & Fashion*, London, 2000

Parker, Rozsika, *The Subversive Stitch: Embroidery and the Making of the Feminine*, London, 1984

Rutt, Richard, *A History of Handknitting*, London, 1987

Vergani, Guido, *The Sala Bianca: The Birth of Italian Fashion*, Milan, 1992

White, Nicola, *Reconstructing Italian Fashion (America and the Development of the Italian Fashion Industry)*, Oxford, 2000

— and Ian Griffiths (eds), *The Fashion Business: Theory, Practice, Image*, Oxford, 2000

Wilson, Elizabeth, *Adorned in Dreams: Fashion and Modernity*, London, 1985

— and Lou Taylor, *Through the Looking Glass: A History of Dress from 1860 to the Present Day*, London, 1989

Exhibition Catalogues and Related Books

Addressing the Century: 100 Years of Art and Fashion, Hayward Gallery, London, 1998

Alaïa, The Groninger Museum, Groningen, 1998

A-POC Making: Issey Miyake and Dai Fujiwara, Vitra Design Museum, Berlin, 2001

Beyond Japan, Barbican Art Gallery, London, 1991

The Cutting Edge: 50 Years of British Fashion 1947–1997 (ed Amy de la Haye), V&A Museum, London, 1996

Droog & Dutch Design, Centraal Museum Utrecht, 2000

Erwin Wurm Kunstverein, Hamburg and Villa Arson, Nice, 1993

Erwin Wurm: One-Minute Sculptures, The Photographers' Gallery, London, 2000

Fabric of Fashion (Sarah Braddock and Marie O'Mahony), British Council, 2000

Fashions by Jürgen Lehl, Gemeentemuseum, The Hague, 2000

Issey Miyake A-UN, Musée des Arts Decoratifs, Paris, 1988; *Issey Miyake Photographs by Irving Penn*, New York, 1988

Issey Miyake Bodyworks: Fashion Without Taboos, V&A Museum, London, 1985

Issey Miyake Making Things, Fondation Cartier pour l'Art Contemporain, Paris, 1998

Issey Miyake Pleats Please, Touko Museum of Contemporary Art, Tokyo, 1990

Issey Miyake Ten Sen Men, Hiroshima City Museum of Contemporary Art, Hiroshima, 1990

Japan Style, V&A Museum, London, 1980

Jouer la Lumière, Musée de la Mode et du Textile, Paris, 2001

Kaffe Fassett at the V&A, V&A Museum, London, 1988

Knit One, Purl One: Historic and Contemporary Knitting from the V&A's Collection (Frances Hinchcliffe), V&A Museum, London, 1985

Knitting: A Common Art (June Freeman), Minories Colchester and Aberystwyth Arts Centre, 1986

Krizia: Una Storia/A Story (Isa Tutino Vercelloni), Il Palazzo della Triennale, Milan, 1995

Looking at Fashion (Germano Celant), 1st Biennale on Fashion and Art, Florence, 1996

Lost and Found: Critical Voices in New British Design (Nick Barley), British Council, 1999

Mil Anys de Disseny en Punt (1000 years of Knitting), Museu Tèxtil, Terrassa, 1997

Mode et Art 1960–1990, Palais des Beaux-arts, Brussels, 1995

The New Knitting (Sandy Black), London College of Fashion, 2000

9/4/1615 Martin Margiela, Museum Boijmans Van Beuningen, Rotterdam, 1997

Radical Fashion (ed Claire Wilcox), V&A Museum, London, 2001

Revelation, The Barbican, London, 1997, and National Museum of Modern Art, Tokyo, 1998

Rosemarie Trockel, Institute of Contemporary Art, Boston, 1991; *Rosemarie Trockel* (ed Sidra Stich), Cologne, 1991

Rosemarie Trockel: Bodies of Work 1986–1998, Whitechapel Art Gallery, London, and Kunsthalle Hamburg, 1998

Satellites of Fashion (Claire Wilcox), Crafts Council, London, 2000

Slipstitch: New Concepts in Knitting (John Allen), Textile Museum Tilburg, 2000

Streetstyle (Ted Polhemus), V&A Museum, London, 1994

Structure and Surface: Contemporary Japanese Textiles (Carla McCarty and Matilda McQuaid), Museum of Modern Art, New York, 1998

The Subversive Stitch: Women and Textiles Today and Embroidery in Women's Lives 1300–1900 (Pennina Barnett), Whitworth Gallery and Cornerhouse Art Gallery, Manchester, 1988

Textural Space: Contemporary Japanese Textile Art (Lesley Millar), Surrey Institute of Art and Design, 2001

Picture Credits

L = Left, C = Centre, R = Right, T = Top, B = Bottom

Jörgen Ahlström, courtesy Artwork p. 17 TL
Mert Alas and Marcus Piggott, courtesy Missoni p. 30
Gregoire Alexandre, courtesy of Twincinc p. 27 R
S. Ansai, courtesy Issey Miyake p. 122
Courtesy Artwork p. 15 R
Doug Atfield p. 133
Courtesy Ballantyne p. 174 B
Courtesy Emily Bates p. 137
Anna Beeke pp. 158 L and R, 159 L and R
Courtesy Heather Belcher pp. 138-9, 139
Sandy Black pp. 58 BL, 61 background, 69 R, 78-9
    background, 80 L, 81 R, 89 R, 99 T, 136, 138 L, 170 L,
    170-1, 173 L, 176 T and C, 177 C and B, 178 C, 180 B
    and collection of Sandy Black pp. 13 TL
Mark Borthwick, courtesy Maison Martin Margiela p. 75 R
Courtesy Cristina Brown p. 165 L
Courtesy Michael Clark p. 153 R
Courtesy Collezioni pp. 25 L, 110-11, 112 R, 160
Miles Comfort pp. 156, 157 T and B
Courtesy Gina Conquest pp. 71-2
Courtesy The Constance Howard Textiles Study Collection,
    Goldsmiths College, London University p. 147 C and R
Courtesy Coogi p. 21 R
Courtesy Courtaulds Textiles p. 14 L
Jonty Davis p. 131 R
Horst Diekgerdes, courtesy Missoni p. 23 L
Courtesy Dolce & Gabbana p. 38
F. Dumoulin, courtesy Sonia Rykiel p. 50 L and R
Chris Dunlop p. 95 T
Courtesy Rebecca Earley p. 76 R
Sean Ellis pp. 40-41
Eric Emo, courtesy Testu pp. 130 L and R, 131 L
Peter Everard Smith pp. 80-81, 84 L, 97 L, 175 B, 177 T
Courtesy Fake London p. 39 L and BR
Robert Ferrier, courtesy Lainey Keogh pp. 34 L, 35 R
Diagrams courtesy Forbes Publications p. 174 T (adapted
    by Karolina Prymaka) and C
Courtesy Shelley Fox p. 59 L
Jens Friis pp. 69 L, 82-3
Mitsumara Fujitsuka, courtesy Issey Miyake p. 119 L
Gry Garness, courtesy Jo Gordon p. 54
Courtesy Lisa Gatherar p. 171 B
Courtesy Jean Paul Gaultier p. 73 C
Ron Geesin pp. 73 R, 88 L, 144 L and R, 145
Courtesy Nichola Gowing p. 169 T
Tim Griffiths p. 41 R
Wade H. Grimbly p. 76 L
Eszter Grurjan p. 56
Courtesy Shirin Guild p. 27 L
Nick Guttridge, courtesy salt p. 172
Courtesy Isabelle Harman pp. 72-3
Friedmann Hauss, courtesy Issey Miyake p. 121 L and R
Frank Hills pp. 64 TL and B, 65, 140, 140-1, 141
Courtesy Hulton Getty p. 12
Courtesy Tracy Hunt p. 74 L
Len Ivins pp. 64-5 background, 147 background
Courtesy Mie Iwatsubo p. 1
Courtesy Jan & Carlos p. 94
Courtesy Mair Joint p. 147 L
Courtesy Adam Jones p. 33 L and R
Ivan Jones pp. 101 L, 124, 125 L and R, 178 B
Courtesy Niki Jones p. 171 T
Jean François José, courtesy Comme des Garçons p. 103 L
Courtesy Tamara Kemoklidse p. 89 L
Neil Kirk, courtesy Elle UK p. 11 and courtesy Vogue Spain,
    p. 67
Tatsuya Kitayama, courtesy Maison Martin Margiela p. 99 B
Réka Kövesdi pp. 52, 53, 169 B
Courtesy Alice Lee p. 72 L and R

Courtesy Marie Lenclos p. 146
Courtesy Nuala MacCulloch p. 87 R
Courtesy Maison Martin Margiela pp. 116 L, 116-17, 117 R
Jean Marc, courtesy salt pp. 172-3
Courtesy Matec p. 126
Courtesy Matta p. 164 L
Michael Maynard p. 95 B
Eammon J. McCabe, courtesy Rowan Yarns pp. 20 R, 36 R
Craig McDean, courtesy Tse p. 17 TR
Niall McInerney pp. 18 L, 19 R, 21 L, 24 L and R, 26, 28 L, 28 R
    (29 L), 29 R, 32, 34 R, 36 L, 37 L and R, 43 L (42 L and R),
    48 L and R, 49 L and R, 51 L and R, 59 R, 77 L, 78 L, 79,
    91 R, 93, 102-3, 103 R, 106, 107 R, 108 L and R, 109, 110 L
    and R, 123 T, 152-3
David McIntyre p. 20 L
Courtesy Alexander McQueen pp. 90, 91 L, 92
Raymond Meier, courtesy Vogue Paris p. 57 BL
Courtesy Simone Memel p. 58 BR
Judy Montgomery, courtesy Stevie Stewart p. 153 L
Chris Moore, courtesy Hussein Chalayan pp. 104 L, C and R,
    105 L and R; courtesy Shelley Fox pp. 19 L, 114 L
Sarah Morris p. 134
Courtesy Georgina Naish pp. 4-5
Courtesy Suzumi Noda pp. 148, 149
Courtesy Hikaru Noguchi pp. 55, 166, 167 T and B;
Courtesy Monika Olszynska pp. 86-7
A. de Parseval, courtesy Issey Miyake p. 77 R
Vikas Patel p. 84 R;
Angelo Pennetta p. 98 TL, TR and B
Courtesy Stephanie Piogé p. 61 T
David Price p. 39 background
Courtesy Pringle pp. 13 R, 15 L
Alan Randall, stylist Georgia Loizou p. 163
Courtesy Rex Features p. 14 R
Linda Rich pp. 154 B, 154-5, 155 R;
Courtesy Freddie Robins p. 135 R
Courtesy John Rocha p. 47 R
Pascal Roulin, courtesy Issey Miyake pp. 118, 119 R
Courtesy Royal College of Art, London pp. 41 L, 87 L
Craig Sanders, courtesy Alan Gallacher p. 57 TL and R
Steve Savage, make-up Christiane Carard pp. 114-15
Bob Seago pp. 68, 70, 81, 82 L, 83 R
Courtesy John Smedley p. 16
Bob Smith p. 85 L and R
Courtesy Marina Spadafora pp. 25 R, 47 L, 78 R
Courtesy Monika Sprüth Gallery, Cologne, Germany p. 142
    background and inset, p. 143
Patrice Stable, courtesy Jean Paul Gaultier p. 43 R
    and courtesy Dries Van Noten p. 22 L and C
Courtesy Lawrence Steele p. 46 R
Chloe Stewart pp. 150-51, 151 R
Courtesy Stoll Knitting pp. 127, 178 T;
Peter Tahl, courtesy Groninger Museum, Groningen,
    Netherlands p. 180 T
Courtesy Tait & Style p. 165 R
Yuriko Takagi, courtesy Jürgen Lehl pp. 44, 62 L and C,
    62-3 background
Eva Takamine, courtesy Jürgen Lehl pp. 45 L and R, 175 T,
    176 B
Courtesy Atsuro Tayama pp. 97 C, 101 R
Mario Testino, courtesy Missoni pp. 2-3, 23 R, 31 L and R
Jamie Thompson p. 135 L
Frank Thurnston pp. 74-5
Courtesy Catherine Tough pp. 162, 164-5
Courtesy Dries Van Noten p. 17 BR
Tessa Verder, courtesy Simone Memel p. 58 TR
Elle Verhagen and Carmen Freudenthal, courtesy Bernhard
    Willhelm p. 100
Courtesy Lynsey Walters p. 62 R
Courtesy Sharon Wauchob p. 115 L and R
Courtesy Rebecca Webber p. 88 R
Bruce Weber p. 175 C

The Wellcome Trust, courtesy Susie Freeman p. 150 L
Kim Weston Arnold, courtesy Tony Glenville pp. 17 BL, 18 R, 22
    R, 35 L, 46 L, 71, 96 L (96-7), 107 L, 111 R, 112 L, 113, 120
Luke White, courtesy salt p. 173 R
Courtesy Bernhard Willhelm pp. 61 B, 63
Courtesy Marcia Windebank pp. 7, 168
Courtesy Wolford pp. 60, 128, 128-9, 129
Courtesy Woolmark (formerly International Wool Secretariat)
    p. 13 BL
Courtesy Erwin Wurm p. 161 L and R
Courtesy Yohji Yamamoto p. 97 R
Yasuaki Yoshinaga, courtesy Issey Miyake p. 123 B

Acknowledgments

This book has been accomplished with the aid of a travel
grant from the Arts and Humanities Research Board (AHRB)
and with the support of the London College of Fashion.
Thanks are due to Elizabeth Rouse and colleagues in the
department, to Caterina Radvan, Martina Steinmetz and
Janice Miller for their invaluable assistance with research.
I would like to thank all the designers, artists, companies
and press officers who provided time, images and
information, including Machiko Agano; Azzedine Alaïa and
Olivier; Artwork; Ian Ewing, Claire Dawson, Clive Brown and
Teresa White at Ballantyne; Maria Blaisse; Stevie Stewart;
Ernestina Cerini; Omar at Hussein Chalayan; Emma for
Clements Ribeiro; Trevor Collins; Haruko at Comme des
Garçons; Julia Lamb at Coogi; Paola Locati at Dolce &
Gabbana; Christian Dufay; Dean at Fake London; Nicole
Farhi; Nora Fok; Shelley Fox; Susie Freeman; Orsola de
Castro of From Somewhere; Alan Gallacher; Lisa Gatherar;
Lionel Vermeil and Léopoldine at Jean Paul Gaultier;
Frances Geesin; Jo Gordon; Marten de Leeuw and Rob
Dijkstra at The Groninger Museum; Shirin Guild; Tracy Hunt;
Elena for Jan & Carlos; Adam Jones; Joseph; Judit Kárpáti-
Rácz; Caroline Randolfi at Kenzo; Lainey Keogh and Cha
Cha Seigne; Alice Smith and Lee Farmer; Jürgen Lehl, Eva
Takamine, and Ricarda Heubel; Winni Lok; Julien Macdonald
and Emma Greenhill; Adeline Cousin at Maison Martin
Margiela; Matta; Amy Witton at Alexander McQueen; Simone
Memel; Deanna Ferretti, Maria and Nina at Miss Deanna;
Chiara at Missoni; Dai Fujiwara and Lydia Phelan at Issey
Miyake; Hikaru Noguchi; Davina Payne, Karen Thompson
and Colin Anderson at Pringle; Victoria Rance; Patricia
Roberts; Freddie Robins; Christine Bryan for John Rocha;
Ann-Louise Roswald; Kathleen Hargreaves at Rowan
Yarns; Jerome Pulis at Sonia Rykiel; Karina Thomas of salt;
Valentina Gentilini at Santoni; Shima Seiki; Julie Skarland;
Jackie Turner at John Smedley; Marina Spadafora; Nick
Vinson at Lawrence Steele; Oliver Vogt, Petra Meyer and
Marten Ligner at Stoll Knitting; Koji Tatsuno; Pascal and
Isobel at Atsuro Tayama; Lilian Haberer for Rosemarie
Trockel at Monika Sprüth Gallery; Jan Truman; Terrence
Charles at Tse; Jean-Luc Dupont for Twincinc and Testu;
Laetitia Rambaud at Dries Van Noten; Sharon Wauchob;
Timothy Clifton Green at Vivienne Westwood; Marilyn at
Bernhard Willhelm; Delphine Wilson; Sidoné at Wolford;
Erwin Wurm and Sandra Frank; Emma Greenhalgh at Yohji
Yamamoto. My apologies to designers who could not be
included due to reasons of space. I would also like to thank
the photographers, in particular Niall McInerney and Ivan
Jones; Inge Cordson of Livingstone Studio London and
Keiko Kawashima of KICTAC, Kyoto, for assistance with
the Japanese research; Ornella Bignami of Elementi Moda
for assistance with Italian research; and Tony Glenville
for generous access to his collection. I am grateful for
comments on the text from Amy de la Haye, Diana Coben
and Vikki Haffenden, and to Rosie Marshall and Annie Black
for additional assistance in gathering material. Thanks also
to Brenda Polan and Suzy Menkes. Special thanks for their
encouragement and support to my husband Morris, and
to Linda, family and friends.

Numbers in *italics* refer to illustrations

Agano, Machiko 136, *138*
Alaïa, Azzedine 28, *29*, 71, 82, 155, *175*, *180*
Alice Lee *72*, *80-1*, *84*, 90, 94, *97*, *175*, *177*, *177*
A-POC 9, 106, 118, *118*, *119*, 120, *120*, *121*, *122*, *123*, *123*, *178*
aran *17*, *39*, *42*, 68, *77*, 152, 176, 179
argyll 15, *17*, *24*, *39*, 176
Artwork *15*, *17*, 68

Ballantyne 15, *174*, 176
Barrie 15
Bates, Emily 134, *136*, *137*
Bayliss, Nadine *154*, *154-5*
beading 12, 28, 79
Belcher, Heather *138-9*, *139*
Benetton 12, 118
Biagiotti, Laura 12
Bigley, Sarah *89*
Bis, Dorothée 12
Black, Sandy *20*
Blaisse, Maria 155, *158*, *159*
blister fabric 88, *176*, *177*; stitch *124*
Body Map 32, *36*, *37*, 152, *152-3*, *153*
bouclé *49*, 180
Bowery, Leigh 152, *153*
Bramwell, Maya 71, *87*
Branquinho, Véronique 90
Branston, Leonie *70*
Brown, Cristina *165*
Bruce, Liza 71

cable *42-3*, *43*, *95*, *115*, 176
Carrick, Kate *82*, *177*
Castra, Orsola de 113
Cerini, Ernestina 90, 94, *112*
Chalayan, Hussein *17*, 90, *104*, *105*, 134
Chanel, Coco 10, *12*, *26*, 32, 40, 52, 57, 152
circular knitting *124*, 174-5
Clark, Michael 152, *152-3*, *153*
Clements Ribeiro 15, *18*, *22*
cloqué, *see* blister fabric
Collins, Trevor *154*, *154-5*, 155
Comme des Garçons 15, 28, 54, 94, *102*, *103*, *177*, *177*
Conquest, Gina *70-1*
Coogi *21*, *177*
Courtaulds Fibres *14*, 152, 179
crochet 32, *33*, 34, *36*, *42-3*, *43*, 47, 52, 53, *63*, *79*, 91, *109*, *111*, 140, 164, 175; mock 175
cut-and-sew fabric 8, 26, 28, *72*, 174, 175, 178

Dallas, Sarah 12
Dior, Christian, 28, *32*, 52, 54, 94
Dolce & Gabbana *38*
Droog Design 164
Duckworth, Susan 12
Dufay, Christian 164, *170-1*
DuPont 179
Dyson, Emily *163*

Earley, Rebecca 71, *76*
elastomeric fibres *82*, 152, 177
embroidery 12, 30, 32, 51, 53, *100*, 175
Expandtex *69*

Fake London *39*, 94, 113
Farhi, Nicole 30, 155
Fendi 52, *57*
Foale, Marion 12
Fok, Nora 53, *64*, *65*, 136, *140-1*, *141*
Fox, Shelley *19*, *59*, 71, 90, 94, *114*, 155
Freeman, Susie 150, *150-1*, *151*, 177
French knitting *156*, *157*
Fujiwara, Dai 120, *123*

Gallacher, Alan *57*
Galliano, John *32*, *35*, 54, 94
Gatherar, Lisa *171*
Gaultier, Jean Paul *17*, 28, *42-3*, *73*, 94, *129*, *129*, 152, 176
Gee, Christine *82*
Geesin, Frances *73*, *88*, *144*, *145*
Genny *18*
Givenchy 40
Gordon, Jo *54*
Gowing, Nichola *169*
Gucci 52, 57
Guild, Shirin 15, *27*, 92

Harman, Isabelle *73*
Høj, Iben 68, *69*, *82-3*
Holah, David 32, 152
Hunt, Tracy *74*

intarsia 18, 20, *21*, 68, 94, *102*, *154*, *154-5*, *174*, *174*, 175-6, *177*, 178; mock 15, 176
interlock fabric 175
Iwatsubo, Mie 53, *62-3*

Jackson, Betty *24*, 30
Jacobs, Marc 15
jacquard 21, *23*, 26, 28, *29*, 32, *37*, 46, 48, *51*, 54, *60-1*, *61*, *74*, *82*, 88, 94, *100*, 127, *129*, 166, *174*, 175, *176*, 177
Jan & Carlos 94
Jansen, Lisa *85*
Joint, Mair *147*
Jones, Adam *33*
Jones, Niki *171*
Jones, Val 155
Joseph 32; Tricot *20*

Kagami, Kei 94, *114-15*
Kagan, Sasha 12
Kárpáti-Rácz, Judit *52*, 53, *53*, *56*, *169*
Kawakubo, Rei 90, 92, 102, 114, 134, 152
Keily, Orla 53
Kemoklidse, Tamara *89*
Kenzo 15, 30, 32, *51*, 52; Jungle Jap 32
Keogh, Lainey 32, *34*, *35*
Kidman, Martin *20*
knitting machines 8, 174-5, *176*, 178; *see also* Matec, Santoni, Shima Seiki, Stoll
Krizia 12, *21*

lace 6, 28, *33*, 34, *35*, *40-1*, *41*, *43*, *46-7*, *47*, *48*, 53, *59*, *70*, 88, 92, *168*, 175, *176*, *176*
Lacroix, Christian 28, *46*, *73*
Lagerfeld, Karl 32, *34*, 40, 52
Lee, Liz *150*
Lee, William 8
Leger, Hervé 71, *129*
Lenclos, Marie *146*
Lehl, Jürgen *44-5*, *62*, *62-3*, *175*, 180
Lok, Winni 92, 104

MacCulloch, Nuala *87*, 176
Macdonald, Julien 32, *34*, *40-1*, 68, *78*, *78-9*, *79*, *111*
macramé 113
Maloney, Emma *83*
Margiela, Martin 68, 71, *75*, *77*, 90, 92, *99*, 113, *116*, *117*
Marni *58*
Marseille, Karen 159
Matec *126*
materials:
  acetate *74*, *80*; alpaca *25*, 179; angora *20*, 50, *85*, 179; calico 88; camel hair *67*; carbon 164; cardboard 80; cashmere 10, *11*, 15, *17*, *18*, *22*, *27*, *39*, 57, *72*, *82*, *85*, 86, 94, *104*, 113,

179; chenille *29*, 34, *43*, *51*, 180, *180*; cotton *45*, *48*, *62*, *77*, *98*, 120, *121*, 147, *167*, *168*, *172-3*, 176, 179; elastane *121*, *130*, 179; flax 179; hair *136*, *137*, 179; jersey 12, 32, *37*, *60-1*, 68, *69*, 71, 75, 92, 94, *103*, *104*, 106, *107*, 152, *153*, 164, 174, 175, *177*, 178, 179, 180; lambswool *62-3*, *124*, *125*, *162*, *165*; leather 71, *80-1*, *81*, 88; linen 10, *125*, 179; Lurex *74*, *138*, 180; Lycra 28, 32, *37*, 71, *82*, *83*, *84*, 89, 94, 114, 152, *154*, *154-5*, 179; Maxxam 71, 152, *180*; merino *19*, 57, 90; mohair *32*, *33*, *47*, 54, *58*, *110*, 179; nylon *47*, 52, 53, *56*, 64, 66, 68, *68*, *74*, *78-9*, *87*, *102*, *110*, *121*, *124*, *136*, *138*, *140*, *140-1*, *144*, *147*, *156*, *157*, *171*, *179*; organsin *171*; paper 66, *138*, *168*; plastic 66, 68, 71, 74, 75, 88; polyester *46-7*, 66, *76*, 71, 92, 179; polyethylene *74*, 180; raffia *48*, *78*; rayon 179, 180; rope 54, *58*, *93*; rubber 59, *125*; satin *58*; shetland *101*, *116*, 176; silicone *70*, 164, *171*; silk 10, *84*, *85*, *167*, 179; stockinette 164, *175*; string *58*; tweed 13, *77*, *89*; viscose *23*, 28, *36*, *40-1*, *41*, 68, *69*, *72*, *77*, *82-3*, 94, *130*, *147*, *154*, *154-5*, *168*, 179; wire 53, *64-5*, 66, *72*, *80*, *84*, 136, *138*, *147*, *169*; wool *24*, *25*, *36*, *38*, *42-3*, *43*, *45*, 47, 49, 53, 59, *62*, 69, *77*, *80-1*, *84*, 89, 90, 92, 94, *101*, *104*, *105*, *108*, *110*, *114*, *115*, *121*, 134, 159, *163*, *164-5*, *166*, *167*, 176, 179
Matta *164*
McQueen, Alexander 68, 90, *90*, *91*, 92
Memel, Simone 54, *58*
mesh 92, *106*, *119*, 175, 178
metallic yarns 42, *70-1*, *72*, *73*, *78*, *79*, *80*, *84*, *98*, *110*, *144*, *145*, 180
Minagawa, Makiko 106
Missoni 8, 12, *23*, 30, *30*, *31*, 52, 180
Miyake, Issey 9, 54, 68, 71, *77*, 90, *106*, *107*, 118, 120, *122*, 132, 152, 178, *178*
Moore, Rosemary 71, 152, *180*
Moschino 10

Noda, Suzumi 136, *148*, *149*
Noguchi, Hikaru 53, *55*, *163*, 164, *166*, *167*
Nuno Corporation 71
Nylstar 179

Olszynska, Monika *86*
Oya, Hiroaki *177*

Parker, Rozsika 132
patchwork 15, *39*, 61, 71, 94, *102*
Pinfold, Karl 71, *80*, *81*
Pinnick, Gina 155
Piogé, Stephanie 54, *61*
plain knitting 175
plating technique *45*, 177
pleated fabric 176
Pleats Please 68, 77, 123, 152
pocket knitting 40, *150*, *151*, *164-5*
Prada 15, *19*
Pringle 10, 12, *13*, 15, *15*
processes:
  bleaching 18, 66; bonding *86*, 88; braiding *58*, 94, *112*; burning 71, 88; coating 66, 70, *70-1*, *71*, *73*, *76*, 164; dip-dyeing 66, 68, *171*; distorting *14*, 68; distressing *18*, 92; electro-deposition 88; embossing *59*, *86*; felting *18*, *19*, 44, 46, 52, 53, 54, 57, 59, *62*, *62-3*, 66, 71, *82*, *84*, *85*, *86*, *89*, *125*, *138-9*, *139*, 159; heat-processing 66, 68, *72*, 75, 76, 88, *88*, *140*, *140-1*, *144*; knotting 52, 53, *56*, 64, *140*, *140-1*, 164, *169*; laminating 66; moulding 68; painting 30; plaiting, *see* braiding; printing 12, 15, 32, *37*, *58*, *68ff.*, *69*, 71, *76*, 77, 86, 88, 94; quilting 26, 46, *177*; recycling 68, 94, *99*, 113; scorching *19*; sequinning *41*, *114*; singeing *19*; space-dyeing *22*, *23*, 180; weaving 34

Radvan, Caterina 120, *124*, *125*
Rance, Victoria 156, *157*
rib fabric 12, *13*, *33*, *48*, 73, 88, *91*, *95*, *108*, *116*, *172*, *174*, 176, 177, *177*, 178, *178*, 180; transfer 71
ribbons 28, *33*, *166*
Roberts, Patricia 9, 12
Robins, Freddie *133*, 134, *134*, *135*
Rocha, John *47*, 176
Roswald, Ann-Louise *58*, 68
Rykiel, Sonia 12, 30, *50*, 155

Saifee, Fatima *84*, 94, *114-15*
salt 164, *172*, *172-3*, *173*
Santoni 118, 127, 129, 175
Schiaparelli, Elsa 52, 132
Sherliker, Clare 155
Shima Seiki 15, 118, 174, 177, 178
short-row knitting 21, *23*, *36*, *37*, *50*, *84*, 94, *97*, *98*, *125*, 155, *177*, *177*
Sissi 160
Skarland, Julie 71, *76*
Smedley, John 15, *16*, 18, 24
Smith, Hilde 32
Spadafora, Maria *25*, 30, *47*, *79*, 94, 176
Sprouse, Stephen 52
Starck, Philippe 118, 129
Steele, Lawrence 46, *67*, 68, *131*
Stewart, Stevie 32, 152, 153
Stoll *127*, 174, 177, 178, *178*
Storey, Helen 134
stretch fabric *28*, 32, *153*, 164
Sui, Anna 61, *112*

Tait & Style *165*
Tatsuno, Koji *66ff.*, *71*, 90, *110*, *111*, 114
Tayama, Atsuro 90, *97*, *101*, *178*
Testu 120, *130*, *131*
Tough, Catherine *162*, 164, *164-5*
Trockel, Rosemarie 132, 134, *142*, *143*, 146
Truman, Jan *64-5*, *147*
Tse *17*
Twincinc by Cinc *27*

Ungaro, Emanuel *73*

Van Noten, Dries 15, *17*, *22*
Verdu, Joaquim *25*
Verhoeven, Julie 52
Vuitton, Louis 15, 52, 114

Walters, Lynsey 53, *62*
warp knitting 8, *24*, *31*, 118, *122*, *123*, *174ff.*, *174*, 178, *178*
Watanabe, Junya 90, *96*, 134
Wauchob, Sharon 68, *69*, *115*
Webber, Rebecca 88
weft knitting 8, 118, *174ff.*, *174*, 178
Weiz, Otto 10
Westwood, Vivienne 14, 15, *24*, 48, *49*, 54, *59*, 61
Whistler, Claire 156, *157*
Whistles 11
Willhelm, Bernhard 53, *61*, *63*, 90, 94, *100*
Wilson, Delphine 90, 92, *95*
Windebank, Marcia *6*, *168*
Wolford *60*, 118, *128*, *128-9*, *129*
Woolmark *13*, 132
Wurm, Erwin 155, *161*

Xuly Bet 94, *113*

Yamamoto, Yohji 90, *91*, 92, *93*, *95*, *97*, *98*, *101*, *108*, *109*, 152, 175, 180